ROUTLEDGE HANDBOOK OF MEDICINE AND POETRY

The *Routledge Handbook of Medicine and Poetry* draws on an international selection of authors to ask what the cultures of poetry and medicine may gain from reciprocal critical engagement. The volume celebrates interdisciplinary inquiry, critique, and creative expansion with an emphasis upon amplifying provocative and marginalized voices.

This carefully curated collection offers both historical context and future thinking from clinicians, poets, artists, humanities scholars, social scientists, and bio-scientists who collectively inquire into the nature of relationships between medicine and poetry. Importantly, these can be both productive and unproductive. How, for example, do poet-doctors reconcile the outwardly antithetical approaches of bio-scientific medicine and poetry in their daily work, where typically the former draws on technical language and associated thinking and the latter on metaphors? How does non-narrative lyrical poetry engage with narrative-based medicine? How do poets writing about medicine identify as patients? Central to the volume is the critical investigation of the consequences of varieties of medical pedagogy for clinical practice.

Presenting a vision of how poetic thinking might form a medical ontology this thought-provoking book affords an essential resource for scholars and practitioners from across medicine, health and social care, medical education, the medical and health humanities, and literary studies.

Alan Bleakley is Emeritus Professor of Medical Education and Medical Humanities at Plymouth University Peninsula Medical School, UK.

Shane Neilson is a poet, physician, and health humanities scholar who teaches at the Waterloo Regional Campus of McMaster University, Canada.

ROUTLEDGE HANDBOOK OF MEDICINE AND POETRY

Edited by
Alan Bleakley and Shane Neilson

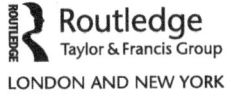

LONDON AND NEW YORK

Designed cover image: Erica Smith

First published 2024
by Routledge
4 Park Square, Milton Park, Abingdon, Oxon OX14 4RN

and by Routledge
605 Third Avenue, New York, NY 10158

Routledge is an imprint of the Taylor & Francis Group, an informa business

British Library Cataloguing-in-Publication Data
A catalogue record for this book is available from the British Library

ISBN: 978-1-032-37762-9 (hbk)
ISBN: 978-1-032-73262-6 (pbk)
ISBN: 978-1-003-34179-6 (ebk)

DOI: 10.4324/9781003341796

Typeset in Times New Roman
by Apex CoVantage, LLC

CONTENTS

Contents

INTRODUCTION

'What's past is prologue'

Alan Bleakley and Shane Neilson

Part one: foraging for metaphors

Medical science abducted by poetry: or, poetry feeds intuitive capacity, that in turn feeds abductive reasoning

In the *Canadian Medical Association Journal* from December 1936, Dr Earle Parkhill Scarlett from Calgary opened an article titled 'Medicine and Poetry' (reproduced here as Chapter 4) with an unreferenced quote: 'A physician should be a kind of poet'. This is not an invitation but an imperative. Scarlett (1936: 676) notes that the arts and biomedicine have drifted so far apart that to link them by equating medicine with poetry would constitute 'an absurdity, a straining of the laudable practice of comparison beyond rational limits. It is not unlike linking the subtle flights of metaphysics and the harsh realities of cold mutton'. While advertising the generally perceived 'absurdity' of trying to link the arts and biomedicine, Scarlett can only achieve this through resort to metaphor and image, beyond the 'rational'. The metaphors for the sublime ('the subtle flights of metaphysics') and the ridiculous ('the harsh realities of cold mutton') are both humorous and striking; more, the phrase about the mutton is a decent line of iambic pentameter free from narrative constraints – simply a spatial, lyrical description inviting a touch of nausea (that cold mutton again). There is a decent analogy here too. The 'harsh realities of cold mutton' and more subtle 'flights of metaphysics' are surely two ends of a spectrum of clinical work: first closely observing a bodily symptom – boil, bruise, swelling, discharge, congestion, lump, contusion – and then speculating as to its cause.

Scarlett notes that Apollo, the Greek god of poetry, is father to Aesculapius, the god of medicine. But Apollo too is linked with reason and science. 'Science and poetry', says Scarlett, 'thus truly dwell together'. Well, it is poor science to jump from a statement to a conclusion without intervening evidence, but Scarlett's intuition is, nevertheless, spot on. Why, in the gods' names, were science and poetry ever separated and opposed in the first place? Not only does one need the other, but we have lived with the fiction that science is rational and poetry irrational (and then the two are naturally opposed) particularly since the Enlightenment and specifically since the chatter around C.P. Snow's (1959) notorious 'Two Cultures' Rede Lecture. Every workaday poet knows that writing poetry is not the mark of divine inspiration but the product of the application of a host

DOI: 10.4324/9781003341796-1

of technical features shaping perceptions. Poetry, then, is 'science-like'. The poet and critic Don Paterson (2023) agrees, claiming that 'Poetry is the science of nuance in language'.

Poetry as science might be seen as the meticulous testing of a hypothesis (as an initial observation, inkling, idea, insight, feeling state, or memory) through the media of formal techniques such as accent, alliteration, metaphor, metre, syncopation, and so forth until the product sings on the page, rings in the ear, and lingers in the mind. This is what the philosopher Charles Sanders Peirce, in the late nineteenth century, called 'abductive reasoning': plumping for the best fit hypothesis given the available evidence. In other words, to ask 'does the poem *work*?' is to also ask '*how* does the poem work?' Where poetry can be cast as 'science-like', science – so often caricatured as rational and objective – can be cast as a socially engineered activity with a high content of imagination and innovation. Science is notoriously hit-and-miss: not in its final force, where reasonable data collection and replicative testing have been carried out, but in its initial speculations and hypothesis-building. Medicine, as science, employs not just inductive and deductive reasoning but abduction: proceeding 'as if' a notion had validity and finding that 'the proof is in the pudding'.

There, we cannot get at what abduction means without a metaphor (in this case an aphorism), where ambiguity is key. Medical practice as a science must work with ambiguity as resource and not as hindrance. Science (and, of course, there are various kinds of science) can be cast as *imaginative reasoning*, necessarily contradictory and ambiguous. The applied science of medicine, as clinical practice, follows this form. Clinical work is not a mass of loose threads (where complexity falls into chaos) but rather a meticulous 'knotworking' (Engeström 2018) of such threads in patterns conforming with carefully wrought hypotheses. This is complexity working at the edge of chaos – with the possibility of reformulating at a higher level of meaning.

Another way of looking at this is that good medicine is never purely instrumental nor functional but engages other value positions such as the ethical, aesthetic, political, and transcendental – then moving from 'information' through 'knowledge' to 'meaning' and 'wisdom' in the poet T.S. Eliot's (1934) formulation (Bleakley 2023). This is because medicine applies generalized science to the unique individual, necessarily making for messy (and sometimes mis-directed) work that is a constant process of knotworking – tying and untying of threads. Poetry works this way too. Instrumental poetry is then a contradiction in terms, as a range of values must be engaged in the process of knotworking. In terms of cognition and meta-cognition (thinking about thinking, or the rules of thinking and how to break them), knotworking's equivalent is Peirce's abductive reasoning.

The common meaning of abduction is to take somebody away by force or deception. The root of this is the Latin *abducere* 'to take away', specifically *ducere* 'to lead'. For Peirce, abductive reasoning is the best use of available clues and cues in terms of grasping an emergent process, necessarily embracing intuition and hunch, and removing it forcibly from any other tinkering or worrying about an ideal of reasoning (the 'perfect' piece of logic or experimental design as an unachievable abstraction from reality). In Peirce's model it is, as it were, not you who is doing the thinking but the overall ecological context for the thinking that abducts you or takes you away from habitual lines of reasoning and logic. It is a hi-jacking of the rational by the imagination, or better, of the literal by the metaphorical. Abduction is inspired 'good enough' thinking, heavy on intuition. Here also habitual thinking is suspended. In this process of side-tracking, you cross wires and trip up, but your line of intention is set fair. Your progress is marked by the multiplication of productive metaphors, and, returning to our mutton and subtle flights of metaphysics, we note that a metaphor is, by nature, embodied (Lakoff and Johnson 1999). While you may be 'spirited away' in moments of inspiration, these are fleshly. Abduction is inspiration tethered to sense.

Such sense itself may be a grounding in embodied language. Carlos Perez (2020) suggests, 'Abduction comes from imagination. But imagination cannot happen without the vocabulary to imagine'. The 'vocabulary to imagine' is primarily that of tropes such as metaphor. We cannot reason abductively without resort to embodied metaphor. Again, as Perez suggests, abductive reasoning is 'inductive thinking but at the meta level'. He suggests that this is an everyday mode of thinking, especially evident where we read text:

> Reading requires a continuous interplay where we create a hypothesis of what the author is attempting to convey and we subsequently test these [sic] against our knowledge and subsequent facts that the author reveals. When we read, a kind of 'progressive disclosure' occurs, where we sequentially grasp the bigger picture via a sequence of words and sentences.

It is, however, 'intuition' that 'automatically allows us to see possibilities'. By intuition, Perez means meta-thinking, or thinking about thinking. As we read, so we work out and question what the author 'means', or implies, as a second-order imagination. The first-order imagination deals with the text as grammar: vocabulary, sentence construction, and so forth. Second-order, or meta-, readings grapple with meanings and possibilities fed by metaphor. Here, hypotheses are constructed and (abductively) both questioned and tested. Thus, Perez notes that where deduction relies on a formal, logical link between hypothesis and conclusion from evidence in the realm of probabilities, intuition works in the realm of possibilities:

> It is only through questioning that we can discover possibilities that we may never have imagined. Peirce's Abduction is commonly understood as hypothesis selection. We often overlook though that a good hypothesis is one that makes obvious the generation of a good question.

'Abduction' – the questioning of what is commonly accepted – is also a common medical term usually used to describe the movement of a limb away from the midline of the body, and this is a useful analogy for what abduction as hypothesis-making does, as a shifting away from the midline (the straight and narrow and the grounded) as an embodied practice. Abduction is a form of tension, or is tense, as a difficult perspective to hold. It is open to slippage to the more familiar, but less complex, induction or deduction. In the poet Emily Dickinson's (1998) words, 'Tell all the truth but tell it slant', for 'The Truth must dazzle gradually'. A blinding truth is surely the hubris of a definitive answer, where a gradually dazzling truth is a series of finely tuned questions in Socratic style. Is the latter not good diagnostic technique and, further, a poetic method?

While medicine is science-based, as theory, in practice it is a science-using activity with a high degree of ambiguity, uncertainty, and contradiction. The practice of medicine is not free from the contamination (for better or worse) of mood. We cannot get away from the conundrum that the observer confounds the experiment. In medicine, the key contradiction again is that the general (guidelines drawn from large-scale clinical trials, typologies) must always be applied to the specific (individual patients, the single case). The fit is rarely perfect. And again, mood intervenes and colours.

Fast forward from Calgary's Dr Scarlett just before World War II to London's Dr John Launer (2014), a celebrated poet–physician (see Chapter 5). Launer read English Literature before studying medicine and so was always interested in the use of language in the consultation. Nothing was more dulling to medical practice for Launer than reducing the language of the clinical encounter to standard technical medical lingo where language tropes were squeezed out:

> I would certainly encourage students and trainees to look out for the times they manage
> to transcend the banal formulas of everyday medical conversations, and find themselves

moving into similes, metaphors, allusions, puns, humour, paradox or other imaginative forms of speech. If they did so, they would discover that medicine can be poetic, in the true meaning of the word.

We heartily concur. Launer says in the same article that he 'rediscovered' William Empson's classic literary analysis text *Seven Kinds of Ambiguity* through reading a 2005 essay on medical ethics by Australian clinician Dr Paul Komesaroff. The essay claimed that tolerance of ambiguity is key to good clinical practice, a fact that is now well known from rigorous medical education research (Bleakley et al. 2011; Bleakley 2014). Indeed, one might claim that it is a scientific fact. Komesaroff bemoans the conservative situation in medicine, described by Launer, 'where one word or phrase is generally believed to represent only a single thing or idea'. Drawing on Komerasoff, Launer says that use of language in clinical practice 'involves the careful, tentative use of the same devices, rhetorical forms, figures and tropes generally eschewed by philosophers and scientists, but embraced by poets and creative writers'. We see this as a journey from closed-circuit linearity, however complicated, to the nonlinear, open nature of medical practice as a dynamic, complex system at the edge of chaos – a creative multiplicity. It is also, again, an embrace of abduction as a method of reasoning.

In the nearly 80 years between the articles of Earle Scarlett and John Launer, many papers and books have been published on the relationships between medicine *and* poetry but little on medicine *as* poetry (or poetry as medicine) – as both Scarlett and Launer posit. Some work comes close to realizing this equation. Joel Weishaus (2006) quotes the North American family physician and poet Peter Pereira: 'the reading and writing of poetry keeps me in touch with my more intuitive and irrational side, and I hope makes me a better listener, to get a closer, more accurate read on patients and their stories'. This reflects a common idea – poetry makes us better listeners. But why should this be? Following Pereira's claim, that poetry makes us both better naturalists and abductive reasoners – observers as much as listeners – we fully agree with Pereira that poetry feeds intuitive capacity that in turn feeds abductive reasoning, but whether poetry makes us better listeners is open to debate. That it may help us to 'read' patients closely, as we might closely read a text, as Pereira also claims, seems to be more on the money.

Why the link between medicine and poetry matters

Medicine is always in danger of regressing to a baseline of technical or instrumental biomedical science explanation, choking the potential release of its metaphoric hoard as 'possibility knowledge' (Engeström 2018). It is in the expansion to embrace ethical, aesthetic, political, and transcendental values that deeper connection with explanatory and exploratory biomedical science, clinical skills, and communication with colleagues and patients occurs. (To this we must add the importance of the historical context.) This makes for an infinitely better medicine. Heightening the productive metaphor count, an indicator of an expanded imagination, makes for a poetic medicine (see Chapter 1 by Laurence J Kirmayer for a full account). But medical education has, historically, failed to grasp the nettle of such a transformative pedagogy.

The poet and physician William Carlos Williams (1962) famously wrote, 'It is difficult/to get the news from poems/yet men die miserably every day/for lack/of what is found there'. People 'die' because they are starved of inspiration and meaning (Socrates's 'unexamined life'). It seems strange then that we should have, historically, starved medical education of inspiration and meaning. Here are seven of medical education's longstanding and interconnected woes:

- Instrumentalism has come to act as a dominant value, reflected in valuing training over education, competence over capability, and linear closed systems over complex, dynamic open systems.
- A chief tool of instrumentalism is intolerance of ambiguity. This is reflected in a preference for authority through hierarchy rather than seeking to establish democratic habits, and in a preference for the indicative (telling) over the subjunctive (debating) mood in speech. Psychoanalysis equates such authoritarianism with unresolved anal fixations (the need to control and be controlled) preventing the development of genitality (mutuality). Poetry educates for tolerance of ambiguity.
- Where medical students typically show empathy decline and cynicism setting in by year three, this may be grounded in habitual, de-sensitizing pedagogical processes.
- Medicine shows unacceptably high rates of iatrogenesis or medical error stemming from systemic issues such as medicine's historically conditioned authority structures that show in poorly performing team settings. Research consistently shows that less hierarchical and more democratic, collaborative interprofessional teams improve patient safety and work satisfaction.
- There is a systematic (mis)education into insensibility, where improving sensibility is the key to close noticing and better diagnostic acumen. Sensibility is dulled through the – often unexamined – common initiation rite of learning anatomy through cadaver dissection and then through emotional insulation as a sharp closing down of the senses and then affect, registering the necessary insults of patients' pains, sufferings, diseases, and deaths. Such de-sensitizing saves from being overwhelmed by emotional flux but is overdetermined.
- Related to the condition above is lack of education in psychological and psychotherapeutic acumen. A by-product of this is the inability to regulate and appropriately employ catharsis. A longer-term effect is cumulative and unattended anxiety, depression, and other mood disorders, often resulting in burnout. Burnout is also due to structural factors such as chronic lack of personnel and resources that must be addressed as an urgent political issue. But within medical culture itself is a history of overdetermination: compulsive overworking and fear of failure. As noted above, hierarchical habits stunt collaborative teamwork, and there is an established culture of individualism, heroism, and self-help that has resulted in lack of supervisory acumen and psychotherapeutic support.

Counter-intuitively perhaps, a close reading of this book, where medicine and medical education are explicitly grounded in poetry, can provide the means to address all the above ills. We harbour grave misgivings about the direction of medical education over the past century plus, since the radical intervention of the Carnegie Foundation's commissioned *Flexner Report* in 1910. While Flexner forced the closure of 'under-performing' (actually, inadequately resourced) medical schools in North America and Canada, these were also the schools that catered for black and women students. The unintended consequence of this intervention has been nearly a century of privileged, all-white, all-male medical education.

While medical education has recently progressed politically – for example, more women than men now enter medical education worldwide – a new set of ruptures has arisen. Medical education has been slow to address, first, lack of ethnic diversity in its population, including opportunities for black, Asian, and minority ethnicity doctors to progress to the most senior positions; and second, pressing contemporary issues such as health consequences of climate change. We have entered an era in which physical diversity, neurodiversity, tolerance for difference, multiple identity formations, trans-nationalisms, trans-gendering, and 'human flow' in terms of displacement through armed and political conflict, ethnic and religious conflict, and environmental disasters are commonly acknowledged and addressed. Yet medical education's response to these issues has been to freeze in the headlights, continuing to export Western-based individualistic models in a largely unacknowledged form of neo-colonialism and failing to grasp the meanings of this changing world for definitions and interpretations of 'health' and 'wellbeing'. The World Health Organization's definition of 'health' as 'a state of complete physical, mental and social well-being and not merely the absence of disease or infirmity' now looks frankly ridiculous as an absolute but of course is relative to context.

Medical education's failure to grasp the nettle on dealing with emergent political dimensions of medicine (such as dealing adequately with forced or voluntary, but 'illegal', immigration and its fallout in post-traumatic stress disorders) is unfortunate. Anyone familiar with the contemporary poetry scene will know that topics concerned with difference, equity, and equality is now standard fare. Aesthetically, politically, and ethically aware poetry offers a consciousness-raising medium as it seeks beauty and justice concurrently. Instrumental medical education dulls consciousness-raising as it seeks mediocrity and a will-to-stability rather than a quest for innovation. Poetry has something to teach medicine, to restore the latter's grace.

We note then that a poetic sensibility appears to be missing in medical education and clinical practice that is part of medicine's heritage. But more, we suggest that medical education is intellectually blunt where it has long lagged behind other academic studies such as cultural studies, critical studies, literary studies, anthropology, history, art criticism, art theory, geography, disability studies, mad studies, gender studies including a variety of feminisms, and race and ethnicity studies, that are entangled with the relationships between, again, aesthetics (qualities), ethics (values), politics (power), and the transcendent (meaning) as these play out in identifications and identity formations. Our concern is that a poetic sensibility (one of close noticing, reflective insight, and sensible embeddedness in the world of objects – reflected as embodied metaphor invention) is largely absent from medical education. Here, it remains a scandal that much curriculum planning has regressed to a largely instrumental and content-driven status, oblivious to aesthetic and process-based pedagogic approaches such as curriculum reconceptualization (Pinar 2019; Bleakley 2021).

For over two decades, critical scholars of medical pedagogy have pointed out that curricula have drifted towards set content and standardized learning outcome models (Bleakley 1998, 2014, 2021; Bleakley et al. 2011). In 1998, one of us (AB) wrote about the decline of learning as an aesthetic practice, where the link between motivation and the creation of beauty is severed:

'Motivation', which entered the English language in the mid-seventeenth century, means to move something to action. Its original reference is to motion: to movement of the limbs, of body, of muscle. This frames motivation as incitement, spur or stimulus – extrinsic motive. Educationists usually see extrinsic motives as less powerful than intrinsic factors such as curiosity, interest and 'desire', a term in use in the English language at least a century before 'motive'. 'Desire' means something wished-for, and returns us directly to matters of the heart, returning us to aesthetics.

This constitutes a drift away from learning through the heart (a matter of desire) to learning by heart (rote). Despite the popularity of problem-based learning approaches that supposedly engender motivation, medical students can be seen to have lost the active, motivational element of learning and are reduced to passive recipients of knowledge and skills (Kusurkar et al. 2012). Further, students only want to learn content and skills that they know will be assessed. Assessment comes to drive learning, and in the absence of rigorous self and peer criteria-based assessment models, such learning is subject to control by another, reducing motivation. The exception to this drift to curricular instrumentalism is the Longitudinal Integrated Clerkship (LIC) model (Bleakley et al. 2011; Norris et al. 2009), where students learn on the job from day one through clinical placements and are active in planning curricular processes tailored to their needs. LIC models work with the general notion of 'the need to know' rather than the instrumental specifics of 'what one needs to know'.

Having diagnosed key symptoms of medical education as these impinge upon consequent medical work, we have also suggested (perhaps too hastily) that poetry may provide a cure for such ailments. Of course, this would be easy to read metaphorically. But we mean it literally, and this opinion, as you will see, is shared in differing ways by the authors in this collection. We are grateful for their contributions, for they collectively point us to a future medicine that is shaped poetically or finds that its means of thinking is isomorphic with patterns of clinical reasoning and judgement (Bleakley and Neilson 2021). This affords a radical manifesto.

A history of the future

In an era when a genetically modified pig's heart has been transplanted into a human recipient (who died two months after the transplant, not from organ rejection but from other complications), a genre of 'near future' literature has also evolved. Near future literature walks the fine line between believability ('science faction') and fantasy ('science fiction') by sketching futures that are clearly grounded in historical realities. In Shakespeare's *The Tempest* (Act 2, Scene 1), Antonio plans the murder of Alonso, the King of Naples, and his advisor Gonzalo so that Sebastian can take the throne. Antonio says to Sebastian: 'Whereof what's past is prologue; what to come, in yours and my discharge'. In other words, knowledge of the past can provide conditions to actively shape the future. It is a matter of reading history appropriately.

Michel Foucault's body of work is the ur-example of this line of thinking. He describes the conditions of possibility for the emergence of modern phenomena such as classification systems, madness, the medical clinic, practices of sexuality, and the modern 'subject' or identity. Foucault even predates contemporary interests in antihumanism (Kirsch 2023) that predict the extinction of the human species through its own follies such as the climate disaster, species extinctions, and nuclear war. We can shape a destiny by better understanding history's consequences as a history of the present. Indeed, close reading of historical circumstance can lead to a paradoxical history of the future. This is advertised by the cutting edge of science in areas such as artificial intelligence, gene splicing and modification, nuclear fusion, neurodynamics, and low-dose psychedelics for mental health. Its primary language is drawn from complexity and chaos theory, while its literary exponents include Don DeLillo and William Gibson.

Understanding the confluence of factors that have shaped not just an authoritative but also an authoritarian modern medicine, patients are better equipped to resist perceived transgressions of that medical authority (such as high levels of medical error). Near future literature provides a form of consciousness-raising in the light of what may seem like autonomous and unaccountable medical advances such as genetic modifications. Poetry too can provide a platform for activism that demands accountability not just for potentially difficult ethical issues but also for the avoidable production of the bland and the biased that avoids aesthetic and political accountability, which we can readily spot in contemporary medical education.

Importantly, poetry can be apprehended as the constant historical companion of medicine that informed and recorded its practices whilst also signalling that which was lacking: an appreciation of beauty both in the abstract and in the specific. In this way, the 'near-future' that medicine might enjoy is always one foretold and told on by the poetry written now, poetry that attests to present conditions. The near-future is one wrought by poetry to make the practice of medicine hospitable to an appreciation of medicine's own beauty. Poetry is not only the fortunate teller of that beauty in medicine but also a significant component of how that medicine is construed.

Part two: our authors imaginatively entwine medicine and poetry

In the immediate near future, you will read the subsequent chapters of this book, which we will briefly summarize now. Our *Handbook* begins with a section intended to quickly orient readers to what the rest of the book will do. 'Toward a poetics of illness and healing', Chapter 1 is a panoptical chapter on metaphor by someone who (among many other things) might be considered the dean of metaphor-related studies in medicine, Laurence J Kirmayer. He explores *poesis* as the means whereby we experience and interpret both illness and healing, along the way offering what could be called a state-of-the-art primer on metaphor theory in medicine. With Laurence having provided our conceptual frame, in Chapter 2 we move to the celebrated poet and German literature scholar and translator Michael Hulse, who provides the practical data and lively story around the prestigious Hippocrates Prize. Michael shares with us how this signal initiative supporting, promoting, and shaping medical poetry came to be and how it preserved its own administrative health. He posits, and answers, the provocative question, 'just what defines *medical* poetry?' Importantly, a model emerges: *contra* the frankly poor poetry that often flows freely from poetry-as-therapy workshops, put on a serious competition with experts at the helm, and you will find that high-quality work emerges.

In Chapter 3, Shane Neilson rounds out the framing section with a succinct account of how time-focused narrative approaches in medicine have come to leave space-focused lyric poetry in the shadows. He makes a plea for reconsidering poetry's subjection to narrative in the context of medical education, where poetry is unlike the mode of language used to both interpret and deploy it in medical education due to the hegemony of narrative in the culture at large. Adding to narrative's misdirection in the context of learning how to practice medicine, there is the additional woe that the infamous 'narrative turn' in culture has taken another turn in the context of medical education where it promotes blunt, instrumental values as it fails to recognize this turn. The chapter argues that through poetry we can recover 'a rich clinical world that is spatial as opposed to chronological', leading to 'a different means to think with patients'. In this sense, poetry in medicine is revolutionary.

In the second section, Chapters 4–8, we consider key historical issues in the associations between medicine and poetry, as both archaeological (significant artefacts dug from the archives) and genealogical (the conditions of possibility for the emergence of certain discourses – as the production of the artefacts we have just dug up). We curate together contributors who speak to the connection between medicine and poetry as categories, be they believers in ideas such as medicine is poetry, or physicians should be poets, or medicine should do something for poetry. As we have already introduced, in Chapter 4, EP Scarlett writes 'Medicine and Poetry' to us from the first part of the twentieth century, using the *Canadian Medical Association Journal* to insist on the place of poetry as both philosophical and anecdotal. Scarlett's sheer encyclopaedic knowledge of practitioners over the history of poetry and medicine offers to any sceptical reader a past reality that we want to bring into being in the near-future – that not too long ago, practitioners lived who thought of medicine and poetry as indivisible and had the receipts to prove it.

Though we have already mentioned John Launer's 'Medicine as poetry', we invoke his Chapter 5 again to be systematic for a reader who wisely skipped our preamble and who wants a quick rundown of the book's contents. Here, we reprint (from the *Postgraduate Medical Journal*) John's appreciation of ambiguity in the clinical encounter with poetry as his means of that appreciation. Out of irritation, in Chapter 6, one of our editors (SN) builds on the argument put forward in Chapter 3, flipping the preferred polarity in medical education in which all learning bends towards instrumentalism. He asks the question, 'What can medicine do for poetry?'

In Chapter 7, Audrey Shafer, an anaesthetist and poet, makes a wonderful comparison: 'Anesthesiology, including the arc of patient care and attention to rhythms and precision, has much in common with the poem, including arcs of thought, rhythms, pauses, and resonances'. She also lists possible functional outcomes of reading and writing poetry such as decreasing stress, enabling reflection, and improving wellbeing. But this latter list of outcomes seems to us to pale in comparison with the poetic notion of the 'arc' of practice, including rhythm and close noticing that forms a poetic gesture as the enactment of medicine. Iain Bamforth in Chapter 8 gives a virtuoso performance in the lyric essay form, mixing medical themes, references, and personages with a laser-like focus on etymology and concluding the essay with an implied metaphor that the practice of medicine, like poetry, invites self-revision.

The third section of the book – '*Poiesis*: metaphor elaborates experience' – focuses on metaphor as subject of study as well as expertly used object, with the section both beginning and closing in the latter fashion, where we meet poems in the flesh. In Chapter 9, Daisy G Bassen, a child psychiatrist, offers eight poems drawn from her clinical experience. Read them carefully: through political rhetoric laced with dark humour, Daisy employs psychoanalytic tropes to display the return of the repressed in medicine's lingering patriarchy.

In Chapter 10, Peter and Christie Stillwell imagine themselves into a poetics of pain management, advocating for the creative use of multidimensional metaphors. In Chapter 11, Daniel Suarez insists on the importance of biocriticism to inform the reading of the poetry of illness and suffering. Poetry is particularly suited to navigating the chaotic experience of illness (and especially so in contrast with medicine's falsely authoritative language), and Daniel illustrates this expertly through a close analysis of the Chilean poet Enrique Lihn's work. In what is a very rare occurrence – there are vanishingly few academic analyses of contemporary physician-poets – Chapter 12 reprints 'Nourished by Experiences' (from the *International Journal of Welsh Writing in English*). This is W Richard Bowen's landmark analysis of the work of popular physician-poet Dannie Abse, bringing biocriticism, religious studies, intersubjectivity, and ethics to bear on the poet's work. In Chapter 13, 'Debriding the moral injury', Nigerian-Canadian physician Tolu Oloruntoba shares some work reprinted from his Governor-General Award and Griffin Poetry Prize-winning collection *The Junta of Happenstance* as well as various other sources. Tolu's work is in conversation with home as it might be constituted medically, and vice versa, creating a discomfiture at the level of identity.

The book builds to a rich fourth section – 'Neurodiversity and the colonizing of the other' – where the special terrain of psychiatry is carefully explored. In what we feel is an exciting development, in Chapter 14, 'Alda Merini and the making of lyrical psychiatry', Marta Arnaldi argues that poetry and science *can* be conceived of as parallel epistemics or ways of knowing. Poetry has a logic and science is imaginative, where translations are invited; through such translations, medical professionals can better appreciate, as well as understand, health and suffering. Marta focuses her argument through the domain of psychiatry as special case and draws on the poetry and life of Italian poet Alda Merini as demonstration. Merini was incarcerated in a mental asylum for 10 years, describing her experiences 20 years later to a fellow inmate who became her lover, in poetry, lyrical prose, and letters.

On a related note, in Chapter 15, Elisabeth Kumar's 'Dear GP' analyzes the poetry contained within two zines to interrogate the expressed inadequacy of mental health care at the level of relationality and intelligibility, but with a true poet's eye, carefully attending to form throughout. The essay similarly considers the other side of the equation, mental health care notes, in its second movement, and anticipates the following chapter by Erin Soros in the process. In Chapter 16, 'The prairies always see you', Erin offers a beautiful and non-didactic lyric essay concerning the poetics of psychosis. The implied injunction is that we should all relate better so that we can approximate (if never reach) understanding.

In Chapter 17, 'The capaciousness of uncertainty', Jiameng Xu takes the baton, applying Gadamer's hermeneutics to two psychiatric encounters to understand how medical work itself is poetic praxis. The author, as both clinician and ethnographer, asks how we can authentically enter the lived experience of an Other who is labelled 'patient'. We love that this chapter experiments with form and voice, moving in and out of poetic and academic registers to enact its argument, showing that the voice of the Other may be lost to academic registers but caught through poetic voices. In Chapter 18, 'Sylvia Wynter and the poetics of psychiatry', Bahar Orang – drawing on traditions of radical psychiatry – deploys Sylvia Wynter's, Aimé Césaire's, and Bedour Alagraa's thoughts concerning anticoloniality to follow various entanglements of language, science, and subjectivity. With a focus on Orang's own location of psychiatric practice in Toronto, Ontario, a rebirth of what used to be called 'anti-psychiatry' and now a 'critical psychiatry' is heralded.

In Chapter 19, 'Psychiatry's turf and poetry's field', Alan Bleakley provides a mini history of such critical psychiatry as he observed its development at first hand in the UK (primarily its poetic origins). Informed by this history, a leap is made to medical pedagogies. An argument is made about how curriculum theorist William Pinar's concept of *currere* can be seen as poetic work, badly required in contemporary medical education. Bleakley draws on UK poet Peter Redgrove's work (and life) as proof of concept.

The penultimate section – 'The intimate soma' – thinks through the intersection of body and time as expressed in metaphors that are often mortal. In Chapter 20, 'Body-related poetry therapy in psycho-oncology', Alfonso Santarpia reviews metaphor theory to delve deeply into certain domains of bodily metaphor that can beneficially influence therapeutics in oncology. Santarpia unabashedly offers a theoretically reinforced and substantiated poetry therapeutics as illustrated by case histories. Chapter 21 provides a useful biocritical terrain for refracting Santarpia's ideas. In 'Oncology and poetry', Martin Dyar considers Irish poet Patrick Kavanagh's experiences as a cancer patient and his representations of illness and treatment, contributing once again another relatively rare scholarly study of a significant poet and his illness.

In Chapter 22, Alastair Morrison presents a novel argument in the context of narrative medicine hermeneutics, proceeding to consider an entire collection of poetry – the collection as 'body' – by Pia Tafdrup, as a unit of narrative. In Chapter 23, Martina Ann Kelly and Megan EL Brown draw on 'big guns' Heidegger and Gadamer to read and apply Paul Celan's metaphors of the 'breath-crystal' and 'timecrevasse', with temporality being a key theme. Here, medicine is informed by conversations between poetry and existential/phenomenological philosophy. The authors critique reductionism and instrumentalism in medicine and medical education to call for more complex values frames through which a richer practice can be conceived. That practice must not stray from the body but must 'think' flesh and its sufferings in innovative ways. For the authors, such thinking is underpinned by startling elisions. We ask, does this afford a new model for clinical reasoning?

The final section of our book – 'Unsettling poetry and pedagogy'- has a purposefully ambiguous title. Poetry and pedagogy are both necessarily unsettling and need to be unsettled. The section focuses on the poetic redress of medical education but also the flawed and thwarted use of poetry in such medical pedagogies. In Chapter 24, 'Medicine, poetry, and Iris Murdoch's invitation towards unselfing', Monica Kidd advocates for attention over authority and hierarchy in medical education, expertly using novelist and philosopher Iris Murdoch's concept of 'unselfing' as it can be demonstrated in the work of Wisława Szymborska.

In Chapter 25, Sarah Fraser and Jessica Chaytor ask, and speculatively answer, a provocative question. Noting that there is evidence of a positive correlation between linguistic complexity and tool use, the authors enact a thought experiment: can poetry enhance surgical skills? In Chapter 26, Sarah de Leeuw conceives of poetry as a potentially anticolonial force, should it not be used in a colonizing way. She brings forward the work of several Indigenous poets and focuses her remarks in a conscientiously local way that is respectful of individual ecologies. Valuable too is de Leeuw's assessment of medicine as an inescapably colonial institution and practice, setting the frame for poetry's limited (but still important) possibility. In Chapter 27, 'When caged birds sing', Thirusha Naidu and Lynne Richards consider the work of feminist poets of colour (Angelou, Lorde, Giovanni, Naidu, Senior, Xaba) as 'a modality of healing both the psyche and the physical body' in prevailing conditions of racism and consequent health inequities. Michael Hanne's Chapter 28, 'Creative writing in medical education', reminds us again that imaginative pedagogy is so often strangled in conventional medical education, where the content of the syllabus (basic science, applied science, clinical skills, communication) is privileged over the process of the curriculum (how we learn also constructing an identity for the learner). Michael is an old hand and seasoned innovator in the field of medical pedagogy and here lets us peek into his classroom. There, we find a pedagogy based on the notion that doctors themselves feel the 'need to write' and it is this urge that must be modelled for neophytes. Consultations require capabilities in both narrative and poetics (where metaphor is central), leading to his argument that both should be taught in a double-barrelled way as 'binocular vision'.

In Chapter 29, 'On the reading list for all trainee medics: *Autobiography of a Marguerite* by Zarah Butcher-McGunnigle', Johanna Emeney close-reads Butcher-McGunnigle's collection of poems to articulate how the writer, as 'patient' suffering from 'an unnamed autoimmune condition', formulates modes of resistance to what she perceives as a patriarchal and controlling medical establishment. Her mother, also named Marguerite, is at her side. How will the 'patient' retain autonomy and identity in the face of 'strategic linguistic choices' by the medical fraternity as Marguerite and her mother seek their own linguistic strategies not just of survival but also identity? Does a body of poetry afford a body of resistance to an authority? Finally, in Chapter 30, scholar Sophie Ratcliffe and physician Andrew Schuman ask, 'Has the poetry of medicine burnt out?' This is a fitting finale to the book, for we do not wish to finish on a triumphant note, but rather on one of caution and realism. Poetry in medical education is, after all, small scale, irregular, hit-or-miss. There is the ever-present problem of production of poor poetry – for what? Entertainment? A welcome break? A salve? Battered by the COVID-19 episode and years of underfunding by government, medicine in the UK and Canada (where the editors are respectively qualified to speak) has become a political football, and the public system is close to collapse.

Sophie and Andrew have years of experience of running poetry inserts within formal medicine curricula, with evident success. Compatible with this anecdotal success is more general published evidence that reading literary texts can counter burnout in doctors, in part because reading in a particular way cultivates a tolerance of ambiguity and uncertainty – qualities endemic in medicine as it is. Should we not therefore consider the value of cultivating a literary imagination through a medical education? However, a spectre looms beyond the machinations of medical pedagogies, and that, in the UK and Canada, is the party politicizing of medicine that has led to such challenging (self-inflicted) structural problems. Can poetry fix a broken health system? Of course not – poetry is not an instrument designed for such purposes. But poetry is expressive of rage, recognises beauty, and shapes sensibilities.

Better perhaps that we think 'what can we do for poetry?' rather than 'what can poetry do for us?', where the purpose of poets is to care for, and add to, the universal body of poetry for the general benefit of the art itself and in turn society. If poetry clarifies things as they are, then medicine can inform and serve poetry in this way by providing its material and work content. Medicine can be seen as it is, which is the first step in any recovery process, and poetry expands its expressive capacity. We are then specialists who treat the body of poetry itself, addressing its symptoms. Is this not expert criticism?

We hope these chapters bring a near-future into being where medicine is not *made* to be poetic but instead is recognized as such, poetry being intrinsic to medicine and its related pedagogies. In other words, and stepping sideways from tautology, medicine and its pedagogies are already poetry if we view them through a poetic imagination. In the democratic spirit of Routledge Handbooks, we include as authors the well-established and internationally respected, as well as voices of new and younger scholars and clinicians with global coverage. We heartily thank all our contributors for their input to create a first in the field beyond the monograph (such as our own *Poetry in the Clinic: Towards a Lyrical Medicine* from 2021): the first collection of academic and creative work to document and critically investigate dialogue between medicine/medical education and poetry. It is then a landmark collection, and you, the reader, its first informed critic.

References

Bleakley A. 1998. Learning as an Aesthetic Practice: Motivation Through Beauty in Higher Education. In: S Brown, S Armstrong, G Thompson (eds.) *Motivating Students*. London: Kogan Page, 165–72.

Bleakley A. 2014. *Patient-Centred Medicine in Transition: The Heart of the Matter*. Dordrecht: Springer.

Bleakley A. 2021. *Medical Education, Politics and Social Justice: The Contradiction Cure*. Abingdon: Routledge.

Bleakley A. 2023. *Medical Humanities: Ethics, Aesthetics, Politics*. London: Routledge.

Bleakley A, Bligh J, Browne J. 2011. *Medical Education for the Future: Identity, Power, Location*. Dordrecht: Springer.

Bleakley A, Neilson S. 2021. *Poetry in the Clinic: Towards a Lyrical Medicine*. Abingdon: Routledge.

Dickinson E. 1998. *The Poems of Emily Dickinson: Reading Edition*. Cambridge, MA: The Belknap Press of Harvard University Press.

Eliot TS. 1954 (originally pub. 1934). Chorus from *The Rock*. In: TS Eliot (ed.) *Selected Poems*. London: Faber & Faber.

Engeström Y. 2018. *Expertise in Transition: Expansive Learning in Medical Work*. Cambridge: Cambridge University Press.

Kirsch A. 2023. *The Revolt Against Humanity: Imaging a Future Without Us*. New York, NY: Columbia Global Reports.

Kusurkar RA, Croiset G, Mann K, et al. Have Motivation Theories Guided the Development and Reform of Medical Education Curricula? A Review of the Literature. *Academic Medicine*. 2012; 87: 735–43.

Lakoff G, Johnson M. 1999. *Philosophy in the Flesh: The Embodied Mind and Its Challenge to Western Thought*. Chicago, IL: University of Chicago Press.

Launer J. Medicine as Poetry. *Postgraduate Medical Journal*. 2014; 90: 302.

Norris TE, Schaad DC, DeWitt D, et al. Longitudinal Integrated Clerkships for Medical Students: An Innovation Adopted by Medical Schools in Australia, Canada, South Africa, and the United States. *Academic Medicine*. 2009; 84: 902–7.

Paterson D. 2023. Poetry Often Involves Obsessive Personalities. Interview with K Kellaway. *The Guardian*, Saturday January 7. Available at: www.theguardian.com/books/2023/jan/07/don-paterson-poetry-often-involves-obsessive-personalities-toy-fights. Last accessed: 12/1/2023.

Perez CE. 2020. What Does Peirce's Abduction Reveal? *4 Min Read*, December 7. Available at: https://medium.com/intuitionmachine/what-does-peirces-abduction-reveal-8dccf5d3decd#:~:text=Peirce%20likely%20derived%20the%20word%20abduction%20as%20the,take%20away%2C%E2%80%9D%20and%20the%20Latin%20ducere%20%20%E2%80%9Cto%20lead%E2%80%9D. Last accessed: 10/1/2023.

Pinar W. 2019. *What is Curriculum Theory?* (3rd ed.). Abingdon: Routledge.

Scarlett EP. Medicine and Poetry. *Canadian Medical Association Journal*. December 1936; 34: 676.

Snow CP. 1993 (originally pub. 1959). *The Two Cultures (Rede Lecture)*. Cambridge: Cambridge University Press.

Weishaus J. The Physician as Poet. Review of P. Pereira *Saying the World. Philosophy, Ethics, and Humanities in Medicine*. 2006; 1: 8. Available at: www.academia.edu/10339526/The_physician_as_poet_review_of_Pereira_Peter_Saying_the_World. Last accessed: 10/1/2023.

Williams WC. 1962. *Asphodel, That Greeny Flower*. Available at: www.poetry.com/poem/39642/asphodel,-that-greeny-flower. Last accessed: 12/1/2023.

PART 1

Conceptual and practical frames

1

TOWARD A POETICS OF ILLNESS AND HEALING

Laurence J Kirmayer

Introduction

Poetry seems to be a special sort of literary activity engaged in by those who seek to fashion objects with words for personal and aesthetic reasons. Yet reflecting on the concentrated language of poetry and the process of *poiesis* – of creating an aesthetic object like a poem – has much to teach us about everyday struggles to give voice to experience in health and illness. And the expressive, bodily, cognitive, and social consequences of *poiesis* may serve the goals of sense-making and healing that are central to medical care.

In this chapter, I want to explore the significance of *poiesis* for how we understand the articulation and elaboration of symptoms and illness experience and their transformation through healing practices. I begin with some reflections on the distinctive nature of poetry and poetic expression and its relation to our capacities for linguistic expression in cognition and communication. At the heart of poetics is metaphor, and the theory of metaphor helps us see the ways that imagination, embodiment, and enactment underlie the processes of poetic expression and transformation. In the sections that follow, I will discuss ethnographic work on illness experience and healing that reveal the ubiquity of metaphor. The languages we use to make sense of illness experience are rooted in existential universals, personal experience, and particular cultural histories. This points to the need to develop a theory of cultural poetics in illness experience.

Any expression of illness experience weaves together personal and cultural sources of meaning. Contemporary work in conceptual metaphor theory and 4E (embodied, embedded, enacted, and extended) cognitive science offers a way to understand this process, and the second section outlines this perspective and its relevance to illness experience and cultural idioms of distress. The third section applies this to a view of medicine as *poiesis*, fashioning new meanings for illness experience. This includes the implicit use of metaphor in the language of medical theory and practice, in the clinical encounter and the processes of diagnosis and treatment. Clinical ethnographic research reveals this hidden dimension of medical care, which is crucial for understanding both the efficacy and failures of medical practice.

The fourth section considers the deliberate use of metaphor and *poiesis* in clinical contexts to foster transformative processes. This may be as simple as offering an alternate metaphor for experience or as elaborate as developing an extended narrative that can be enacted through ritualized

      DOI: 10.4324/9781003341796-3

performance. The final section turns to poetry proper to discuss what reading or listening and writing or performing poetry afford us in terms of specific types of knowledge, insight, aesthetic experience, self-transformation, and rhetorical power. Poetry allows us to explore intimate experiences, reveal hidden connections, and push back against structures of oppression to enlarge our imagination of the possible in the lives of our patients, ourselves, and our communities.

The origins and immanence of poetic language

We are language animals: it is language that makes us distinctive, allowing our imagination almost boundless scope, enabling the construction of complex social worlds, the richness of our cultures and histories, and the intricacies of our relationships with each other (Taylor 2016). Language enables us to construct our sense of self through organizing autobiographical memory into a narrative arc and to generate expectations for what comes next that are the basis of action, perception, and adaptation (Bouizegarene et al. 2022). While language opens onto infinite worlds of possibility – the subjunctive 'what if' or 'could be' that can be extended as long and as far as we have the breath to continue a sentence with 'and then' – language is rooted in particular cultural histories and worlds of experience. This grounding of words comes from experiences that are always a blend of existential universals – desire, love, loss, pain, suffering, mortality – and the unique circumstances of individual biographies, histories, and positioning in a local world.

The everyday uses of language include both cognitive and social functions. Language allows us to coordinate our relationships with others, plan, make commitments, and, in the case of performative utterances and rhetorical influence, not simply describe situations but bring them into being (Di Paolo et al. 2018). In addition to these basic adaptive functions, there is a wide range of creative and expressive uses of language in literature and the arts including novels, plays, poetry, and other forms. What is distinctive to poetry is the use of attention to language itself to create an aesthetic object that concentrates thought and feeling in a moment of awareness. As Vladimir Nabokov (1967: 218) put it, 'while the scientist sees everything that happens in one point of space, the poet feels everything that happens in one point of time . . . all forming an instantaneous and transparent organism of events, of which the poet . . . is the nucleus'. For the reader, the poem invites an embodied experience in which all the facets of language – sound, sense, order, physical representation, and abstract meaning – work together to link multiple complementary and competing associations between ideas and experiences. The result is not a single image or message that can be concisely paraphrased but an endlessly generative process of meaning-making:

> Through poetry's concentration great sweeps of thought, emotion, and perception are compressed to forms the mind is able to hold – into images, sentences, and stories that serve as entrance tokens to large and often slippery realms of being.
>
> (Hirshfield 1997: 6–7)

Poetic language, then, uses the medium of everyday communication but arranges it in ways that create parallels, layers, and connections in meaning, sound, and form that heighten attentiveness and evocativeness:

> If we take the ideas of a poetic language seriously, it can be defined first as a language in which the sound of words is raised to an importance equal to that of their meaning, and also equal to the importance of grammar and syntax . . . a nonsensical statement may, simply

because of its music, seem to present some kind of truth, or at least to *be* something – even, in a certain way, to be memorable.

(Koch 1998: 44)

Semantic meaning, music or prosody, and syntactic structure all contribute to intensify the emotionally evocative power of poetic language (Johnson-Laird and Oatley 2022).

In addition to this deliberate attention to sound, music, and other material facets of language, poetry has a special relationship to the generative capacities of language enabled by metaphor:

Poetry is made of metaphor. It is a collision, a collusion, a compression of two unlike things: A is B. The term metaphor comes from the Latin *metaphora*, which in turn derives from the Greek *metapherein*, meaning 'to transfer', and, indeed, a metaphor transfers the connotations or elements of one thing (or idea) to another. It is a transfer of energies, a mode of interpenetration, a matter of identity and difference. Each of these propositions about the poem depends upon a metaphor.

(Hirsch 1999: 13)

Metaphor is not simply simile or analogy but an active process of finding new connections by juxtaposition or comparison. The source and target domains of a metaphor interact to generate links based on based on analogies or associations:

For poetry, representation is organized starting with what one might call ontic comparison (the comparison of the already present with the already-present), from which arise figures of images, 'metaphors and other tropes', all the turns of phrase that allow a certain use of language to be defined as 'poetic'.

(Lacoue-Labarthe 1986: 48)

In this way, poetry breaks out of the constraints of conventional narrative to discover new possibilities in and through language. As Edward Hirsch (1999: 10) explains,

[t]he poem is an act beyond paraphrase because what is being said is always inseparable form the way it is being said. Osip Mandelstam suggested that if a poem can be paraphrased, then the sheets haven't been rumpled, poetry hasn't spent the night.

While metaphor is central to all linguistic meaning and can drive narrative reasoning and imagination by foregrounding metaphor and giving it free rein, poetic language intensifies emotional meaning and allows for wider and wilder exploration and invention (Lakoff and Turner 2009). This can not only provide entertaining excursions into the unknown or provocative ways of looking aslant at the familiar but also reveal what may be present yet unsaid or even hitherto unsayable. As Donald Hall (2004: 4) elaborates, poems give embodied expression to experience in all its tensions and contradictions:

Poetry . . . wants to address *the whole matter of the human* – including fact and logic, but also the body with its senses, and above all the harsh and soft complexities of emotion. Our senses, excited by sound and picture, assimilate records of feeling that are also passages to feeling. Poems tell stories; poems recount ideas; but poems *embody* feeling. Because emotion is illogical – in logic opposites cannot both be true; in the life of feeling, we love and hate together – the poem exists to say the unsayable.

Through its ability to bring together conceptual opposites, including embodied feelings that pull us in different directions, poetic expression can be truer to experience than a narrative paraphrase because it captures some of the complexity of an experiential moment. Indeed, the conjunction of opposites and the intensity of conflictual feelings are central to the existential predicament of our experience of consciousness and our sense of being in the world:

> the world is a can of contents under pressure;
> a human being should have a warning label on the side
> that says, *Beware: Disorganized Narrative Inside;*
> *Prone to frequent sideways bursting*
> *of one feeling through another*

(Hoagland 2015: 48)

The narrative that aims to impose a simple order on experience is pressurized and disorganized by the complexity of feelings that accompany life's most signal experiences. Lyric poetry allows us to confront this experience and explore its texture and dimensions, and in so doing, it enlivens and, sometimes, enlightens.

Embodiment, enactment, and *poiesis*

Poiesis refers to making or fashioning, and in the case of poetry, this creative work is done with words. However, it involves words taken in a somewhat different way than their everyday instrumental use to navigate the world. Many of the poetic uses of language are the same as these everyday uses: to formulate and express a point of view, desires, or concerns and elicit from others an appropriate (helpful or desired) response. However, poetry has additional interests or goals that include evoking a perspective or experience, finding a new way of expressing things and achieving new insight, or appealing to the aesthetic pleasures of language, music, and song. These goals involve engaging with language as a material medium with bodily grounding and discursive meaning that is realized through participation in particular cultures and communities. This participation means that poetry allows a kind of *worlding*, in which the places conjured through language create a world that may be experienced as complete and self-contained, even as it clearly draws from the stuff of everyday life (Hayot 2011; Lukács 2023). This world can be local and familiar or expansive and connected to the great diversity the world contains, something celebrated by the post-colonial poet, philosopher, and critic Édouard Glissant (2020) in his notion of the *tout-monde* in which the encounter of different languages creates fertile hybridity through a 'Poetics of Relation'.

The bodily grounding and worldedness of language are revealed in the developmental history and cognitive semantics of metaphor. Lakoff and Johnson (Lakoff and Johnson 2008) explored how metaphors emerge from basic bodily engagements with the world. The infant learns the meaning of words through sensory experiences with important objects and bodily events. The theory of grounded cognition argues that our basic lexicon of concrete nouns is learned through sensory experiences with specific objects and events (Barsalou 2008, 2010). Concrete nouns are the names of specific objects that are generalized to produce more abstract categories. The category retains associations and connotations that point back to the first instances or exemplars on which it is built.

This developmental scaffolding applies not only to objects but also to relationships. Relational terms like 'in' and 'out', 'in front' and 'behind', 'on top' and 'under' are learned through physical actions with objects. These can then be combined following syntactic rules to construct more elaborate phrases and can be extended through metaphor to generate descriptions of new objects, actions, and situations. As the scaffold of meaning is built up, metaphors come to underpin more abstract terms and models that are treated as literal descriptions of the world. They become 'dead' metaphors, whose metaphoric basis is treated as a matter of etymology (Lakoff 1987). As the literary critic Owen Barfield (1973: 63) insisted,

> [e]very modern language, with its thousands of abstract terms and its nuances of meaning and association, is apparently nothing from beginning to end, but an unconscionable tissue of dead or petrified metaphors. . . . A man cannot utter a dozen words without wielding the creation of a hundred named and nameless poets.

Yet it is easy to show that the underlying metaphoric structure is present and influences the connotations of words and the directions of thought. This occurs whether or not we are explicitly aware of the metaphoric origins of our words. In a sense, then, metaphors are never really dead but only hidden, implicit, and sometimes dormant. This recognition has led to the development of conceptual metaphor theory, which shows how pervasively metaphors structure experience, thought, and action (Gibbs 1994, 2005; Thibodeau et al. 2017; Kövecses 2020).

Of course, all language begins and ends in the world we share with others – though we could equally say it begins and ends in our imaginative constructions (Dor 2017). Since the process of languaging is circular, how we describe the beginning and end of this cycle depends on our goal, for example to describe historical or developmental origins, processes of mediation, or outcomes from the point of view of our own or an other's agency and subjectivity. As Marjorie Perloff put it, '[S]ubjectivity always depend[s] on a language and a language belongs to a culture before it belongs to me' (Perloff 1996: 20). Recognizing the social origins and ends of language encourages us to look at how our choice of metaphors reflects a cultural context with its own history, institutions, and practices.

While attention to language would seem to underscore the mediated nature of experience, poetic language often gives us a sense of immediacy even as it draws attention to its own artifice. This duality of vivid presence and deliberate artifice is part of the unique capacity of poetry to move beyond pointing to the world to constitute an experience of worldedness in itself. Phenomenology, cognitive semantics, and 4E cognitive science have revealed some of the secrets of how metaphor mediates the immediate by focusing on processes of embodiment, embedding, enactment, and extension (Gibbs 2005; Gallagher 2017).

Phenomenologically, poetry returns us to elemental experiences of presence through language. From infancy, we are spoken to (and learn to speak) in the crucible of our most intimate and intense relationships and dependencies. Initially, there is no gap between the words we acquire to draw others near (or move them in ways that matter) and the thought or desire itself: evocation/invocation are primary and are part of material reality. Thought itself – and much of feeling and sensation – rests on this footing in language and its gestural and communicative possibilities.

The theory developed in 4E cognitive science outlines how metaphor – and by extension poetry – depends on linguistic capacities that involve embodiment and enactment. Our imagery and evocative language are built on scaffolding of early and essential bodily experiences. Many of these experiences are affectively charged. And whereas much of language, in its everydayness and taken-for-grantedness, lets this scaffolding remain in shadow, poetry deliberately reveals it, sometimes by drawing attention to its own artful construction but most basically through its bodily expression in voice and song. As Pinsky (1998: 8) observes,

> [p]oetry is a vocal, which is to say a bodily, art. The medium of poetry is a human body: the column of air inside the chest, shaped into signifying sounds in the larynx and the mouth. In this sense, poetry is just as physical or bodily an art as dancing.

The embodied, imagery-laden, and sensual nature of poetry animates its language, making it alive and able to move us with its power. It is that efficacy, more than any specific form, that renders language poetic. In its physicality, spoken poetry carries with it always the reality of the body, even when it aspires to evoke and inhabit a disembodied, transcendental realm.

In addition to this physical, embodied basis, metaphor (and poetic language more generally) draws from larger discursive structures – everyday conversational practices, the formulae of performative utterances, ritual, myth, and the grand narratives that encode, justify, and maintain collective history, identity, and cultural institutions. This cultural history and context come to us not just in fully formed versions that we can deploy in the way a storyteller or musician quotes a theme or passage but also as *affordances*: structured patterns and possibilities that are ready to hand (or ear or eye) and that can be used to improvise new narratives or performances. These affordances include ways of attending to the social world (Ramstead et al. 2016). To be enculturated is to learn to read these cultural affordances effortlessly or automatically and experience them as natural, commonsensical, or inevitable.

The overarching discursive structures that constitute a culture, worldview, or tradition may have begun as simply extensions of a metaphor or moment in a brief arc of narrative, but they get elaborated over time, drawing together multiple strands shored up by memory and image, the whole closing in on itself in ways that become a self-sustaining loop. The cultural affordances in a situation, niche, or landscape are produced and maintained by the collective activity of a group or community. In accessing these affordances, we participate in that community, strengthening its presence, ratifying its primacy, and contributing to its lived reality. Culturally grounded thinking – which is most of what we do and recognize as essentially human – is *thinking through other minds* (Veissière et al. 2020). At the same time, we need not be tightly coupled to others in every moment, and we can invent new metaphors or mine even well-worn metaphors for new meaning. Metaphors are inventions that foster inventiveness:

> Effective metaphors are always more complicated than we suppose. Their bright, singular quality, that endorphin-like impact, which strikes so swiftly and so hard, like a happy blow on the head, makes us believe that they are simple. Also, their nature as equations misleads us to suppose that they are the servants of logic. Snow = Sahara. Dead man = fallen nation. A fine metaphor exceeds logic in odd ways.
>
> (Hoagland 2006: 24)

It is precisely because metaphors can precede and exceed logic that they serve as the vehicles for making sense of the new, unfamiliar, and unsettling, including experiences of illness and affliction. In doing so, they do not simply mirror experience but elaborate, enrich, and extend it with new meaning and qualities.

Cultural idioms and the poetics of illness experience

Faced with illness, people across cultures use language to make sense of symptoms and suffering, ask for help, navigate the local health care system, negotiate treatment, and adapt to challenges and limitations. This occurs through everyday conversational practices that initially may be tentative and improvised but that eventually may be consolidated into narratives that provide meaning and coherence to illness experience (Kleinman 1988; Mattingly and Garro 2000). Clinical interventions may work with or against these narratives and in some cases explicitly work to change the symptom or illness narratives in ways that aim to be helpful to the person. Narrative medicine and psychiatry encourage clinicians to listen to patients' stories and employ them to deepen empathy and understanding and to identify resources for coping and healing (Charon 2008; Lewis 2011; Kirmayer et al. 2023). Reading poems and stories can serve important pedagogical goals by enhancing empathy and understandings of illness experience.

The narrative turn in medicine has foregrounded this process of meaning-making through stories but may also exaggerate the coherence and elaborateness of everyday illness narratives (Kirmayer 2000; Woods 2011). Ethnographic studies of illness narratives reveal that they are complex, hybrid assemblages of multiple models that draw from diverse sources of information, including past experiences and knowledge from family or friends, popular media, and medical systems (Kirmayer and Bhugra 2009). In a study of illness explanations in rural Ethiopia, for example, Young (1981, 1982) observed that people used at least three different types of knowledge to assemble illness narratives: (i) sequences of events organized by contiguity or metonymy; (ii) prototypes, based on their own or others' previous experiences or exemplars available in popular media; and (iii) explicit explanatory models drawn from biomedicine or other local, ethnomedical systems. In practice, these are assembled in jury-rigged ways that can be characterized as 'bricolage'; only when challenged by dominant cultural models or medical authority are the gaps and contradictions worked over to create a more seamless and consistent whole. Young's work led to the development of the McGill Illness Narrative Interview, which aims to elicit these narrative strands (Groleau et al. 2006). Although they are usually thoroughly intertwined, temporal narratives, prototypes, and explanatory models can be identified in interview transcripts (Stern and Kirmayer 2004).

The building blocks of illness narratives are metonymic and metaphoric structures that are rooted in personal, cultural, and professional models of symptoms and affliction. The effort to make sense of and communicate complex symptom and illness experiences that are initially inchoate leads to a plethora of diverse and divergent metaphors that may be based on different facets of experience and that may be competing or contradictory (Gibbs 2023). Over time, certain metaphors may come to dominate the way symptoms are expressed and exert effects on both experience and understanding (Kirmayer 1992, 1994). Such dominant metaphors may provide relief or aggravate distress, not simply because they are more or less accurate but because of their personal meaning and connotations as well as their meanings to others in the sufferer's family, community, or the health care system.

If, as Beardsley (1958) suggested, every metaphor is a poem in miniature, and given that metaphors can easily be extended to yield images or scenarios that prompt particular descriptions, trajectories, or stories, we could also say that metaphor is narrative in waiting. Of course, the way that a metaphor is interpreted or unpacked depends on context: both the conversational or discursive context in which the metaphor is introduced and the larger contexts provided by cultural history and creative imagination. Metaphor thus may come before, during, and after narrative: before narrative, when it generates implications that become part of a longer story; during, when the story prompts new metaphors based on how we inhabit it and imagine it forward; and afterward, when the story is stabilized and becomes the basis for new metaphors – that may be intelligible only to those who know the story or catch its drift.

A metaphor offers a way of looking at the world through a particular lens or taking hold of the world in a particular way. Given the complexity and polysemous nature of what the world (and our bodies and thoughts) affords us, any given situation provokes a wide range of metaphors. From moment to moment, sentence to sentence, and, indeed, within any given utterance, we may deploy multiple metaphors that are mixed in their sources, levels of abstraction, and implications. Most of these are conventional or 'throwaway' expressions chosen because they are formulaic or ready to hand or they follow from some stray association in the ongoing streams of language and experience.

Some metaphors may be strikingly novel or idiosyncratic. Both conventional and novel metaphors may be central to our thinking, serving to organize perception, action, and experience; evoking important associations; generating predictions; and producing longer narratives. What makes a metaphor recurrent, central, or dominant in the sense that it serves to organize multiple subordinate metaphors (in a schema) and/or draws more aspects of longer stretches of experience and narration under its dominion? Answering this question can make an important start on answering the related questions of when and how a poem, phrase, or story grips us and promotes change. But the impact of these larger structures of meaning depends vitally on other dimensions including affect, context, the dynamics of relationships, and pragmatic goals of expression and communication.

The metaphoric mediation of illness experience

We use metaphor to make sense of the world; our selves; and our experiences of illness, adversity, and healing. Poetry makes explicit use of metaphor, but metaphoric logic is evident even in mundane language, where basic forms of *poiesis* serve to articulate and elaborate experience. Everyday stories and poetic expressions serve mainly to invoke conventional images and attitudes; employing conventional, formulaic language creates a sense of familiarity and reinforces the ordinary and taken-for-granted nature of daily life. This use of language sustains our routines and, when we are challenged with unfamiliar, threatening, or chaotic situations like illness, helps to organize the inchoate and show a way forward.

Symptom experience is mediated by metaphors: a *killing* pain, a *crippling* fear, a *dark cloud* of depression; all are natural metaphors for embodied experiences of particular forms of distress (Kirmayer 2008). The metaphors not only describe that experience but also evoke associations, sensory images, and thoughts that elaborate on the experience and, in so far as they feedback into bodily processes, may act to maintain or amplify it. Of course, specific metaphors capture only part of any experience; the experience and potential meaning of any symptom or illness always exceeds any particular metaphor – that is why we use many and mixed metaphors in trying to articulate experience. But metaphor too has its own generativity, and once a metaphor is deployed, it opens up new possibilities and ways of seeing that can be mobilized for problem-solving, coping, healing, and growth or transformation.

Illnesses too have metaphoric mediation and elaboration. The metaphors used to talk about illness convey features of the condition as well as the stance that the person takes towards it (Kirmayer 1992; Schuster et al. 2011; Sinnenberg et al. 2018). Asking the patient, 'What does this illness mean to you?' (Carter 1989: 162) can open up a conversation about the metaphors, models, and associations that situate that illness experience in the patient's life and social world.

For some people, high blood pressure is 'hyper-tension', associated with subjective feelings of tension that arise from being 'hyper', too active and reactive to stress (Blumhagen 1980). Diabetes is 'sugar' illness, and in the metaphoric imagination, too much sugar in the blood makes it thick and syrupy, blocking its flow (Naemiratch and Manderson 2007). Cultural models are key to the choice of metaphor, and depending on the associated disease ontology and ethnomedical system, particular instances of metaphoric language may be viewed either as colourful exclamations or literal descriptions of mechanisms. For example, in a mixed-methods study of help-seeking for medically unexplained symptoms, Vietnamese immigrants in Montreal described *phong thấp* (rheumatism) as an illness caused by exposure to winds and cold that results in joint pain (Groleau and Kirmayer 2004). Living in a cold climate and experiencing the emotional chill of a shrinking family in which children have moved away to pursue their careers were also described as causes of the condition.

The functions of clinical diagnosis can also be understood from this perspective. Patients and physicians want coherent explanations that categorize and explain, transforming the unknown into the named and orderly. At the same time, diagnostic labels have connotations that arise from their origins and use in medicine but also in wider cultural spheres; this can include idiosyncratic meanings that clinicians are unaware of but that have powerful effects on patients' experiences. For example, when a nephrologist tells a patient that her low-functioning kidney is 'dead', she imagines it as a dark, black, inert mass in her flank and favours that side for years (Kirmayer 1994). The clinician's offhand remark meant to clarify creates a persistent image and alteration of bodily experience. Every aspect of clinical language has metaphoric connotations or surplus meaning that can lead to unintended consequences (Kirmayer 1988, 1992; Bleakley 2017). For example, Fuks (2021) describes how the frequent use of metaphors of war in medicine serve to mobilize public support for research and hearten patients who feel under attack by disease but may also create conflictual situations that elide other elements of patients' predicament and experience.

In clinical encounters, physicians use metaphors to convey diagnoses, explain symptoms, and prescribe interventions (Bleakley 2017). Even when clinicians think they are using literal language, talk of blood and guts is thick with metaphoric connotations and implications. These metaphors reflect underlying values or attitudes that may be idiosyncratic to the physician, implicit in medical theory, or part of a deliberate effort to find words that speak to patients' concerns. The ways that these metaphors are heard and interpreted depend on patients' pre-existing knowledge and associations and cultural background knowledge, as well as the expectations and framing of the immediate conversation and clinical context. These associations may determine whether metaphors offer hope or lead to cycles of pain and perplexity. In interviews with patients with persistent medically unexplained symptoms, for example, we found they had repetitive narratives that centred on particularly arresting images and/or enduring grievances and a sense of moral injury and injustice (Kirmayer et al. 2004). Compelled to tell the same story over and over, they were unable to move on. The insistent metaphor served to truncate narrative, blocking the subjunctive function of story-making as a generator of possibility.

The clinical encounter itself is undergirded by metaphors for the helping relationship (Carter 1989). The clinician may be seen in diverse ways: as a technician or mechanic whose job is to repair the body; as a teacher or guide who gives health instruction and advice; as a helper, carer, or nurturer who succours the suffering patient and stands by them through adversity; as a wounded-healer, whose knowledge stems from his or her own illness experience; and as a guide who mobilizes the patient's own self-healing capacity (Kirmayer 1988, 2003). Each of these metaphors reflects cultural models and constellates a particular type of relationship that governs the clinical interaction with consequences for the ethics and efficacy of interventions.

Faced with the negative connotations of some metaphors for illness, some have advocated for more careful use of language (Sontag 1978). Certainly, the critique of dominant metaphors is essential for uncovering the hidden values that govern medical practice (Kirmayer 1988). However, given the ubiquity of metaphor in illness experience and emotional expression – as well as in conceptual thinking, problem-solving, and creativity – there is no hope of eliminating metaphor in favour of more literal or 'precise' language. Instead, we need to learn to listen to the metaphors at play in clinical conversations, diagnostic formulations, and interventions. In addition to the ideas that they are intended to convey, these metaphors may have unintended implications through their connotations, surplus meaning, and emotional undertow.

In addition to challenging negative or disabling meanings of metaphors, critique can prompt new metaphors or alternate interpretations. Even conventional metaphors are polysemic and can be extended in novel and unexpected ways that can open up new ways of seeing and new possibilities for action (Törneke 2020; Wohlman 2022). Listening for the evocative meaning of metaphors requires a kind of openness and attentiveness to the body and the other that can foster both empathy and creative imagination (Cox and Theilgaard 1997). A poetics of illness experience that clarifies the personal, social, and cultural roots of the metaphors with which both laypeople and professionals frame symptoms, illness, and afflictions can enable clinicians to more clearly hear and respond to the predicaments that are patients' central concerns (Katz and Shotter 1996; Kirmayer 2023). This response can go beyond recognition and acknowledgement to include the co-construction of new metaphors that allow patients to find ways out of their impasse (Witztum 1988; Siegelman 1993; Törneke 2020).

Poetry and the writing cure

There are many approaches in contemporary medicine, psychiatry, clinical psychology, and expressive arts therapy that aim to use poetry and other forms of creative writing for therapeutic benefit and to promote resilience and wellbeing (Bolton et al. 2004; Connolly Baker and Mazza 2004; Knill and Atkins 2020; Bleakley and Neilson 2022; Kirmayer et al. 2023). Poetry can be used therapeutically in different ways: as bibliotherapy to acknowledge, engage, and enlarge patients' experience (Peterkin and Grewal 2018); as a vehicle for practitioners' education and self-care (Joshi et al. 2022); as a method of reflection on the therapeutic process (Anthony 2004; Phillips 2010); and as a form of creative activity prescribed to patients to mobilize their own self-healing capacities (Collins et al. 2006; Mazza 2021).

There is substantial evidence from experimental research that writing about an emotionally distressing or traumatic experience can lead to improvements in both physical and mental health (Pennebaker and Beall 1986; Niles et al. 2014). This benefit occurs when the narrative recounts negative feelings but also includes positive experiences and provides a coherent story or allows the person to stop ruminating or suppressing the painful memory and put it aside (Pennebaker and Seagal 1999). Interestingly, this benefit may not require that another read or hear the narrative; the act of constructing the narrative itself is beneficial, whether or not there is someone who listens and responds. This work has led to the development of expressive writing as a clinical and health promotion intervention (Pavlacic et al. 2019).

Writing poetry might be expected to have the same benefits. However, there is some evidence that professional poets have poorer mental health than other kinds of writers and artists or the general population (Kaufman and Sexton 2006).[1] The authors suggest that this might be because writing poetry may not include the key elements thought to be beneficial in writing narratives. To the extent that writing poetry intensifies a negative focus on the self and amplifies painful feelings, it could contribute to poor health outcomes, including suicidality (Stirman and Pennebaker 2001). However, Kaufman and Sexton (2006) note that studies of therapeutic writing workshops suggest that writing poetry can have positive effects and that the lack of a narrative (in lyric poetry) does not seem to impede these benefits. They suggest that this potential benefit points to the importance of context in the practice of expressive arts therapies in which the therapist 'holds', maintains, and modulates the space of creation for and with the client. The limitations of current studies also indicate the need for other ways of assessing the coherence-creating, meaning-making, and affect-regulating properties of poetry than those currently used in studies of expressive writing. A closer look at how poetry (and metaphor) work to transform experience can suggest ways that this work could be refined.

Poetics of healing

If metaphor inevitably accompanies clinical language providing a poetic subtext and 'under-thought', it can be harnessed to promote positive therapeutic change. There are many potential ways in which poetic expression can heal, each of which works both within the person to change embodied cognition and consciousness and in communication between people to change relationships:

- *Giving form to cognition and experience*: creating order by organizing the inchoate or reorganizing what has a harmful, disruptive, or disorganizing effect into a coherent, meaningful, and aesthetically satisfying configuration. Metaphors order experience under a particular description and so create coherence. This may involve finding an apt image that captures salient features of experience or creating a higher-order structure that augments, contains, reframes, or transforms experience.
- *Conferring meaning and value* on affliction, pain, suffering, and loss by linking them to predicaments or events that explain why the person got sick or clarifying their personal and cultural significance. This may involve reframing experience as part of a narrative that gives it a larger meaning. This can also serve to maintain coherence and belief in a social order, value system, or cosmology.
- *Creating aesthetic distance from suffering*. The poetic rendering of suffering and affliction may afford the person a sense of separateness from their distress, both by transforming the experience through spatial or other metaphors and by invoking other competing thoughts and feelings associated with aesthetic imagery, art, and play (Nachmanovitch 1991). This may allow us a measure of self-regulation but also facilitate expression.
- *Giving voice to experience*, communicating, and connecting to others. Expressive language is social even in its most basic form as a kind of exclamation, registering presence and urgency and calling forth a response from others, like an infant's cry. The most basic aim is eliciting that desired response: basic cognition, acknowledgement, solidarity, or some specific forms of remedy or restitution. But expression may also be directed back to the self, as we comfort ourselves with our expressions of shared language.

Each of these forms of healing through *poiesis* can occur in spontaneous, idiosyncratic, improvised forms or as part of formal practices in art therapies or other therapeutic frameworks as well as in culturally prescribed forms of ritual and artistic performance. These ritualized practices add further dimensions to healing by mobilizing shared meaning, affirming cultural institutions, and engaging others who are also the target of intervention. Healing rituals in many cultures employ language, gesture, music, dance, and other media to engage the patient and those in their family, community, or entourage (Kirmayer 1993, 2004). In many instances, the ritual may be judged therapeutically successful if others are helped and social values and institutions are affirmed, even if the individual continues to be ill.

Poetic form itself can contribute to the healing process. Compared with everyday language, poetry is characterized by its careful construction and arrangement which find or create order along many dimensions: metre, rhyme, assonance, alliteration, spatial arrangement on the page. In so doing, it strengthens the evocative and order-making functions of metaphor and imagination. As Gregory Orr (2002: 16–7, italics in original) suggests, this is a basic human faculty:

The awareness of disorder generates in the human mind a spontaneous ordering response. This ordering response is innate, a natural power – all human minds possess it. Why not call it 'imagination' and recognize it as a fundamentally human cognitive capacity?

This order-making function is what Jung (1916/1969) called the *transcendent function*, the self-organizing or healing capacity of the psyche, which uses imagery, fantasy, dreams, internal dialogue, or active imagination to create symmetry, balance, completeness, and closure to restore wellbeing (Miller 2004). Poetry can provide an arena for this symbolic dialogue through the process of reverie, imagination, and the emergent construction of a poem or text. This inner work is facilitated when the poem is not constrained by narrative but can follow the evocative associations of image, sound, and word through to new discoveries and encounters with the self, as Orr (2002: 22) argues: 'In the personal lyric, the self encounters its existential crises in symbolic form, and the poem that results is a model of this encounter'.

Our interest here is especially in lyric poetry, which differs from the extended narrative of epic or other forms. Hirsch (1999: 242) suggests that '[P]oems are lyrical precisely because they interrupt or interfere with narrative', forcing us to stop, look, and listen. Lyric presents a concentrated reflection or exploration of a moment of time or stretch of consciousness. As such, lyric has particular dynamics that differ from those of longer narrative forms (Bleakley and Neilson 2022); these dynamics reside in part in the nature of metaphor and in the ways in which a poem can enact a metaphor not only in a sequence of images but in its overall structure.

Metaphors draw attention to neglected elements of experience. A poem can provide a metacognitive frame that attends to neglected elements or possibilities that allow us to break the grip of a narrow view, affording greater cognitive and affective flexibility (Hinton and Kirmayer 2017). Through metaphor, a poem allows us to look at the world or a facet of experience in a new way. What we see that surprises us teaches us something about how language shapes our perception of the world and the ways we take hold of it. Poet-philosopher Jan Zwicky (2014: 33) describes this unsettling process as 'what the world acquires/From the strangeness of the way we see'. This 'making strange' enriches and enlivens our imagination, making even ordinary experience an object of intense interest (Perloff 1996).

One way to understand the cognitive and meaning-generating functions of metaphor and *poiesis* is through the notion of conceptual blending, in which metaphors (and narratives) evoke imaginal spaces formed from the interaction of words and images (Turner 1996; Fauconnier and Turner 2008). These spaces are not static but provide a scene one can enter, inhabit, and transform through metaphoric action.

Metaphors then create movement. Poetry evokes metaphoric landscapes that allow movement through sensory, affective, and imaginative space. This movement can occur in myriad ways, but its significance can be illustrated with four kinds of movement: inward and downward, to explore the self; outward to engage the world; between self and other, to engage with alterity; and along a vertical axis, 'upward' to transcendence.

Descending into the self: spelunking the soul

Poetry can be a vehicle of self-exploration, creating and nourishing a sense of depth and interiority. The metaphor of depth suggests exploration, mystery, weight, and profundity, as Antonio Machado's (2012) aphoristic poem makes plain:

> Mankind owns four things
> That are no good at sea:
> Rudder, anchor, oars,
> And the fear of going down.

The sense of interiority comes from the nature of embodiment and perspective: we have private experience by virtue of our physical boundedness, but where we draw the boundaries of the self reflects cultural constructions of personhood (Kirmayer 2007a). We have circles of intimacy or privacy into which we may invite others, and we are also mysteries to ourselves in some ways.

The process of reading and writing can lead us to new insights, new places, and hitherto unrecognized, unacknowledged, or even unsuspected aspects of the self. Everyday experiences of illness and health can be imbued with layers of meanings that come from this process of self-exploration. Visiting these interior places, uncovering forgotten memories or inner secrets, deepens our sense of self and complexity, and, while it may risk self-estrangement, when governed by the right attitude and receptiveness, it can lead to self-acceptance and, ultimately, connection to others in our common humanity and unique experience. As Dean Young (2010: 83–4) suggests, '[P]oetry's greatest task . . . is to foster a necessary privacy in which the imagination can flourish. Then we may have something to say to each other'.

Reaching out to the world: materiality and the imagination of matter

Poetry can connect us to the world in especially vivid ways, evoking a sense of kinship and connection with all that is outside us, beyond our mundane human concerns, allowing us to recognize the ways in which we are part of nature. This happens through images that evoke the bodily grounding of experience. The sensory qualities of imagery and imagistic language provide sensual pleasure and emotional connection to what matters (Abram 1996). As Blake (1975) put it in *The Marriage of Heaven and Hell*,

> Body is a portion of Soul discern'd by the five Senses
> the chief inlets of Soul in this age

At the same time, sensory imagery through the invocation of objects and experience in the world allows us to imagine *with* matter, to draw from the materiality of experience in ways that open new imaginative possibilities (Bleakley 2020). The prose poems of Francis Ponge (1972) show how through close attention to the sensory and sensual qualities of objects (including the objects of medical inquiry and care), we can engage them not as static entities but as vehicles of imagination and transformation. This is the alchemical dimension of *poiesis* in which the world is a mirror of the soul (Bleakley 2023).

The work on reverie and the imagination of elements by the philosopher Gaston Bachelard (1964, 1969, 1971; Smith 2016) explores this potential for thinking with and through matter. His poetic excursions reveal the thorough intertwining of existential universals, shared cultural meaning, and personal idiosyncrasy in the choice of tropes and the tracing of their implications. Engagement with the sensual qualities of the material world acts as a counter to our tendency to retreat when wounded or confronted by illness and adversity. Though medicine confronts us with stark realities of bodily injury and pathology, Bleakley (2020) shows how openness and attentiveness to sensory experience can humanize medical education and practice.

Recognizing the other: the politics of alterity

As much as we share a common humanity, we are also mysteries to each other. We can affirm a basic solidarity by ignoring this gap – appealing to our common experience and shared existential predicaments – but a more profound kind of connection comes from recognizing and accepting our differences. Poetry can invite us into the embodied experience of difference, whether it is manifested in a gendered body, a divided self, or a particular kind of experience of illness and suffering.

Reading poetry provides an opportunity to learn about different ways of being human, across variations in gender, embodiment, social position, and both personal and collective histories. In clinical work, this allows us to imaginatively engage the other, recognizing both our similarities and differences not just from a third person perspective but, more intimately, as felt experience, habitus, and habitation. The philosopher Emmanuel Levinas (2003) argued that this recognition of the Other as fundamentally 'other' is the basis of ethical awareness. This recognition of otherness is basic to medical care (Clifton-Soderstrom 2003; Irvine 2005), while literature and poetry provide important pedagogical tools in medical education for learning about the Other (Kirmayer et al. 2023).

The poet Paul Celan struggled long and hard with this challenge of alterity, which was made inescapable by the horrors of the Shoah (Felstiner 1995, 2001; Celan and Hamburger 2007; Kirmayer 2007b). He adopted a recondite vocabulary and extreme concision in his later poems to explore extremities of experience that could only be conveyed through language that demanded intense focus. At the same time, he rejected claims that he was a 'hermetic' writer whose meanings were obscure. On the contrary, while differences and divides between people are inevitable, he saw each poem as an opening and invitation to a sincere encounter. As he put it, 'I cannot see any basic difference between a handshake and a poem' – provided the writer has 'truthful hands that write true poems' (Celan 1986).

Encountering otherness through poetry can open new ways of being with people who differ from us in their background and life experience. Of course, illness itself constitutes a primordial 'Other' that may be located within us, a manifestation of the autonomy of the body that that the early psychosomaticist Georg Groddeck (1991) called 'the It'. Illness can be experienced as a strange other within us with its own agency and agenda. Cancer may be imagined as a crab clawing at one's insides (Demaitre 1998) or a malevolent entity that invades and colonizes the body even as it is attacked by the army of the immune system (Williams Camus 2009). Infectious diseases are also invaders that must be defended against and vanquished, but people with the stigma of a disease that is perceived as infectious (even when it is not) are themselves tainted with the negative emotional valences of the disease (Curtis 2013). We keep our distance from the presumed carrier of disease for fear of contamination or infection. Fear of contagion, disfigurement, pain, suffering, and mortality, as well as the varied metaphorical meanings attached to disease, all can contribute to stigmatization. The afflicted person then can suffer social exclusion, marginalization, and self-estrangement.

Poetry can capture the intensity of this self-estrangement and, in some instances, transform this primal experience for the sufferer and for others who accompany them. Here is an example of how poet Max Ritvo (2016), drawing on metaphors of dust and cleansing, confronted and transfigured his relationship to his own tortured body during the long struggle with the cancer that ended his life in his twenties (extract from 'The End'):

> The moon was dark
> like it had taken too many pills
> to produce light.
> . . .
>
> Heaven was a vacuum –
> the earth, a dirty carpet.
> . . .
>
> Perhaps He is using my body
> to remake His
> into a kind of thinking dust.

For Ritvo, who brought extraordinary expressive and reflective abilities to bear on his experiences of extremity, the body in illness is the Other that, in epiphanic vision, can connect him with the ultimate other of God – or remind him of the possibility of choice and agency even in the face of mortality. In the same poem, Ritvo (*ibid*.) says 'God may have many images/He may want even more', while there is 'no madness but the one of life'.

The opposition of self and illness as other is still more challenging in the case of psychiatric conditions in which the very experience of self is altered or undermined; this is so both for the afflicted person and for others close to them. The poet David Ignatow (1993) wrote of this other in his experiences with his son, who suffered from schizophrenia. In *Sunday at the State Hospital*, he describes the painful ruptures in body and time he and his son experience, as his son eats his 'visit sandwich', his 'past is sitting in front of' him, trying unsuccessfully 'to bring the present to its mouth'. Ignatow (1973) struggled with guilt over his son's illness and his own desire to devote himself to writing. Yet poetry also allowed Ignatow a way find power and meaningfulness in his son's experience and, through a shared epiphany, a path towards acceptance that he describes in his poem *The Rightful One*:

> I heard my son burst out of his room
> and shout, he is here, dad. He is here.
> I understood and I managed to stand up,
> melting within, and walk the hall
> between our rooms to meet Him
> whom I had neglected in my thoughts

The hallucinatory presence of God or Christ, as an archetype of the wounded-healer, brings forgiveness, enjoins the father to bless his son, and leaves him with 'a power to feel free'. His epiphany speaks to the parents of any child with grave affliction who struggles make sense of the meaning of suffering. It also speaks to those who directly experience such challenges, as the poet and health practitioner Paul White (2014: unpaginated) has eloquently described:

> I was diagnosed a paranoid schizophrenic at age seventeen. The poetry of David Ignatow helped to save my life. I carried his little red book of selected poems wherever I went. My hands began to wear the colors off the covers. His book was like a talisman to ward off anxiety. If I could only stop and read for a moment, I'd be okay. In general, people do not want to know about schizophrenia. When I would try to tell people about my experience, it was as if a brick had fallen out of my mouth and landed on their foot. I learned to keep my mouth shut. David Ignatow's notebooks are full of desperation and anguish in dealing with a mentally ill son. Even though I never met him, David Ignatow became like a spiritual father to me.

White found validation for his experience in Ignatow's poems and notebooks and could identify with both the afflicted son and the anguished father. The content of the poems provided moments of recognition and the act of writing itself a path forward.

Poets' accounts of their own suffering serve as anchors and affirmations of solidarity with others who wrestle with similar states of extremity. Jane Kenyon (1992) wrote of her own depression in *Having It Out with Melancholy*:

> When I was born, you waited
> behind a pile of linen in the nursery,
> and when we were alone, you lay down
> on top of me, pressing
> the bile of desolation into every pore.

A long recitation of drugs taken to treat her recurrent episodes of depression ends with an epiphany. Kenyon is 'High on Nardil and June light' when she wakes early eager for the 'first note of the wood thrush'. She is 'overcome//by ordinary contentment' and wonders what has hurt her so badly throughout her life until this epiphany:

> How I love the small, swiftly
> beating heart of the bird
> singing in the great maples;
> its bright, unequivocal eye.

Connection to the world, recognizing the sentience of the bird in its 'bright, unequivocal eye', brings a moment of equipoise and connection that makes past hurts distant and less unavailing.

Reaching upward: poetics of wholeness and transcendence

Poetry can express feelings of hope and yearning, a sense of immanence or presence, and the experience of transcendence. Reading and writing poems can do this because the poem creates a house in time that we can inhabit and that, on entering, transforms body, self, and person. The poetic moment involves what Gaston Bachelard (Bachelard and Lescure 2013: 173) calls 'the principle of an essential simultaneity in which the most scattered and disunited being achieves unity'. As

Richard Kearney (2008: 38) notes, 'Bachelard claims that every "real" poem signals a stopping of ordinary clock time, introducing instead a dimension of "verticality," in depth and height'. The poetics of presence and transcendence reflect not simply the content of poems, which may talk explicitly or obliquely about the quest for or encounter with the sacred, but especially the ways that the poem invites a kind of participation in the moment through attentive reading or listening and active imagination, which allows words and images to take flight.

Poetry provides the kind of transcendence possible in an instant of perception of the connectedness of all things – not as something we own or encompass but as all that we can be in living relation to. This transcendence is present in Kenyon's (2005) poem 'Briefly It Enters, and Briefly Speaks', which stands as a clear counterpoint to her poem about her experiences of depression discussed earlier and amplifies that poem's epiphany. In the poem, Kenyon rings the changes of personae as, amongst a host of delectable objects, a blossom pressed in a book found after 200 years; a maker, a lover, and a keeper; food on a prisoner's plate; water filling a well-head and spilling from a pitcher; a patient gardener of a 'dry and weedy' garden; from a musk rose that opens to the world unattended. As a poet should, she catches the reader by surprise for here objects of utility are equally praised (a hinge, a latch, a stone step) and surprise too where she is a 'heart contracted by joy' – and not, as we might expect, a heart expanded. Here is the site of love and courage pulled in on itself. Finally,

> I am the one whose love
> overcomes you, already with you
> when you think to call my name

The poem is not simply the recollection and record of a timeless moment of transcendence but, by building towards that through a series of common objects and experiences, is an invitation to the reader to feel more fully present and replete in life. The poem thus shows us a way to enact a contemplative stance through aesthetic awareness.

While the process of reading a poem unfolds in linear time, the images it evokes layer one on another to create a moment dense with meaning. Absorbed in this experience, we may become unaware of its duration, existing outside the ordinary flow of time. The poem can play with time, moving back and forth across a lifespan but making each memory or recollection feel present, and invoke mythic time, which is eternal, by holding us in immanence:

> I think this feeling of transformation, of an action taking place in real time, the time it takes to read the poem, is what we crave from poetry, even if a poem spends most of its energy recounting an event that has already happened. To crave change is to court mortality, the event toward which all change points, but poems afford us the opportunity to experience loss as gain, absence as presence: our experience of the language fulfills us even as we are asked to inhabit the future perfect – the knowledge that one day we will have been.
>
> (Longenbach 2013: 157)

This transformation of temporality is one of the most profound effects of poetry because it allows us to confront the experiences of duration that are central to suffering and the sense of limitedness that is the burden of mortality. This confrontation is not a rejection or negation of the existential facts of illness, suffering, and death but their transmutation, through grief, into sources of presence, empathy, solidarity, and creative imagination.

The poem then provides a way to transform experience, to change the meaning and significance of memories and our perceptions of the world by mobilizing alternate images, frames, and ways of attending. The poetic moment distils that movement of transformation, of containing the ineffable in a configuration that includes the tensions and contradictions of life within a supervening aesthetic order. The poem provides a kind of liminal space, a threshold where disorder meets order, as Orr (2002: 53) suggests: 'At [that] threshold, linguistic, imaginative, and emotional energies are vastly heightened'. This heightened meaning and emotional energy or activation mean that poetry may provide not a static state of completion and order but a ferment of possibility, an invitation to disorder in which imagination is poised at the edge of chaos:

> The essential point is that for a poem to move us it must bring us near our own threshold. We must feel genuinely threatened or destabilized by the poem's vision of disordering, even as we are simultaneously reassured and convinced by its orderings.
>
> (ibid.: 55)

The threshold between aesthetic order and disorder depends on our own mental state, personal history, and cultural resources. This disordering effect of poetry occurs especially when it engages with violence, transgressive imagery, and experience. Writing of his own profound traumatic loss and the ways in which poetry served to provide a way forward, Orr (*ibid.*: 92) attests to this potential for poetry to address even the most extreme experiences, where 'the enormous disordering power of trauma needs or demands an equally powerful ordering to contain it, and poetry offers such order'.

To account for this ordering power, Orr (*ibid.*: 94) further suggests that 'there are three abiding and primordial powers that shape language into poems regardless of the culture: story, symbol, and incantation'. Story allows us to reframe experience as part of a larger structure of meaning. Symbol concentrates meaning in evocative images, where '[T]he incantatory power . . . [of] repetitions loosen[s] the intellect for reverie' (Hirsch 1999: 22). It is in the addition of techniques of densely layered or linked symbols (images, metaphors) and the music and rhythm of incantation (and song) that lyric poetry achieves unique effects not typically present in prose.

Incantation can bring us into our bodies in a way that gives meaning to momentary experience but links us to a larger arc. Here is Orr's (2021: 54) recognition of the everyday miracle of embodiment:

> Talk about miracles!
> How I take empty air
> Deep in my lungs,
> Warming it there,
> Extracting from it
> What my blood needs,
> Then breathing it back
> Out as sound
> I've added meaning to.

The poem celebrates the life-giving mechanisms of the body, tracing the path of air into the lungs and back out into the world as sounds imbued with meaning and intention. Breathing draws in air for sustenance but also turns it into the vehicle for meaningful communication and connection to others.

The metaphor of breath and the possibility of transcendence made possible by this movement between inside and outside are explored with poignancy in the memoir of the neurosurgeon Paul Kalanithi (2016), *When Breath Becomes Air*, who died of cancer at the age of 37. Tracing the arc of life from his passion for literature to his embrace of the vocation of medicine, Kalanithi reflects on the existential challenges at the heart of the clinical encounter that can guide ethical practice. His memoir is also a record of his own insights as a wounded-healer as he struggles to come to terms with his impending death. In an essay on the narrative self in terminal illness, de Muijnck (2019) describes the ways in which Kalanithi's narrative serves to articulate, affirm, and stabilize the many strands of his identity as physician, lover of literature, writer, husband, father, and friend. As Kalanithi (2016: 39) put it,

> I had come to see language as an almost supernatural force, existing between people bring-ing our brains, shielded in centimeter-thick skulls, into communion. A word means some-thing only between people, and life's meaning, its virtue, had some to do with the depth of relationships we form. It was . . . human relationality . . . that undergirded meaning.

Although Kalanithi treasures his memories and longs for an unreachable future, his openness and imagery and the lyrical quality of his prose invoke a timeless present even as he confronts the hard stop of mortality. This is captured in the metaphor of his title, which locates us at the cusp between life and death, the place where we can live fully even as we are dying.

The politics and praxis of healing

The healing potential of writing and reading lyric poetry stems from its capacity to organize expe-rience in ways that imbue it with meaning, contain or transform suffering and symptoms, enrich our imagination with possibilities, and enliven our engagement with the world. Of course, poetry shares this with narrative and other art forms, but it can achieve these effects with concision and immediacy. As Orr (2002: 405) puts it,

> [h]uman culture 'invented' or evolved the personal lyric as a means of helping individu-als survive existential crises represented by extremities of subjectivity and also by such outer circumstances as poverty, suffering, pain, illness, violence or loss of a loved one. This survival begins when we 'translate' our crisis into language – where we give it symbolic expression as an unfolding drama of self and the forces that assail it. This same poem also arrays the ordering powers our shaping imagination has brought to bear on these disorder-ings. Thus the poem we compose (or respond to as readers) still accurately mirrors the life crisis it dramatizes, still displays life's interplay of disorder and order. But in the act of mak-ing a poem at least two crucial things have taken place that are different from ordinary life. First, we have shifted the crisis to a bearable distance from us: removed it to the symbolic but vivid world of language. Second, we have actively made and shaped this model of our situation rather than passively endured it as lived experience.

One function of a poem – as with other kinds of artistic activity – is that it can create aesthetic dis-tance: one is confronted with emotional evocative stimuli but in a somewhat distanced or diluted form, strong enough to evoke strong emotion but not so strong as to be overwhelming or (re) traumatizing. This distancing can be beneficial when it is offered or presented by a particular form of aesthetic activity that allows a measure of control by the listener/viewer (who can let their mind wander or be riveted to the experience), in which case it becomes a limited form of agency over experiences that are otherwise beyond our control. Scheff (1979) describes the ways in which ritual and artistic performances manipulate aesthetic distance to find an optimal position that allows catharsis: experiencing and expressing emotion freely but without re-injury. Aesthetic form itself may allow a helpful distance from pain, conflict, and confusion, as Doty (2010: 80) notes: '[M] etaphor's distancing aspect may allow us to speak more freely'.

In his moving compendium of poems of loss and grief, Hirsch (2021) describes the personal context of the poems, their emotional presence and rhetorical power, and technical aspects of their construction. The personal and historical background to the poems intensify their meaning and resonance. When discussing elements of craft and technical devices, however, Hirsch enacts a kind of aesthetic distancing, exemplifying the multilevel awareness that the act of reading can afford. And in offering this instruction to the reader, he provides a guide to creating such distance and order in one's own writing. Hirsch brought this aesthetic power to bear on his own grief in his book-length poem and elegy for his son, *Gabriel* (2014), which wrestles with his irresolvable pain and confusion, even as it insists that the irremediable nature of loss is an essential act of remembering.

Beyond emotion regulation, poetry involves other forms of language as 'doing' and active reshaping of the world, first in imagination, then in our bodily engagements, and finally in the lived experience of a community. This can involve reconfiguring our modes of self-understanding and the ways we present ourselves to others, but it can also change our families, social niches, and larger societal contexts. It also holds the promise of building bridges to others who have different identities, histories, cultural backgrounds, and social positions.

An encounter with poetry can build bridges to worlds of experience that are otherwise barred to us. We can experience moments of embodied knowing and new forms of relatedness to others whose experiences are radically different from our own. This can allow us to begin to understand the powerful forces that shape our unique experiences and positions in the world that vary with age, gender, sickness, trauma, structural violence, and racialized or other stigmatized identities that give rise to discrimination. Understanding these larger contexts of affliction is crucial to structural competence in medicine and healing (Metzl and Hansen 2014; Tsevat et al. 2015).

Many poets have offered vivid portraits of the reality of racism through works that capture the sweep of history, the personal impacts of violence, or the microcosm of moments of everyday misrecognition and exclusion (Derricotte 2019; Brand 2022). While poetry cannot resolve the enduring forms of structural violence and systemic racism, it can kindle an awareness that begins a process of personal transformation (Stepakoff 1997). As Derricotte (1999: 18) suggests, 'We are all wounded by racism, but for some of us, those wounds are anesthetized. None of us, black or white, wants to feel the pain that racism has caused. But when you feel it, you're awake'. Allowing ourselves to be opened and reshaped by these encounters with the other enlarges our imagination and, with that, the possibilities for empathy, solidarity, and healing. Through confronting mortality, loss, grief, and pain in their shared and unique expressions, poems can allow us to become more fully awake and to mobilize the ethical stance and power of the wounded-healer (Kirmayer 2003).

Conclusion

A poetics of medicine starts with recognizing the ubiquity of metaphor and imagination in illness experience and healing practices. Ghalib (in Hirshfield 1997: 5) says, 'For the raindrop, joy is in entering the river –/Unbearable pain becomes its own cure'. Attention to metaphor in illness narratives and clinical interventions has many potential benefits. Listening to patients' metaphors provides a way into their self-understanding and ways of coping. Similar attention to the metaphors of medical literature and clinical practice can reveal the (often unintended) metaphoric connotations of the clinical diagnosis and interventions. With this awareness, we can begin to move beyond technical and instrumental goals to explore aspects of meaning and embodied experience that are crucial for wellbeing and effective care. Finally, we can develop a clinically applied poetics that makes strategic use of metaphor in therapeutic interventions to elicit beneficial placebo effects, altering symptom experience and helping patients make sense of suffering.

Poetic language – in everyday communication and in the deliberate construction of poems – has the power to connect us to each other, to the texture of experience and the unique positions we each occupy in the world. As such, a poetics of medicine can serve basic pedagogical goals of enhancing empathy and understanding. Learning to listen to the poetics of language is an essential tool for medical communication; it reveals the bodily, emotional, and cultural formations that underlie clinical conversation. A poetics of illness experience and healing offers tools for taking hold of experience and transforming it by generating alternate metaphors and creating forms and frames that allow aesthetic distance and imaginative transformation. Active engagement with *poiesis* opens onto a politics of knowing that acknowledges the other in our common humanity and essential alterity. And as the epigram by the eighth-century Urdu poet Ghalib declares, at times, poetry can bring a profound shift in perspective that transforms pain, suffering, and demoralization into the kinds of insight, aliveness, and belonging that are medicine for the human condition.

Note

1 The studies showing this disadvantage are methodologically limited, with multiple confounds and an inability to resolve causal direction. They tend to focus on famous artists present in the literary and historical record, confounding fame and success with activity per se. They also tend to employ crude proxy measures of mental health. Most importantly, such studies examine lifetime correlates without resolving causal direction, leaving it unclear whether poetry writing precedes (and hence might contribute) to poor mental health or follows (and hence might be a consequence of or even an effort to mitigate) mental health problems. For example, it is unclear whether people are drawn (or driven) to artistic activity or vocations because of pre-existing mental health problems (in which case the activity could still be helpful compared with what the outcome might have been without such engagement). Finally – as Kaufman and Sexton (2006) note – poetry (like mathematics) is an area where some achieve great success early in life, increasing the chances that if they die young, they will have left a meaningful legacy that increases their likelihood of being included in retrospective studies.

References

Abram D. 1996. *The Spell of the Sensuous: Perception and Language in a More-Than-Human World*. New York, NY: Vintage Books.

Anthony E. 2004. Third Person Song: The Poetics of Response. In: BL Moon, R Schoenholtz (eds.) *Word Pictures: The Poetry and Art of Art Therapists*. Springfield, IL: Charles C Thomas Publisher.

Bachelard G. 1964. *The Psychoanalysis of Fire*. Boston, MA: Beacon Press.

Bachelard G. 1969. *The Poetics of Space*. Boston, MA: Beacon Press.

Bachelard G. 1971. *The Poetics of Reverie: Childhood, Language, and the Cosmos*. Boston: Beacon Press.

Bachelard G, Lescure J. 2013. *Intuition of the Instant*. Evanston, IL: Northwestern University Press.

Barfield O. 1973. *Poetic Diction: A Study in Meaning*. Middletown, CT: Wesleyan University Press.

Barsalou LW. Grounded Cognition. *Annual Review of Psychology*. 2008; 59: 617–45.

Barsalou LW. Grounded Cognition: Past, Present, and Future. *Topics in Cognitive Science*. 2010; 2: 716–24.

Beardsley MC. 1958. *Aesthetics*. New York, NY: Harcourt, Brace World.

Blake W. 1975. *The Marriage of Heaven and Hell*. Oxford: Oxford University Press.

Bleakley A. 2017. *Thinking with Metaphors in Medicine: The State of the Art*. Abingdon: Routledge.

Bleakley A. 2020. *Educating Doctors' Senses Through the Medical Humanities: "How Do I Look?"*. Abingdon: Routledge.

Bleakley A. 2023. *Psychotherapy, the Alchemical Imagination and Metaphors of Substance*. Berlin/Boston: Walter de Gruyter GmbH.

Bleakley A, Neilson S. 2022. *Poetry in the Clinic: Towards a Lyrical Medicine*. Abingdon: Routledge.

Blumhagen D. Hyper-Tension: A Folk Illness With a Medical Name. *Culture, Medicine and Psychiatry*. 1980; 4: 197–227.

Bolton G, Howlett S, Lago C, Wright JK. 2004. *Writing Cures: An Introductory Handbook of Writing in Counseling and Therapy*. Hove: Brunner-Routledge.

Bouizegarene N, Ramstead M, Constant A, et al. 2022. Narrative as Active Inference: An Integrative Account of the Functions of Narrative. *PsyXiv*. 10.

Brand D. 2022. *Nomenclature New and Collected Poems*. Durham, NC: Duke University Press.

Carter AH. Metaphors in the Physician-Patient Relationship. *Soundings*. 1989; xx?: 153–64.

Celan P. 1986. *Collected Prose*. Riverdale-on-Hudson, New York: The Sheep Meadow Press.

Celan P, Hamburger M. 2007. *Poems of Paul Celan*. London: Anvil Press Poetry.

Charon R. 2008. *Narrative medicine: Honoring the Stories of Illness*. New York, NY: Oxford University Press.

Clifton-Soderstrom M. Levinas and the Patient as Other: The Ethical Foundation of Medicine. *Journal of Medicine and Philosophy*. 2003; 28: 447–60.

Collins KS, Furman R, Langer CL. Poetry Therapy as a Tool of Cognitively Based Practice. *The Arts in Psychotherapy*. 2006; 33: 180–87.

Connolly Baker K, Mazza N. The Healing Power of Writing: Applying the Expressive/Creative Component of Poetry Therapy. *Journal of Poetry Therapy*. 2004; 17: 141–54.

Cox M, Theilgaard A. 1997. *Mutative Metaphors in Psychotherapy: The Aeolian Mode*. London: Jessica Kingsley Publishers.

Curtis V. 2013. *Don't Look, Don't Touch: The Science Behind Revulsion*. Oxford: Oxford University Press.

de Muijnck D. 'When Breath Becomes Air': Constructing Stable Narrative Identity During Terminal Illness. *Colloquy*. 2019; 38: 44–69.

Demaitre L. Medieval Notions of Cancer: Malignancy and Metaphor. *Bulletin of the History of Medicine*. 1998; 72: 609–37.

Derricotte T. 1999. *The Black Notebooks: An Interior Journey*. New York, NY: WW Norton & Company.

Derricotte T. 2019. *I: New & Selected Poems*. Pittsburgh, PA: University of Pittsburgh Press.

Di Paolo EA, Cuffari EC, De Jaegher H. 2018. *Linguistic bodies: The continuity between life and language*. Cambridge, MA: MIT press.

Dor D. From Experience to Imagination: Language and Its Evolution as a Social Communication Technology. *Journal of Neurolinguistics*. 2017; 43: 107–19.

Doty M. 2010. *The Art of Description: World into Word*. Minneapolis, MN: Graywolf Press.

Fauconnier G, Turner M. 2008. *The Way We Think: Conceptual Blending and the Mind's Hidden Complexities*. New York, NY: Basic Books.

Felstiner J. 1995. *Paul Celan: Poet, Survivor, Jew*. New Haven, CT: Yale University Press.

Felstiner J. 2001. *Selected Poems and Prose of Paul Celan*. New York, NY: WW Norton.

Fuks A. 2021. *The Language of Medicine*. Oxford: Oxford University Press.

Gallagher S. 2017. *Enactivist Interventions: Rethinking the Mind*. Oxford: Oxford University Press.

Gibbs Jr RW. 1994. *The Poetics of Mind: Figurative Thought, Language, and Understanding*. Cambridge: Cambridge University Press.

Gibbs Jr RW. 2005. *Embodiment and Cognitive Science*. Cambridge: Cambridge University Press.

Gibbs Jr RW. How Metaphors Shape the Particularities of Illness and Healing Experiences. *Transcultural Psychiatry*. 2023; 60: 770–780.

Glissant E. 2020. *Treatise on the Whole-World*. Liverpool: Liverpool University Press.

Groddeck G. 1991. *The Book of the It*. New York, NY: Vintage Books.

Groleau D, Kirmayer LJ. Sociosomatic Theory in Vietnamese Immigrants' Narratives of Distress. *Anthropology & Medicine*. 2004; 11: 117–33.

Groleau D, Young A, Kirmayer LJ. The McGill Illness Narrative Interview (MINI): An Interview Schedule to Elicit Meanings and Modes of Reasoning Related to Illness Experience. *Transcultural Psychiatry*. 2006; 43: 671–91.

Hall D. 2004. *Breakfast Served Any Time all Day: Essays on Poetry New and Selected*. Ann Arbor, MI: University of Michigan Press.

Hayot E. On Literary Worlds. *Modern Language Quarterly*. 2011; 72: 129–61.

Hinton DE, Kirmayer LJ. The Flexibility Hypothesis of Healing. *Culture, Medicine, and Psychiatry*. 2017; 41: 3–34.

Hirsch E. 1999. *How to Read a Poem: And Fall in Love With Poetry*. Boston, MA: Houghton Mifflin Harcourt.

Hirsch E. 2014. *Gabriel: A Poem*. New York, NY: Knopf Doubleday.

Hirsch E. 2021. *100 Poems to Break Your Heart*. Boston, MA: Houghton Mifflin.

Hirshfield J. 1997. *Nine Gates: Entering the Mind of Poetry*. New York, NY: HarperCollins.

Hoagland T. 2006. *Real sofistikashun: Essays on Poetry and Craft*. Saint Paul, MN: Graywolf Press.

Hoagland T. 2015. *Application for Release From the Dream*. Minneapolis, MN: Graywolf Press.

Ignatow D. 1973. *The Notebooks of David Ignatow*. Chicago: Swallow Press.

Ignatow D. 1993. *Against the Evidence: Selected Poems, 1934–1994*. Middletown, CT: Wesleyan University Press.

Irvine C. The Other Side of Silence: Levinas, Medicine, and Literature. *Literature and Medicine*. 2005; 24: 8–18.

Johnson-Laird PN, Oatley K. How Poetry Evokes Emotions. *Acta Psychologica*. 2022; 224: 103506.

Joshi A, Paralikar S, Kataria S, et al. Poetry in Medicine: A Pedagogical Tool to Foster Empathy Among Medical Students and Health Care Professionals. *Journal of Poetry Therapy*. 2022; 35: 85–97.

Jung CG. 1969 (originally pub. 1916). The Transcendent Function. In: H Read, M Fordham, G Adler (eds.) *The Structure and Dynamics of the Psyche. Collected Works of C. G. Jung*. Vol. 8. London: Routledge & Kegan Paul, 67–91.

Kalanithi P. 2016. *When Breath Becomes Air*. New York, NY: Random House.

Katz AM, Shotter J. Hearing the Patient's 'Voice': Toward a Social Poetics in Diagnostic Interviews. *Social Science & Medicine*. 1996; 43: 919–31.

Kaufman JC, Sexton JD. Why Doesn't the Writing Cure Help Poets?. *Review of General Psychology*. 2006; 10: 268–82.

Kearney R. Bachelard and the Epiphanic Instant. *Philosophy Today*. 2008; 52 (Supplement): 38–45.

Kenyon J. Having It Out With Melancholy. *Poetry*. 1992; 161: 86–89.

Kenyon J. 2005. *Collected Poems*. Minneapolis, MN: Graywolf Press.

Kirmayer LJ. 1988. Mind and Body as Metaphors: Hidden Values in Biomedicine. In: M Lock, D Gordon (eds.) *Biomedicine Examined*. Dordrecht: Kluwer, 57–93.

Kirmayer LJ. The Body's Insistence on Meaning: Metaphor as Presentation and Representation in Illness Experience. *Medical Anthropology Quarterly*. 1992; 6: 323–46.

Kirmayer LJ. Healing and the Invention of Metaphor: The Effectiveness of Symbols Revisited. *Culture, Medicine and Psychiatry*. 1993; 17: 161–95.

Kirmayer LJ. Improvisation and Authority in Illness Meaning. *Culture, Medicine and Psychiatry*. 1994; 18: 183–214.

Kirmayer LJ. 2000. Broken Narratives: Clinical Encounters and the Poetics of Illness Experience. In: C Mattingly, LC Garro (eds.) *Narrative and the Cultural Construction of Illness and Healing*. Berkeley: University of California Press, 153–80.

Kirmayer LJ. Asklepian Dreams: The Ethos of the Wounded-Healer in the Clinical Encounter. *Transcultural Psychiatry*. 2003; 40: 248–77.

Kirmayer LJ. The Cultural Diversity of Healing: Meaning, Metaphor and Mechanism. *British Medical Bulletin*. 2004; 69: 33–48.

Kirmayer LJ. Psychotherapy and the Cultural Concept of the Person. *Transcultural Psychiatry*. 2007a; 44: 232–57.

Kirmayer LJ. Celan's Poetics of Alterity: Lyric and the Understanding of Illness Experience in Medical Ethics. *Monash Bioethics Review*. 2007b; 26: 21–35.

Kirmayer LJ. Culture and the Metaphoric Mediation of Pain. *Transcultural Psychiatry*. 2008; 45: 318–38.

Kirmayer LJ. The Cultural Poetics of Illness and Healing. *Transcultural Psychiatry*. 2023; 60: 844–51.

Kirmayer LJ, Bhugra D. 2009. Culture and Mental Illness: Social Context and Explanatory Models. In: IM Salloum, JE Mezzich (eds.) *Psychiatric Diagnosis: Patterns and Prospects*. New York, NY: John Wiley & Sons, 29–37.

Kirmayer LJ, Gómez-Carrillo A, Sukhanova E, et al. 2023. Narrative Medicine. In: J Mezzich, W James Appleyard, P Glare et al. (eds.) *Person Centered Medicine*. Dordrecht: Springer, 235–55.

Kirmayer LJ, Groleau D, Looper KJ, Dao MD. Explaining Medically Unexplained Symptoms. *The Canadian Journal of Psychiatry*. 2004; 49: 663–72.

Kleinman A. 1988. *The Illness Narratives: Suffering, Healing, and the Human Condition*. New York, NY: Basic Books.

Knill MF, Atkins S. 2020. *Poetry in Expressive Arts: Supporting Resilience Through Poetic Writing*. London: Jessica Kingsley Publishers.

Koch K. The Language of Poetry. *New York Review of Books*. 1998; 45: 44–47.

Kövecses Z. 2020. *Extended Conceptual Metaphor Theory*. Cambridge: Cambridge University Press.

Lacoue-Labarthe P. 1986. *Poetry as Experience*. Stanford, CA: Stanford University Press.

Lakoff G. The Death of Dead Metaphor. *Metaphor and Symbol*. 1987; 2: 143–47.

Lakoff G, Johnson M. 2008. *Metaphors We Live by*. Chicago, IL: University of Chicago Press.

Lakoff G, Turner M. 2009. *More Than Cool Reason: A Field Guide to Poetic Metaphor*. Chicago, IL: University of Chicago Press.

Levinas E. 2003. *Humanism of the Other*. Champaign, IL: University of Illinois Press.

Lewis B. 2011. *Narrative Psychiatry: How Stories Can Shape Clinical Practice*. Baltimore, MD: Johns Hopkins University Press.

Longenbach J. 2013. *The Virtues of Poetry*. Minneapolis, MN: Graywolf Press.

Lukács G. 2023. Issues of Mimesis II: The Path to the Worldedness of Art. In: *The Specificity of the Aesthetic*. Vol. 1. Leiden: Brill, 381–461.

Machado A. 2012. *Times Alone: Selected Poems of Antonio Machado*. Middletown, CT: Wesleyan University Press.

Mattingly C, Garro LC. (eds.) 2000. *Narrative and the Cultural Construction of Illness and Healing*. Berkeley, CA: University of California Press.

Mazza N. 2021. *Poetry Therapy: Theory and Practice*. London: Routledge.

Metzl JM, Hansen H. Structural Competency: Theorizing a New Medical Engagement With Stigma and Inequality. *Social Science & Medicine*. 2014; 103: 126–33.

Miller JC. 2004. *The Transcendent Function: Jung's Model of Psychological Growth Through Dialogue With the Unconscious*. Albany, NY: SUNY Press.

Nabokov V. 1967. *Speak, Memory*. New York, NY: Vintage.

Nachmanovitch S. 1991. *Free Play: Improvisation in Life and Art*. Harmondsworth: Penguin.

Naemiratch B, Manderson L. Lay Explanations of Type 2 Diabetes in Bangkok, Thailand. *Anthropology & Medicine*. 2007; 14: 83–94.

Niles AN, Haltom KE, Mulvenna CM, et al. Randomized Controlled Trial of Expressive Writing for Psychological and Physical Health: The Moderating Role of Emotional Expressivity. *Anxiety, Stress, & Coping*. 2014; 27: 1–17.

Orr G. 2002. *Poetry as Survival*. Athens, GA: University of Georgia Press.

Orr G. 2021. *The Last Love Poem I Will Ever Write: Poems*. New York: WW Norton & Company.

Pavlacic JM, Buchanan EM, Maxwell NP, et al. A Meta-Analysis of Expressive Writing on Posttraumatic Stress, Posttraumatic Growth, and Quality of Life. *Review of General Psychology*. 2019; 23: 230–50.

Pennebaker JW, Beall SK. Confronting a Traumatic Event: Toward an Understanding of Inhibition and Disease. *Journal of Abnormal Psychology*. 1986; 95: 274–81.

Pennebaker JW, Seagal JD. Forming a Story: The Health Benefits of Narrative. *Journal of Clinical Psychology*. 1999; 55: 1243–54.

Perloff M. 1996. *Wittgenstein's Ladder: Poetic Language and the Strangeness of the Ordinary*. Chicago, IL: University of Chicago Press.

Peterkin A, Grewal S. Bibliotherapy: The Therapeutic Use of Fiction and Poetry in Mental Health. *International Journal of Person Centered Medicine*. 2018; 7: 175.

Phillips J. Poetry as Self-Supervision for Mental Health Professionals: The Use of Poetry to Process and Understand Clinical Work. *Journal of Poetry Therapy*. 2010; 23: 171–82.

Pinsky R. 1998. *The Sounds of Poetry: A Brief Guide*. New York, NY: Farrar, Strauss & Giroux.

Ponge F. 1972. *The Voice of Things* (B Archer, trans.). New York: McGraw Hill.

Ramstead MJ, Veissière SP, Kirmayer LJ. Cultural Affordances: Scaffolding Local Worlds Through Shared Intentionality and Regimes of Attention. *Frontiers in Psychology*. 2016; 7: 1090.

Ritvo M. 2016. *Four Reincarnations*. Minneapolis, MN: Milkweed Editions.

Scheff TJ. 1979. *Catharsis in Healing, Ritual, and Drama*. Berkeley, CA: University of California Press.

Schuster J, Beune E, Stronks K. Metaphorical Constructions of Hypertension Among Three Ethnic Groups in the Netherlands. *Ethnicity & Health*. 2011; 16: 583–600.

Siegelman EY. 1993. *Metaphor and Meaning in Psychotherapy*. New York, NY: Guilford Press.

Sinnenberg L, Mancheno C, Barg FK, et al. Content Analysis of Metaphors About Hypertension and Diabetes on Twitter: Exploratory Mixed-Methods Study. *JMIR Diabetes*. 2018; 3: e11177.

Smith RC. 2016. *Gaston Bachelard: Philosopher of Science and Imagination*. Albany, NY: State University of New York Press.

Sontag S. 1978. *Illness as Metaphor*. New York, NY: Farrar, Straus and Giroux.

Stepakoff SS. Poetry Therapy Principles and Practices for Raising Awareness of Racism. *The Arts in Psychotherapy*. 1997; 24: 261–74.

Stern L, Kirmayer LJ. Knowledge Structures in Illness Narratives: Development and Reliability of a Coding Scheme. *Transcultural Psychiatry*. 2004; 41: 130–42.

Stirman SW, Pennebaker JW. Word Use in the Poetry of Suicidal and Non-Suicidal Poets. *Psychosomatic Medicine*. 2001; 63: 517–23.

Taylor C. 2016. *The Language Animal: The Full Shape of the Human Linguistic Capacity*. Cambridge, MA: Harvard University Press.

Thibodeau PH, Hendricks RK, Boroditsky L. How Linguistic Metaphor Scaffolds Reasoning. *Trends in Cognitive Sciences*. 2017; 21: 852–63.

Törneke N. Strategies for Using Metaphor in Psychological Treatment. *Metaphor and the Social World*. 2020; 10: 214–32.

Tsevat RK, Sinha AA, Gutierrez KJ, DasGupta S. Bringing Home the Health Humanities: Narrative Humility, Structural Competency, and Engaged Pedagogy. *Academic Medicine*. 2015; 90: 1462–65.

Turner M. 1996. *The Literary Mind: The Origins of Thought and Language*. Oxford: Oxford University Press.

Veissière SP, Constant A, Ramstead MJ, et al. Thinking Through Other Minds: A Variational Approach to Cognition and Culture. *Behavioral and Brain Sciences*. 2020; 43: e90.

White P. 2014. *Poetry Unites Winner: Paul White*. Available at: https://poets.org/text/poetry-unites-winner-paul-white. Last accessed: 2/6/2023.

Williams Camus JT. Metaphors of Cancer in Scientific Popularization Articles in the British Press. *Discourse Studies*. 2009; 11: 465–95.

Witztum E, Van der Hart O, Friedman B. The Use of Metaphors in Psychotherapy. *Journal of Contemporary Psychotherapy*. 1988; 189: 270–90.

Wohlman A. 2022. *Metaphor in Illness Writing: Fight and Battle Reused*. Edinburgh: Edinburgh University Press.

Woods A. The Limits of Narrative: Provocations for the Medical Humanities. *Medical Humanities*. 2011; 37: 73–78.

Young A. When Rational Men Fall Sick: An Inquiry into Some Assumptions Made by Medical Anthropologists. *Culture, Medicine and Psychiatry*. 1981; 5: 317–35.

Young A. Rational Men and the Explanatory Model Approach. *Culture, Medicine and Psychiatry*. 1982; 6: 57–71.

Young D. 2010. *The Art of Recklessness: Poetry as Assertive Force and Contradiction*. Minneapolis, MN: Graywolf Press.

Zwicky J. 2014. *Wisdom & Metaphor*. Edmonton, Alberta: Brush Education.

2

THE HIPPOCRATES INITIATIVE 2009–2022

Michael Hulse

In January 2009, I was approached by a Warwick University colleague, Professor Donald Singer of the medical faculty, to help with judging a poetry competition he had arranged for staff at University Hospital Coventry, where he was a consultant. Donald proved to be a well-organized, soft-spoken man with a ready smile, a courteous manner, and a pragmatic approach to problem-solving, and I took to him instantly. Some time later, once the judging was done, we discussed the arresting fact that 38 poems had been submitted by those who worked at a single hospital and wondered whether there might be a future for a nationwide or even international prize for poems on medical themes. That was the hour in which the Hippocrates Prize for poems on medical subjects was born, in March 2009, and during the spring of that year, the idea ramified, so that our nascent plan soon envisaged two competitions in tandem, one for UK medical professionals (present or past) and full-time students of medicine, the other for anybody anywhere in the world. To these an annual symposium was soon added at which the interactions of the two disciplines of poetry and medicine might be explored, and a publishing wing was a further addition the following year, when the desirability of an anthology of prizewinning and commended poems brought the Hippocrates Press into being. To the triad of prize, symposium, and press we gave the umbrella name the Hippocrates Initiative.

Particularly over the past century, there have been a number of substantial poets who have also been doctors, from Gottfried Benn to Miroslav Holub to Peter Goldsworthy, and in our first year, we secured as a judge of the Prize competition the UK's most eminent doctor-poet then living, Dannie Abse (see Chapter 12). Our second judge was one of the most distinguished members of the medical profession, Professor Sir Bruce Keogh, at that time medical director of the National Health Service. For our third judge, Donald and I had agreed that it would be strategically helpful to have a figure influential in the media, and that first time we were fortunate to recruit the veteran broadcaster James Naughtie. The deadline for entries had been set for the end of January 2010; some 1600 poems were submitted from more than 30 countries; and on 10 March 2010, the three named judges met Donald and me at the Medical Society of London in Chandos Street to agree on the major prize winners and the commended runners-up in the very first Hippocrates Prize for Poetry and Medicine.

At that point the poems were still anonymous, but as the judges' debate proceeded, one poem that was emerging as a favourite in the open category left me increasingly certain that I could guess

DOI: 10.4324/9781003341796-4

its author. Written in the voice of Catullus, it spoke of recovery from a stroke, and my thoughts flew to an old friend of mine, the pre-eminent New Zealand poet, novelist, and critic C.K. Stead, who had frequently adopted the persona of Catullus in his poems and had also suffered a stroke not long before. Sure enough, the confident and engaging monologue titled 'Ischaemia' turned out to be Karl's, and that poem remains one of the finest pieces ever seen among the Hippocrates Prize winners. Karl Stead subsequently agreed to join the Hippocrates Initiative's advisory board, while the London-based poet Wendy French, winner in the medical professional category, went on to publish collections of poetry with the Hippocrates Press and to serve as a competition judge herself in 2016.

Wendy, daughter of one of the first generation of doctors to serve in the UK's National Health Service, had worked in the service herself and now offered writing workshops to medical professionals. She struck everyone as an ideal winner in her category, and at the first annual symposium that April of 2010, she gave a powerful reading of her winning poem at the award ceremony that closed the day, while Karl Stead contributed from Auckland a video of his own reading. That symposium, held at Warwick University, laid down the template that Donald and I were to follow in essential outline in every subsequent year, with papers (chiefly from literature scholars) on medical poetry filling the morning, a poetry reading or keynote address by a distinguished guest following lunch, papers (chiefly from medical practitioners) on poetry in medical contexts filling the afternoon, and the prize-giving event concluding. That year, papers on A.D. Hope's poem 'On an Engraving by Casserius', on William Carlos Williams as exemplar of the doctor-poet, and on the poison used to murder Hamlet's father were among those given in the morning; Peter Goldsworthy, visiting the northern hemisphere, gave a keynote talk on 'The Physiology of Literature'; and subjects of afternoon papers included a poetry residency at Cheltenham Hospital's oncology unit and the use of poetry in sensitizing medical students at Imperial College, London. Dannie Abse, the poet judge, gave a short reading from his own work to introduce the awards; James Naughtie, ever a friend to literature, gave a warm welcome to a prize conjoining these two unusual disciplines (hailing it as 'one of the most original prizes that has come along for a long time', a phrase that naturally found a lasting place in our promotional materials); while Bruce Keogh diffidently disavowed any knowledge of poetry before showing himself to have noted with patent acumen the key features and phrases of every poem he spoke of. The new competition had attracted interest and strong winning poems, and the first symposium had been well attended and found to be a success, so after its first year the venture plainly had potential. But what exactly was the point of it?

From the outset, Donald and I were agreed that our venture should pursue a number of aims. First and most straightforwardly, it should draw attention to a substantial strand of writing within the total corpus of poetry: poems written on medical themes. This first aim involved identifying and answering questions of definition. Second, it should establish a database relating to the practical uses to which poetry might be put in clinical contexts, if any. Third, it should collect materials for an authoritative historical and international anthology of poetry on medical themes.

The first of these aims wears a deceptive appearance of simplicity. A convention upheld more assiduously by publishers than by scholars has been the collection of poems by subject matter – love poetry, war poetry, religious verse, and so forth – in an Oxford Book, Penguin Book, or similar. Love and war and the worship of gods have incontrovertibly been a part of the human experience since time immemorial, and the surviving poetry on these themes similarly reaches back thousands of years. Whether the same can be said of medical poetry, however, is self-evidently a moot point. The human creature has been born, has suffered ailments, and has died, but poetry on birth was arrestingly uncommon in the past, poetry on illnesses and afflictions was almost as infrequently encountered, and only death left a substantial and significant trail, in the form of the elegiac tradition. That tradition took little interest in the medical nature of a death: it would be fatuous to look for a clinical account of the body's experience of drowning in Milton's 'Lycidas'. Elegy laments the dead in a spiritual or existential mode and is unconcerned with medical minutiae since the fact of loss and grief is of far greater human consequence than how precisely the loss occurred. Moreover, Dylan Thomas, urging those facing death to rage against the dying of the light, does not offer advice on preparations to soothe inflammations of the joints, nor does he recommend regular exercise or the installation of a stair-lift.

Consideration of poems as 'medical' presupposes an agreed-upon understanding of what medical poetry might be, but we found ourselves in a field where no such consensus obtained. It is certainly possible to outline the characteristics one might rationally expect it to have. If a poem speaks of the course and symptoms of a condition; of medicine; of hospital, doctors, nurses, and the instruments they use (etcetera), it takes on a 'medical' character which a poem that makes no mention of these will not have. If a poem begins by identifying a condition or disease or injury as its subject and gives an account of it that conveys a reasonably clear and concrete sense of how it might feel to the sufferer, then it is fair, no matter how many flourishes and images may oil the rhetorical progress of the piece, to describe it as 'medical'. Poems on insomnia by Sylvia Plath, Attilio Bertolucci, and Julia Darling are of this kind; poems on blindness by Milton, Baudelaire, Rilke, and Borges are all arresting, whether the author was himself blind or not; Nazim Hikmet's 'Angina Pectoris' bears the poet's characteristic political imprint but is plain-spoken concerning the medical condition; and C.K. Stead's Hippocrates Prize-winning 'Ischaemia' is unambiguous about the experience of a stroke even as it moves confidently into broader dimensions.

To these fundamental thoughts on medical poetry, others on what might constitute a corpus of such writing in the world's poetry are quickly added. Just as the evolution of the medical profession was historically slow – with many conditions unidentified or ill understood until recent times, treatments based on little more than guesswork, and everything lacking that is now considered essential to medical practice (from basic hygiene and suitable instruments to appropriate and rigorous medical training) – so too the poetry of medical experience was conspicuous by its relative absence until the last three or four centuries. Medical poetry evolved at the same pace as medicine itself: medical understanding quite simply needed to broaden and to deepen. As the common experience of treatment by doctors acquired a modern character and was accompanied by more widely disseminated familiarity with medical diagnostics, procedures, and contexts (such as modern hospitals), so the medical literacy of populations, and poetry on medical subject matter, grew as well. It was of course still possible and proper for a great elegiac poem, Kenneth Slessor's 'Five Bells', to be written in the twentieth century with as little reference to the clinical nature of death by drowning as its seventeenth-century model, 'Lycidas'. On the other hand, the poems written in the twenty-first by Rebecca Goss in response to her first child's death from a congenital heart defect are steeped in the experience of consultation in hospital rooms, confrontation with an unfamiliar specialist vocabulary, and other features of modern medical experience that have come to be staples of medical poetry as now understood. The expectation of modern humanity worldwide is that medical experience now happens in practices, hospitals, and similar settings, and much medical poetry takes this for granted.

In addition to a sense of the historical evolution of medicine and of the popular understanding of medicine, medical poetry requires of the reader alertness to the principal modes in which it is written. The first such mode deals with the course of an illness (or other medical experience) from the perspective of the patient and is written in the first person by the patient. Poems on cancer by Marilyn Hacker, Yannis Ritsos, and John Updike are examples. The second mode deals with conditions from an outside, non-patient perspective, usually that of an intimate: Les Murray's verse portrait of his autistic son, Robert Gray's 'In Departing Light' (on his 90-year-old mother with Alzheimer's), or Philip Gross's poems about his father suffering aphasia are of this kind. Many poems submitted for the Hippocrates Prize have been of this sort too, frequently written by the surviving, grieving partner or parent or offspring of a person who has died (all too often of cancer – poems on cancer from a detached, non-intimate perspective, such as Lesley Saunders' 'Peccant Atoms', on Fanny Burney's mastectomy, or those in Peter Reading's *C*, are less common). A third major strand in medical poetry has less to do with authentic experience and is concerned instead with inquiry into the nature of medical science; its history, progress, and key figures; and its defining characteristics. Poems of this kind range from Hope's already mentioned to Larkin's 'Ambulances' and 'The Building'; intriguingly, among the numerous figures taken as subjects of Hippocrates Prize entries, the wives of Sigmund Freud and Wilhelm Röntgen were favourites.

It rapidly became clear to Donald and me that the Hippocrates Initiative was considered a success. In the first three years, in addition to C.K. Stead and Wendy French, major prize winners included Michael Henry, Siân Hughes, Nick Mackinnon, and Pauline Stainer, names familiar or at least recognizable to anyone who followed poetry in the UK, and the hitherto unknown Paula Cunningham, first prize winner in 2011, quickly went on to take the Aldeburgh Prize for a First Collection. Mark Lawson, then presenter of Radio Four's *Front Row* and our media judge in 2011, wrote a full page on the project in *The Guardian* (advertising on a scale we could never have afforded), and his enthusiasm was matched by that of poets Gwyneth Lewis, Marilyn Hacker, Jo Shapcott, Philip Gross, and Kit Wright as well as of Sir Robert Francis QC (who chaired the inquiry into the Mid Staffordshire NHS Foundation Trust) and Sarah Crown (then editor of Mumsnet and subsequently literature director of Arts Council England), all of them judges in the first five years.

In 2011, as an afterthought in an undisturbed hour at the office, I entered the Initiative in the *Times Higher Education* Awards, and to my astonishment we took the Award for Excellence and Innovation in the Arts that autumn. Martha Kearney, our media judge in 2012, gratifyingly featured the Hippocrates Prize on *The World at One*, Radio Four's lunchtime news programme, where she was joined for discussion by Robert Francis. Entries to the Prize continued to come from every part of the globe, and while there were always some that were written in crayon and all in capitals, familiar to anyone who has ever judged a poetry competition, the standard of the poems that rose to the top, both from familiar names and from unknowns, spoke for itself. (When Donald and I originally decided on two Prize categories, it was out of a misplaced anxiety that health professionals writing in their spare time might be at a disadvantage when pitted against full-time writers, but the quality of winning entries in what began as the NHS category and later embraced health professionals from anywhere in the world was fully equal to that of Open category winners.)

The second symposium, in 2011, was again held at Warwick University, but in 2012, we moved to the Wellcome Collection in London, where the symposium remained in 2013 before transferring to the Royal Society of Medicine for 2014. These were years of consolidation, during which the reputation of the Hippocrates Initiative grew rapidly and substantially. Top prizes continued to be won by poets with established reputations (Rafael Campo in 2013; Jane Draycott in 2014) as well as by unknowns. In 2013, we added a third category to the Hippocrates Prize, for younger poets aged 14 to 18. Symposium papers, though chiefly contributed by UK and US scholars, were also given by speakers from Denmark, France, Spain, Greece, and Russia, and for 2012, our keynote speaker was Greek Cypriot poet, paediatric physician, and MEP Eleni Theocharous. In 2013, we also added a three-day workshop in Venice that was happily attended by Karl Stead, on an extended visit to Europe, with whom it was possible to have lengthy debate over finer points of Thom Gunn's AIDS poems in a way that the symposium did not permit.

In 2013, thanks to a twelvemonth of additional support from Warwick University, Donald and I had the services of an excellent assistant, Nicola Williams, and her efficient ability to relieve us of burdensome chores was a reminder of the key importance of funding. We had begun the Hippocrates Prize with £5,000 as the first prize in each category, and essential annual expenditure (the prize pot, the judges' fees and expenses, hire of a symposium venue, and much more) totalled £30–40,000. In addition to the annual Prize anthology, the Hippocrates Press was now publishing volumes of poetry, beginning with *Born in the NHS*, a collaborative venture by Wendy French and Jane Kirwan, and *Rupture* by 2014 Prize winner Ellen Storm, a Merseyside doctor-poet; and poetry publishing is notoriously loss-making. The income from Prize entries, delegate fees, and book sales was far from sufficient, so the Hippocrates Initiative depended for its existence on the munificence of sponsors. While we were always fortunate in finding generous sponsors, several were part of the venture for a brief period only, and it was left to two, the Fellowship of Postgraduate Medicine (FPM) and the Cardiovascular Research Trust, to prove long-haul, dependable supporters. During 2015/2016, a time of anxiety ensued, when internal disagreement in the FPM placed a question mark over its continued funding. Donald and I reduced the competition first prize from £5,000 to £1,000 and retreated for the symposium to the Medical Society of London premises, which were more affordable than the Wellcome or RSM venues we had recently used. Happily, this anxious interval was soon overcome, thanks to Donald's diplomatic skills.

Our second aim from the outset was to identify the uses to which poetry might be put in clinical contexts, and our initial assumption was that we were likeliest to find it in therapeutic or palliative care, where the use of music, painting, and craftwork has an established record. At the 2010 symposium, this intuition had been confirmed by one paper describing the use of poetry in Cheltenham Hospital's oncology unit, but another had told of its deployment in teaching medical students at Imperial College, London. The 2011 symposium pursued both strands, with papers on poetry and dementia and poetry and adolescent health but also a deeply interesting presentation on poetry in nurse education; we accordingly made poetry in therapy and education the focus of the health professional wing of the 2012 symposium. We heard papers from the UK and US on poetry and the rediscovery of a lost sense of self and poetry in alcohol addiction recovery programmes, but we also heard papers from Brighton and Sussex Medical School and from Texas, on poetry and training medical students, doctors, and nurses, and from Kent came a paper on poetry as a tool for reflective learning in GPs.

What was emerging from discussion of the education and training of medical professionals was the startling notion that, highly intelligent though these people were, they could also be surprisingly insensitive towards the human dimensions of their work. Poetry, it appeared, was of genuine use in quickening the sensitivity they might lack. If that were indeed the case, one could only wish that its use would become more widespread. The authentic usefulness of poetry in other clinical contexts seemed more in doubt, however, until an unforgettable moment at the Venice workshop in 2013.

An Englishwoman resident in Connecticut, Clare Wilmot, who had become a dedicated follower of the Hippocrates Initiative, travelled to Venice to describe her own gradual recovery from a long battle with cancer. Her Connecticut hospice offered a choice of music, painting, or poetry, and choosing poetry led her to a profound engagement with the art, so impassioned that her entire week centred on the 90-minute visit of the poet in residence and his opinion of her writing. After a few weeks of this, she began to gain weight. When Clare said this, every medical professional in the room leaned forward. Patently she had recovered the will to live, and the part that that pivotal moment plays in patient progress can be immense. In that Venice palazzo room, it was as if a switch had been thrown, and the passive attentiveness of the medical experts instantly became active. The gaining of weight told them everything.

For Donald and me, that moment brought back remarks made by Professor Sir Bruce Keogh in 2010 when we had discussed with him the possibility of making a case to the NHS, in due course, for adopting poetry as one of its tools in certain contexts. Clearly poetry cannot be more than an adjunct to mainstream medicine. The odds against its acceptance were clear since many serious hurdles would need to be overcome. Additionally (though in 2010 this fear had yet to become a reality), the NHS was about to enter the deepest and most prolonged period of financial constraint in its history and would not be open to any but the most efficacious and economically viable proposals. But Bruce's comment was simplicity itself: everything depended on the evidence. If there was sufficient strong evidence to support the case, it could be made and would always get a fair hearing.

In truth, moments such as that produced by Clare Wilmot in Venice proved rare. While Donald and I listened to numerous papers from around the globe in the 13 years covered by this essay (chiefly from the US, the UK, and Australasia) describing the helpfulness of poetry in medical care as well as in education, we were never in a position to make a serious case to the NHS for its adoption, or even to assemble a suitably wide-ranging and substantial compilation of symposium papers for publication by a university press. This was something of a disappointment because it felt as if one of our goals on beginning the venture had not been realized.

Once the financial impasse had been negotiated, the Hippocrates Initiative continued to extend its range. In the UK, it steadily evolved a programme of reading events at libraries, schools, and universities, and in 2017, it moved overseas both for the annual symposium and for launches of *The Hippocrates Book of the Heart*. Rafael Campo, the most distinguished living doctor-poet in the US, had become a friend to the Initiative since his 2013 Prize win and had himself served as a judge in 2016, the year in which the Hippocrates Press also published his selected poems, *Comfort Measures Only*. Now the symposium transferred to Harvard, where Rafael taught in the medical school, and the programme expanded to include events at the Boston Museum of Fine Arts and at the Massachusetts Poetry Festival over a three-day period. For me, it was a time of renewing old connections, since Harvard's Houghton Library had bought some of my manuscripts and I had a number of writer friends in greater Boston, but it also brought a new friend in Sydney pulmonologist Andrew Dimitri, who took second prize in that year's Health Professional category, made the long journey, and impressed audiences with the moving clarity of poems written out of his experience of crisis zones with *Médecins sans Frontières*. Another impressive doctor-poet, Andrew went on to publish *Winter in Northern Iraq* with the Hippocrates Press in 2019.

The year 2017 also saw the publication of *The Hippocrates Book of the Heart*, a substantial collection of commissioned poems together with short essays by medical experts. The book was launched in Sydney and Auckland that September, in Toronto in November, and in London in December, Donald being present in Toronto (where Roo Borson and Kenneth Sherman were among half a dozen contributors reading) and I in Sydney (where Geoff Lehmann and Stephen Edgar appeared with Andrew and myself) and Auckland (where Elizabeth Smither joined me). The following year, despite the complications introduced into the preparation process by the need to collaborate with a university organizing committee, Donald and I returned to the US, holding the 2018 symposium at Northwestern University in Chicago. Mark Doty followed Jorie Graham as US poet on the judging panel, and events were programmed at the Poetry Foundation as well as the university. The sense that the Hippocrates Initiative had become a global brand, desirable in the eyes of serious partners, was reassuring but also posed a risk: though one or two who could afford to do so travelled from the UK to Harvard or Northwestern, the core following remained in

Britain, and it seemed neither wise nor kind to alienate them. So, the decision was easily made to hold the tenth symposium, which would have a celebratory anniversary quality, in the UK once more, and our choice fell on Newcastle University, since we had repeatedly been asked to hold the event in the north for a change.

Newcastle in 2019 was to prove (at the time of writing this essay) the last symposium held as an in-person gathering. Luz-Mar González-Arias, a fine Spanish scholar who had given no fewer than three papers on Irish women poets, was to host the 2020 symposium at Oviedo University, but COVID-19 intervened, as it did once again in 2021 when Andrew Dimitri was to host at the University of New South Wales in Sydney. Both Luz-Mar and Andrew were in Newcastle and spent the eve of the 2019 symposium on the banks of the Tyne, dining and planning with Donald and me, unmindful of what famously happens to the best-laid plans.

The tenth symposium was satisfyingly substantial, with papers from American, British, French, Spanish, and Australian speakers and a colloquium on the work and legacy of Newcastle's Julia Darling, to which five poets who had known Darling contributed. Two experts on medical poetry spoke, Tony Daniels – the polymath who used to write a *Spectator* medical column as Theodore Dalrymple and was now launching an erudite but lightly written collection of short essays published by the Hippocrates Press, *Illness as Inspiration* – and Michael Salcman, editor of *Poetry in Medicine*, whom Donald and I had met at Harvard and were eager to hear on the making of his anthology. Michael joined Carolyn Forché to give another of the notable readings for which the symposia had become known.

The third of the aims we had kept in mind from the outset was the compilation of an authoritative anthology of poetry on medical themes. This was work which devolved upon me, as I had already co-edited the best-selling anthologies *The New Poetry* (in 1993, with two others) and *The Twentieth Century in Poetry* (2011, with one), and I knew from the experience of the second of those books, which had taken seven years to assemble (or, considered differently, a lifetime), that this order of undertaking required diligence and stamina. Since I had an extensive historical and international personal library of poetry, and a university library as back-up, Donald was always content for work on poetry to be done by me, just as I left medical labours to him. Our intention was to produce a book that would prove attractive for a publisher with the reach of (say) Penguin.

Compiling an anthology of poems on medical subjects presents self-evident difficulties. If a poet is commissioned to compile a book of love poems, there are already numerous pieces that serve as points of orientation in the field: it would be a curious anthologist who omitted (say) Marvell's 'To His Coy Mistress', Donne's 'The Sun Rising', Elizabeth Barrett Browning's 'How Do I Love Thee', and one or two sonnets of Shakespeare's. No comparable mapping of the terrain has yet been done for medical poetry. Very quickly, once a handful of outstanding pieces by Martial or Heine, by Milton or Larkin, by Hope or Gwen Harwood or Richard Wilbur (the delicious 'Pangloss's Song') have been noted with satisfaction, the long labour begins of sifting volume after volume with an altered attention, a new set of criteria. There is no such thing as an unfilled quarter-hour if the time can be used to leaf through a favourite or neglected book in seemingly endless quest. Collections one had thought familiar suddenly yield unsuspected medical poems. The mind reads with wishes, needs, and pigeonholes open: if Lucretius, Thomas Nashe, Keki Daruwalla, and Jeffrey Harrison have written on plague, can any of these texts be thought the outstanding poetic word on the subject, or is there not an unguessed-at masterpiece on the plague hidden away in *this* book? A self-evident risk in assembling such an anthology is that one may read for the subject matter of poetry rather than for the poetry of poetry.

It seemed to me that the task might easily occupy many years, but in 2014, during the twelve-month in which we had an assistant, Donald and I agreed that publication of such a book, even if it was (as I felt) far from finished, would help advance research in the field. The book could be published by our own press, and Nicola Williams set to work clearing permissions. Some months into the process, we found ourselves stalled by the failure of some copyright holders to respond and our own failure to locate a number of others; Nicola's contracted period of employment came to an end; it was not at all clear that the funds we currently had were equal to the task, and, not altogether unhappy that the first attempt was being halted, I agreed with Donald that the compilation process needed more time and that we would do well to abide by our first intention of winning over a major publisher with the resources to tackle problems that might arise.

The following year, it became clear that we would not be the first to publish a substantial and well-researched anthology of medical poetry when Michael Salcman's *Poetry in Medicine* was published in the USA in 2015. A Baltimore doctor-poet, Salcman had cast his net wide, across periods and provenances, and had given useful thought to categories in which one might think of medical poetry. When Donald and I held Salcman's superb book in our hands, the chagrin we'd been tempted to feel was quickly dispelled by relief and delight: relief because almost incredibly, the contents of his book and our unfinished book overlapped by barely a dozen poems and the two publications would therefore be complementary (he was understandably stronger on US poets, we on the UK and Commonwealth and translated poetry) and delight because the implication was that medical poetry really was a very large and substantial field and the work of charting it was in hand. We met Salcman at Harvard in 2017, invited him to speak in 2019 at our Newcastle symposium, and were pleased to find in him a fellow labourer in the vineyard.

I write this in 2023, after the peak period of the COVID-19 pandemic and after the untimely death of Donald Singer. Retired now from university life and with my own health and energy diminished, I think it possible that the anthology Donald and I planned may not be completed. In 2021, the Hippocrates Press published *Storm Brain*, a book of commissioned poems and essays about the brain and its ailments, a successor and companion to *The Hippocrates Book of the Heart*. In 2020, the Press also published *Once Upon a Time in Aleppo* by Syrian doctor-poet Fouad M. Fouad, and *Days of Wonder*, a cycle of poems written between March 2020 and March 2021 in response to the pandemic by Lesley Saunders in collaboration with artist Rebecca Swainston. The symposia did not take place in those years, and neither did any other Hippocrates events, but the Initiative's following gathered regularly online for poetry, in meetings attended by 50 to 150 people – meetings timed for nine in the UK evening so that the Americas could join (at what was mid-afternoon for them) and Australasia (early the next morning). Surely our most dedicated follower was the medical professional in the Philippines, a commended poet in the Hippocrates Prize, who would rise at four in the morning to join the Zoom gatherings.

For two years during COVID-19, Donald and I did not meet in person, and the first time I saw him again was also to be the last, three weeks before he died in June 2022. We met in Roman ruins near Lichfield and for 15 minutes talked of Roman sites around Europe before adjourning to a pub a field's-breadth away for lunch in the sunshine. Thirteen years had deepened a professional relationship into a sturdy friendship, in which mutual professional respect always remained at the heart. Donald valued my knowledge of poetry, my editorial skills, and my address book: decades on the international reading circuit had brought me friendships with poets around the world, and Donald could be as delighted as a child seeing the rabbit pulled from the hat when I enlisted as judge a Jennifer Clement (then president of PEN International) or the Indian poet and novelist Keki Daruwalla, who, Donald realized (raising an eyebrow), had occupied a senior position in India's intelligence services.

I for my part savoured Donald as one who not only knew his medical calling inside out but had a deep love of music, history, poetry, the comedy of the world's cultures, tennis, birds, and very much more. When I first lived in Cologne, a new neighbour moved into the adjoining apartment, and within hours I heard through the wall the flute part of a Mozart quartet being practised: she proved to be a student of medicine but a person of parts, and I have had the pleasure in life of knowing a number of such renaissance medics, the latest being Donald. Often, we would meet at his Leamington home for a working lunch; at intervals, I joined him at his home-from-home in London, The Athenaeum, where he liked to entertain a Dannie Abse, Rafael Campo, or Tony Daniels; and in Boston, he took me to the club on Commonwealth Avenue which was twinned with The Athenaeum. Undoubtedly, he loved the good things, but he was also one of the least self-important people I have known, a down-to-earth man who would find a solution when problems arose rather than looking for others to fix them.

Thirteen years of probing poetry and medicine with Donald served not only as an education in the inter-relations of the disciplines but also as a constant reminder of the gulf between them. On too many occasions to count, I found myself told by a well-meaning medical professional that he planned to take up poetry when he retired. In his mind, an art that had given humanity some of its greatest achievements thousands of years before medical science attained its maturity was little more than a pastime, and every time I heard this, I struggled hard not to reply that, for my part, I planned in retirement to take up brain surgery (a quip introduced by Margaret Atwood). The reality is that poetry and medicine know very little of each other. When I guested at the FPM's annual conference, feeling like the tolerated jester as I presented medical poetry to an assembly of the world's finest medical researchers, I was shocked to listen to one of them calmly predicting that the ceiling of life expectancy would keep on being raised, as intervention upon medical intervention made it possible to extend life indefinitely. Had this man not heard of the real world, in which there are neither the armies of medical staff nor the infinite resources to perform the untold numbers of interventions he spoke of? Or, had he no sense of the social tensions that would attend new regimens available only to the wealthiest few? For that matter, had he not come across *taedium vitae*? Had he not read Swift and reflected on the struldbruggs? Answers on a postcard.

A season of uncertainty followed Donald's death that ended when the two of his three middle-aged children who followed him into medicine opted to take his place in the Hippocrates Initiative. As I write, its full spectrum of work is set to resume in 2024, with the Hippocrates Prize awarded once more after a year's hiatus and the symposium convening at Oviedo in Spain. What did it achieve in its 13 years under Donald and me? It helped give form and solidity to an under-defined and indistinct field of study, it tacitly demonstrated that that field was of more value in its practical than in its theoretical manifestations, it brought a quantity of excellent poetry into print, it gave pleasure and instruction, and it catalysed a commonalty among the many disparate sensibilities that came together in its name. A growing body of knowledge was shared among a large number of people who 13 years ago did not care one way or the other what poetry could do for medicine, or medicine for poetry, and who think very differently now. To have been a force in effecting that change is not to be sneezed at, as Fernando Pessoa might have put it.

i.m. Donald Robert James Singer (1954–2022)

3

MARKING TIME: POETRY AS SUBJECT TO NARRATIVE IN MEDICAL EDUCATION

Shane Neilson

Notwithstanding the long history of practising physician poets – see EP Scarlett's (1936, 1937) encyclopaedic list spanning two long articles in the *Canadian Medical Association Journal*, with over 100 physicians in the UK–USA–Canadian traditions discussed (see Chapter 4) – there is also a long history of the use of poetry in Western medical education that perhaps begins with Sophocles participating in the healing cult of Aesculapius in 420 BC (Connolly 1998). A large and ever-expanding number of published studies attest to the efficacy of poetry in improving educational outcomes (Shapiro and Stein 2005; Marthouret 2016; Wietlisbach et al. 2023). Yet Scarlett's account and the quasi-experimental studies all resort to a different (and default) method to explain their findings: narrative. And how could it be otherwise?

A lyric testimony of an experimental study is a category error, and even if medical historians like Scarlett tried to list their subjects as if composing a list poem, the project would tilt ever narrative-ward as dull biographical details (birth and death dates; location of practice; names of book titles) would structurally overwhelm the poetic telling. Critically, any information a reader might like to glean about the use of poetry in medical education would only be obscured if it were conveyed in the form of lyric poetry, making for both a paradox and tension. Poetry pulls against (and cannot completely resist) any narrative sense one might want to make of it, and yet any reader hoping to learn about poems in medical contexts will do so in narrative, experiencing the linearity imposed so as to tame the artifice of poetry, or what the Russian Formalist Viktor Shklovsky (2009) defined as *ostraniene*: 'language that draws attention to itself'. Over two centuries before, Aristotle (1898) identified the same quality in *The Poetics* when he wrote,

> but nothing contributes more to produce a clearness of diction that is remote from commonness than the lengthening, contraction, and alteration of words. For by deviating in exceptional cases from the normal idiom, the language will gain distinction; while, at the same time, the partial conformity with usage will give perspicuity.

To consult medical journals concerning poetry's use in medical education in the manner of language 'deviating in exceptional cases from the normal idiom' would be, of course, silly. My argument here is simple, though novel in the extant health humanities literature: *poetry is unlike the mode of language used to both interpret and deploy it in medical education due to the hegemony*

DOI: 10.4324/9781003341796-5

of narrative in the culture at large. Poetry is inexorably wrenched into narratological interpretation in medical contexts not only because of an instrumental bias in the profession but also because of the gravitational pull of narrative in wider culture.

Consider the very influential narratologist H. Porter Abbot (2008), author of many texts on narratology, who in *The Cambridge Introduction to Narrative* defines narrative as 'the representation of an event or a series of events'. After writing of the developmental fact of narrative as intrinsic to how humans interpret the world from the point of acquiring a functioning grammar, he clinches the case by writing, 'Narrative is so much a part of the way we apprehend the world in time that it is virtually built in to the way we see'. He then lives up to the conceptual imperialism of his scholarly subject by prying the lyric from lyric poetry when examining Ben Jonson's poem 'To Celia'. He boldly states his case at the start:

> If you look at any of the so-called non-narrative genres, like, say, the lyric poem, which is frequently featured as pre-eminently a static form – that is, dominated not by a story line but by a single feeling – you will still find narrative. 'Drink to me, only, with thine eyes', wrote Ben Jonson in the first line of his 'Song: To Celia', and already we have a micro-narrative brewing – 'look at me' – overlaid by another micro-narrative which acts as a metaphor – 'drink to me'.

To point out that verbs provide the hinge for narrative in the form of action, as Porter Abbott does, is to recapitulate Aristotle (1898) when he wrote that verbs are for 'marking time'. Yet what phrase or series of lines could cohere without verbs? One discerns a 'gotcha' technique in which a narratologist detects verbs gainsaying the relabelling of lyric into a species of narrative. Notwithstanding this transgenre capture move, which strikes me as a practising poet as bizarre – as Williams (1986) said in 'Asphodel, that Greeny Flower', 'you can't get the news from poems, but men die miserably every day for lack of what is found there'; or, in perhaps the clearest taxonomic distinction yet made, Northrop Frye (1971) wrote that poetry is words in space and prose is words in time – I arrive at a more powerful reason why poetry in medical education finds its subsumption into narrative: hermeneutics. After transcribing Jonson's poem in its entirety, Abbott (2008) *analyses it* from the point of view of narrative:

> Here you have a poem dedicated to the expression of a powerful feeling, erotic love (threaded with irony and good humor), but the poem as a whole is structured by two narrative situations. The first is a series of micro-narratives, in the conditional mode, involving looking, kissing, and drinking. The second, beginning midway through, tells a more elaborate story of flowers that were sent, breathed on, returned, and now flourish, smelling of his beloved.

In case you think Porter Abbott is an isolated case amongst the narratologists, J. Hillis Miller does the same transgenre trick as well as dutiful narrativistic interpretation on as ridiculous a prospect as A.E. Housman's 'The Grizzly Bear' in his chapter 'Narrative' from Lentricchia and McLaughlin's (1995) influential *Critical Terms for Literary Study*. One can therefore forgive the many published studies mentioned before on the use of poetry in medical education as well as books like poetry-promulgating medical educator Joanne Shapiro's (2009) well-known thematic investigation *The Inner Lives of Medical Students*. Rather than consider poetry as poetry, the narratologists steamroll it into linearity.

Just as the use of narrative for hermeneutic purposes is demanded by narratology no matter what genre presents itself, the dominant player in medical education pedagogy when it comes to arts-based methods, Rita Charon's narrative medicine, habitually resorts to narrative to interpret poetry. To start, poetry is less than an afterthought in Charon's programme. Her first textbook from 2006, *Narrative Medicine: Honouring the Stories of Illness*, featured exactly zero poems transcribed, excerpted, or quoted from. The multi-authored follow-up textbook, *The Principles and Practice of Narrative Medicine* (Charon et al. 2017), comported itself somewhat better, with poems by Lucille Clifton and David Ferry analysed but only to derive their meaning – that familiar grade-school exercise notoriously responsible for killing most students' appreciation of poetry. Abstracting out a narrative is the quarry of poetry in medical education because narrative medicine is a field of narratology, plain and simple. The point of studying and practicing narrative medicine is – famously – to develop 'narrative competence', defined by Charon (2006) as facility with

> a combination of textual skills (identifying a story's structure, adopting its multiple perspectives, recognizing metaphors and allusions), creative skills (imagining many interpretations, building curiosity, inventing multiple endings), and affective skills (tolerating uncertainty as a story unfolds, entering the story's mood).

The point is *not* the development of poetic competence. The objective is to do as the narratologists do when in the land of perpetual narrative: use narratology to transgenre-ify the poem.

An instrumental rationale is touted by the narrativists in medicine. For example, David Morris's (2008) 'Narrative Medicines: Challenge and Resistance' repeatedly refers to narrative as a clinical 'instrument'. Furthermore, the title tells all in Milota et al.'s (2019) 'Narrative medicine as a medical education tool: A systematic review'. Charon (2006) asserts that narrative medicine is

> bound to enhance clinical effectiveness, not only by guiding choices of treatment interventions but also by alerting doctors to all considerations that might help or hinder patients from following medical recommendations and becoming true partners in achieving and maintaining the best health within their reach.

Yet it is this very instrumentalism – an 'applied humanities', if you will – that reinforces the inherent cultural bias towards narrative itself, for in the field of narrative medicine one kind of hermeneutics (narratology) is wedded to outcomes, pulling narrative forward to purpose. Lyric poetry has nothing to say to plot, and as it is currently deployed in the narrative medicine tradition, lyric poetry has little to say to poetics. This leaves a relatively vast potential for the unexplored relational potential of poetics with regards to patient care. Letting go of the narrative yoke might result in the development of new ways to engage with patients.

I therefore call for a recalibration of the use of narrative in medical education. By subscribing to the view of the narratologists, who consider the entirety of existence story-dependent, we miss much of a rich clinical world that is spatial as opposed to chronological. We miss out on a different means of thinking with patients. We miss out on developing a poetics of medicine. It is time to liberate poetry from the tyranny of narrative in medical education and consider poetry on its own terms.

References

Abbott HP. 2008. *The Cambridge Introduction to Narrative* (2nd ed.). Cambridge: Cambridge University Press.
Aristotle. 1898. *XXII: The Poetics of Aristotle* (SH Butcher, trans.). London: MacMillan.
Charon R. 2006. *Narrative Medicine: Honoring the Stories of Illness*. Oxford: Oxford University Press.

Charon R, DasGupta S, Hermann N, et al. 2017. *The Principles and Practice of Narrative Medicine*. Oxford: Oxford University Press.

Connolly A. Was Sophocles Heroised as Dexion? *The Journal of Hellenic Studies*. 1998; 118: 1–21.

Frye N. 1971. *Anatomy of Criticism*. Princeton, NJ: Princeton University Press.

Lentricchia F, McLaughlin T. 1995. *Critical Terms for Literary Study* (2nd ed.). Chicago, IL: University of Chicago Press.

Marthouret T. Medical Humanities in the English Classroom: Building Students' Professional Identity Through Poetry. *ASp*. 2016; 70: 65–85.

Milota MM, van Thiel GJMW, van Delden JJM. Narrative Medicine as a Medical Education Tool: A Systematic Review. *Medical Teacher*. 2019; 41: 802–10.

Morris DB. Narrative Medicines: Challenge and Resistance. *Permanente Journal*. 2008; 12: 88–96.

Scarlett EP. Medicine and Poetry: Being an Account of Those Sons of Æsculapius Who Have on Occasion Paid Homage to the Elder God, Apollo. Part I. *Canadian Medical Association Journal*. 1936; 35: 676–82.

Scarlett EP. Medicine and Poetry: Being an Account of Those Sons of Æsculapius Who Have on Occasion Paid Homage to the Elder God, Apollo. Part II. *Canadian Medical Association Journal*. 1937; 36: 73–79.

Shapiro J. 2009. *The Inner World of Medical Students: Listening to Their Voices in Poetry*. Oxford: Radcliffe Publications.

Shapiro J, Stein H. Poetic License: Writing Poetry as a Way for Medical Students to Examine Their Professional Relational Systems. *Families, Systems & Health*. 2005; 23: 278–92.

Shklovsky V. 2009. *Theory of Prose*. Dallas, TX: Dalkey Archive Press.

Wietlisbach LE, Asch DA, Eriksen W, et al. Using Poetry to Elicit Internal Medicine Residents' Perspectives on Wellness. *Postgraduate Medical Journal*. 2023; 99: 428–32.

Williams WC. 1986. Asphodel, That Greeny Flower. In: C MacGowan (ed.) *The Collected Poems of William Carlos Williams*. Vol. II. New York, NY: New Directions.

PART 2

Archaeology and genealogy

IN CELEBRATION OF THE WORD

Introduction to EP Scarlett's
'Medicine and Poetry'

Shane Neilson and Alan Bleakley

In December 1936 and January 1937, Earle Parkhill Scarlett (1896–1982) published a two-part article, meticulously researched, titled 'Medicine and Poetry'. Outwardly, the article catalogues physicians who were also major or minor poets, but read closely, Scarlett's glosses on such poets reveal an uncanny psychological insight into a form of sensibility. Physicians educated in reading the body could also read the world. In other words, they were experts in close noticing, and their medium for such sensate work was the abstraction of the metaphor. Not quite 'abstract', for metaphors are always embodied, but the transition from the literal to the metaphorical is cognitive – and not, say, the work of the surgeon's knife to which John Keats refers in Scarlett's careful reading of the English surgeon who abandoned medicine for the Word. As Keats said to a friend,

> my last operation was the opening of a man's temporal artery. I did it with the utmost nicety, but, reflecting on what passed through my mind at the time, my dexterity seemed a miracle, and I never took up the lancet again.

The opening of the temporal artery may have prevented loss of vision in Keats' patient, but this moment provided Keats with a vision and a confirmation of calling as a poet. The Word became Keats' patient that he treated with extraordinary care and sensuality.

Scarlett too was a distinguished physician and writer, serving as Chancellor of the University of Alberta from 1952–58. Born in Manitoba and gaining his medical qualifications at the University of Toronto, Scarlett first practiced in North America (where he specialized in cardiology) and then moved to Calgary, where he established his reputation and eventually died. Scarlett was the first fully trained cardiologist to practice at Calgary, where his post was accompanied by the clinic's first ECG machine. Scarlett's personal life was shaped by a serendipitous meeting with William Osler, regarded as the father of modern medical education. During World War I, Scarlett survived both a mustard gas attack and a life-threatening shrapnel injury to his neck. He met Osler during his rehabilitation, after which Scarlett decided to study medicine.

In time, Scarlett developed an interest, and became a leading scholar, in the history of medicine, retiring from clinical practice in 1959 to become a full-time academic. He produced an impressive number of articles on poetry and literature along the way, published mostly in the *Archives of*

 DOI: 10.4324/9781003341796-7

Internal Medicine, including a regular column titled 'Doctor out of Zebulon: Gleanings from the Commonplace Book of a Medical Reader', that title taken from an obscure phrase in the Old Testament's *Book of Judges* – a very poet thing to do. Identifying as a keen observer, he states in his own words that he was ever 'the bemused boy, sitting in the back row of the cosmic theatre . . . listening and making notes – and wondering'. We are not certain if Scarlett ever wrote that wonder out as poetry. We could not find any, though our search was not exhaustive. We do, however, strongly suspect that he did, and we may undertake this inquiry sometime in the future.

When medical students or practising physicians ask what they can gain from studying poetry, we might ask them to read between the lines of Scarlett's two-part essay reproduced here. Pare away the factual history, the lists of achievements of the physician-poets considered, and passing references to their cultural contexts, and we are left with Scarlett's close reading of their work. Here, he digs into the strata of poetry and cleans out the adhering soil to present us with extracted gems – the right words; in other words, he has an eye and an ear for quality. He shows sensory discrimination, or again close noticing, of the kind that you want from your cardiologist – a heart doctor with heart who notices stuff. A heart doctor who notices that poetry, the Word, provides the heartbeat for the world.

We like to think something was in the water around the turn of the twentieth century in Canada when it comes to eminent physicians. The number of physician-authors and -editors associated with the journal is impressive. We already mentioned the grandaddy of them all, Sir William Osler, Regius Professor of Medicine as well as author of *The Principles and Practice of Medicine* but more important to us, physician to Walt Whitman (Osler both consulted for and contributed pieces to the journal). Second only to the very great distinction of Osler's patient–doctor relationship with Whitman, one of the greatest poets of the nineteenth century, are Osler's exhortation to physicians to read poetry as well as his frequent quoting of it.

Many other Canadian names continue to carry weight today, including John McCrae, who published on pathology in the *Canadian Medical Association Journal* (*CMAJ*) and whose most famous contribution to posterity is 'In Flanders Fields'. Maude Abbot – famously, one of the first female physician graduates from a medical faculty, the first member of the Montreal Medical-Chirurgical Society's, and a world expert on congenital heart disease, as well as responsible for producing the tremendously influential *Atlas of Congenital Cardiac Disease* – served as editor-in-chief of the *CMAJ* during part of the First World War while some of the (male) editorial cohort travelled overseas to fight. Abbott also routinely wrote poems in her journals. One of the *CMAJ* editors who fought in that war, Andrew MacPhail, himself published *The Book of Sorrow*, an anthology of poems on the eponymous subject that included his own work. For his part, as we have mentioned, Scarlett fought in the war and based partly on his experience with Osler decided to practice medicine, a case of the art encouraging entry into the profession. The point we are making here is obvious: one commonality amongst this grouping (and there are other names we could add) is that their lives were in close contact with poetry as informant and artistic expression.

The metaphor we used earlier is wrong, though. There wasn't something 'in the water' for eminent physicians around the turn of the century for Canada. Really, poetry had, for millennia, been either a part of medical practice or a spiritual overseer of it, signpost and interpreter, lamentation of the art or celebration of same. Prior to the Second World War's acceleration of the biomedical turn, poetry was intrinsic to the lives for a good many Western physicians insofar as they actually produced poetry, some of them gaining entry to the English canon. Thus, there was something 'in the water' concerning the institution of medicine itself, how it was historically conceived of as both art *and* science.

Even so, we argue that there was something quite special happening at the turn of the twenti-eth century based on the eminent contributions of the aforementioned physicians to both science and poetry. We believe – though can hardly prove – that the capacity for poetry itself underwrote, or somehow contributed to, their other noteworthy achievements. The likes of this phenomenon haven't been seen since in Canada, making us believe further that it was the density of poetry practice in this locale that led to a kind of critical mass of excellence. Further, a reductive Victorian lens of cultural refinement does not adequately explain the literary-scientific flowering described.

EP Scarlett lacks our perspective in the early twenty-first century, of course. We can focus our attention in this brief introduction on a single concentrated node of poetry in Canada thanks to the sifting and sorting of time. Scarlett practised and wrote contemporaneously with the period described, producing an impressive number of scientific publications himself. Yet Scarlett's gen-eral case in 'Medicine and Poetry' elaborates on our specific one: his argument is simple – 'science and poetry truly dwell together' – but his evidence is impressive, contributing an encyclopaedic gathering of physicians who also wrote poetry, the preponderance of whom have properly faded into time but whose names nevertheless collectively attest to the historical validity of the thesis that poetry and medicine are, in some way, interdependent. Time tells us that this was so; but where are we now in our vaunted perch atop the present day? Why does poetry seem so far away from contemporary medical practice?

The truth is, it isn't; it can't be. That is an argument that this Handbook makes convincingly, repeatedly. For now, enjoy Scarlett's obsessive (for all poets are obsessive) catalogue for the fact of its emphatic bulk but also for his enthusiasm concerning his favourites, his quotations from poems that have registered in his mind. That Scarlett was there, compiling names and quoting his darlings in the *CMAJ*, makes one editor in particular (SN) quite proud of both profession and nation, notwithstanding the obvious critiques medicine then, as well as now, deserves. But even more than pride, both editors of this Handbook are simply glad and humbled on behalf of the art itself. That it is proven that poetry mattered throughout the history of the practice of medicine means that poetry itself is honoured – that poetry was given due recognition and respect rather than capitalized upon as per present-day medical pedagogy. And so, from the vantage point of almost a century later, we grandiloquently adopt the role of avatar and thank Scarlett on behalf of both arts. And, as this text argues throughout, on behalf of their shared epistemes of a range of sciences.

4

MEDICINE AND POETRY

EP Scarlett

BEING AN ACCOUNT OF THOSE SONS OF AESCULAPIUS WHO HAVE ON OCCASION PAID HOMAGE TO THE ELDER GOD, APOLLO.
  'A physician should be a kind of poet'.
  Calgary

Part I

At first glance, at least to modern eyes, any attempt to relate poetry and medicine appears to be almost an absurdity, a straining of the laudable practice of comparison beyond rational limits. It is not unlike linking the subtle flights of metaphysics and the harsh realities of cold mutton, so far has specialization destroyed our perspective in the modern world. But a little speculation reveals a different story. These two activities of the human spirit are closely linked historically, and in tradition they emerged from the same shrine in the temple of the gods. Apollo, the god of poetry, was the father of Aesculapius, the divinity of the healing art, and in Greek times those practising medicine were dignified as 'the children of Apollo'. The figure of Apollo, the supreme god of medicine, together with the Muses and the serene goddess Pallas Athene, the immortal exemplar of Reason and Discipline, are the ancient personifications of the great intellectual virtues which have raised us from the barbaric state. Science and poetry thus truly dwell together, and in any rounded philosophy of life they find full and mutual expression.

Both poetry and medicine go back to the childhood of the race. For while 'poetry, like Beatrice, was born under a dancing star', medicine came into being with the first struggles for existence under the noonday sun, and under the fear of the terror that walketh by night. They have been man's spiritual companions all down the long journey. This kinship between poetry and science has been expressed by many writers. Poetry, says Bacon, 'doth raise and erect the mind, by submitting the shows of things to the desires of the mind; whereas reason doth buckle and bow the mind unto the nature of things'. Wordsworth in his preface to *Lyrical Ballads* describes the relation even more adequately – 'Poetry is the breath and finder spirit of all knowledge; it is the impassioned expression which is in the countenance of all Science'. The business of science is to accurately observe and describe – 'To express what then I saw'; this done, poetry's function is to 'add the gleam,/The light that never was, on sea or land,/The consecration, and the Poet's dream'.

DOI: 10.4324/9781003341796-8

To revert to our title and set it forth in more accurate fashion, while physic requires no definition, poetry, like many of the best things in life, defies definition. The only way to know what poetry is is to read it. The appreciation of poetry has been bedevilled by the too generally accepted idea, brewed in some witch's cauldron of folly, that poetry is a rather pallid cult of abnormal or weirdly intellectual persons. The truth of the matter is that poetry is natural to man. This fact may be abundantly proved by watching any group of men who are not necessarily under the spiritual instancy of alcoholic nectars lustily roar some current song or ballad and with emotional fervour and a far-off expression in their eyes. And, if poetry eludes definition, it may be set forth by example in a thousand ways. For instance, modern science proclaims that, in the scale of the universe as we know it, man is a mere speck, an impotent creature. But only poetry can state this fact adequately:

> One generation passeth away, and another generation cometh: but the earth abideth forever –
> Then I looked on all the works that my hands had wrought, and on the labour that I had laboured to do: and behold, all was vanity and vexation of spirit, and there was no profit under the sun. – *Ecclesiastes* I: 1–11.

Or again,

> Tomorrow, and tomorrow, and tomorrow,
> Creeps in this petty pace from day to day,
> To the last syllable of recorded time,
> And all our yesterdays have lighted fools
> The way to dusty death. Out, out brief candle!
> Life's but a walking shadow, a poor player
> That struts and frets his hour upon the stage
> And then is heard no more: it is a tale
> Told by an idiot, full of sound and fury
> Signifying nothing. – *Macbeth*, V, 5.

Definition or no definition, that is poetry!

The relation of science and poetry recalls two notable passages which incidentally set forth the nature and function of poetry. The first is from the *Defence of Poesy* by Sir Philip Sidney:

> Now, therein, of all sciences (I speak still of human, and according to the human conceit) is our poet the monarch. For he doth not only show the way, but giveth so sweet a prospect unto the way as will entice any man to enter into it. . . . He beginneth not with obscure definitions, which must blur the margins with interpretations and load the mind with doubtfulness; but he cometh to you with words set in delightful proportion, either accompanied with, or prepared for, the well-enchanting skill of music; and with a take, forsooth, he cometh unto you – with a tale which holdeth children from play and old men from the chimney corner: and, pretending no more, doth intend the winning of the mind from wickedness to virtue, even as a child is often brought to take most wholesome things by hiding them in such other as have a pleasant taste, which, if one should begin to tell them from the nature of the aloes or rhubarbum they should receive, would sooner take their physic at their ears than their mouth. So it is in men – most of whom are childish in the best things till they be cradled in their graves.

The other passage is from an essay written by Matthew Arnold fifty-four years ago:

> More and more mankind will discover that we have to turn to poetry to interpret life for us, to console us, to sustain us. Without poetry, our science will appear incomplete; and most of which now passes for religion and philosophy will be replaced by poetry. Science, I say, will be incomplete without it . . .. Wordsworth finely calls poetry the breath and finer spirit of all knowledge . . .. The day will come when we shall wonder at ourselves for having trusted to them, [current philosophy and religion] for having taken them seriously, and the more we perceive their hollowness, the more we shall prize *the breath and finer spirit of knowledge* offered to us by poetry.

But, you say, this is all very well, but to a man whose ear is tuned to the exact phrases of science, poetry means nothing. He can find no satisfaction in reading poetry; his fate is not unlike that of Darwin who after years of science lost his appreciation of music. The answer to such a plaint is – 'why did you ever give up reading poetry? You used to enjoy it'.

> London Bridge is broken down,
> Dance o'er my Lady lee,
> London Bridge is broken down
> With a gay lady.

For, as Lynd says, every child is a poet from the age at which he learns to beat a silver spoon on the table in numbers. And later at every great hour of his life – hours of love or sorrow – his deeper emotions find no expression in common speech and at such times he must be inarticulate or find speech in poetry.

For, indeed, poetry is infinite in its variety. It may proceed from the lowest to the highest. Let us try to set out such a gradation.

> Tom he was a piper's son
> He learned to play when he was young,
> But all the tunes that he could play
> Was, *Over the hills and far away.*

Childish, you say; but the last line is the stuff of pure poetry. Poetry, too, depends not only on verbal music but also on the association of the words employed. Sir John Squire, a modern master of parody, illustrates this by devising a set of lines in which the names of diseases conjure up music if we could forget their association. Thus:

> So forth then rode Sir Erysipelas
> From good Lord Goitre's castle, with the steed
> Loose on the rein; and as he rode he mused
> On knights and ladies dead; Sir Scrofula,
> Sciatica, he of Glanders, and his friend
> Stout Sir Colitis out of Aquitabe,
> And Impetigo, proudest of them all,
> Who lived and died for blind Queen Cholera's sake . . .
> And then once more the incredible dream came back,

How long ago upon the fabulous shores
Of far Lumbago, all of a summer's day,
He and the maid Neuralgia, they twain,
Lay in a flower-crowned mead, and garlands wove,
Of gout and yellow hydrocephaly . . ..
Cirrhosis and that wan, faint flower
The shepherds call dyspepsia. Gone, all gone:
There came a night he cried, 'Neuralgia!'
And never a voice to answer. Only rang
O'er cliff and battlement and desolate mere
'Neuralgia!' in the echoes' mockery.

A higher example still, its appeal depending on alliteration, is Coleridge's verse in *The Ancient Mariner*:

The fair breeze blew, the white foam flew,
   The furrow followed free;
We were the first that ever burst
   Into that silent sea.

Proceeding, here is a stanza sounding the sad wisdom of life which has long satisfied the average man – a stanza from Gray's "Elegy":

The boast of heraldy, the pomp of power,
And all that beauty, all that wealth e'er gave,
Awaits alike th'inevitable hour:
The paths of glory lead but to the grave.

And so by degrees we come to poetry in its highest expression, sounding a requiem on man and all his works. Prospero's last speech from *The Tempest*:

And like the baseless fabric of this vision,
The cloud-capped towers, the gorgeous palaces,
The solemn temples, the great globe itself,
Yea, all which it inherit, shall dissolve
And like an unsubstantial pageant faded
Leave not a wrack behind. We are such stuff
As dreams are made on, and our little life
Is rounded with a sleep.

There is no occasion to pursue the thought further. It is worth remembering, however, that one of the reasons why the bible is cherished by man is for the poetry which it contains – its thoughts are expressed in memorable verse:

Or ever the silver cord be loosed, or the golden bowl be broken, or the pitcher be broken at the fountain, or the wheel broken at the cistern. Then shall the dust return to the earth as it was: and the spirit shall return unto God who gave it. *Ecclesiastes*, XII: 6–7.

Set me as a seal upon thine heart, as a seal upon thine arm: for love is strong as death, jeal-ousy is cruel as the grave: the coals thereof are coals of fire, which hath a most vehement flame. *Song of Solomon*, VIII: 6.

Where wast though when I laid the foundations of the earth? Declare, if thou hast under-standing. Who hath laid the measures thereof, if thou knowest? or who hath stretched the line upon it? Whereupon are the foundations thereof fastened? or who hath laid the corner stone thereof; when the morning starts sang together, and all the sons of God shouted for joy? *Job*, XXXVIII: 4–7.

Without indulging in any ethereal generalizations, enough, I think, has been said to suggest what we mean by poetry. We are concerned just now with the relation between the writing of poetry and the practice of physic, not of course in any philosophical sense. It has indeed been said that 'a physician should be a kind of poet', on which aphorism Sir Clifford Allbutt remarked: 'A hard saying, but to their patients what are the most scientific physicians if they know all things save the human heart?' Our task is rather to consider those physicians who have written poetry, not the mere talented dabblers in verse of whom there have probably been thousands, but those men who have achieved a measure of distinction in poetry, the most difficult of all the arts. It has been claimed by Mitchell Banks that medicine stands foremost among the professions in the number of distinguished literary men who began life in its ranks. In Renaissance times and during the following century the relation between literature and medicine was close. Those were the days of the scholar – physicians such as Linacre – and medicine was in a very special sense one of the learned professions. With the advance of specialization of knowledge, however, the connection has become less intimate, and today medicine suffers because of this fact.

When we come to review the contributions of medical men to poetry we find that there are few who have distinguished themselves in both fields. The talents required to do first-rate work in medi-cine are widely divergent from those essential in the writing of great poetry. Only a genius of the most varied and universal character, such as Goethe, can be preeminent in poetry and science. And, besides, divided allegiance is not infrequently fatal to personal or popular success. Physicians, therefore, who have written poetry have treated it as an oblique pursuit or have practised little med-icine. Some have qualified as doctors and then abandoned the profession for some other pursuit. The list, however, is an interesting one. In 1916 Dr. C.L. Dana, in a treatise called *Poetry and the Doctors*, compiled a catalogue of poems written by doctors, comprising the names of 162 medical men. In 1925 Sir Humphry Rolleston, in an address on *Poetry and Physic*, mentioned over eighty medical men or medical students who had written notable poetry. And in the *Bibliotheca Osleriana* there are ninety medical men represented by their poetry, two-thirds of whom wrote prior to 1801. We purpose considering some of these names, arbitrarily following a chronological order.

The identity of sympathy existing between medical men and literature has its roots far back in the early centuries of the medieval period, when students of medicine wandered through the medi-cal schools of Europe under the spell of the great humanist tradition of letters. The 'Guadeamus igitur' still sung in universities is a remote echo of the eleventh and twelfth centuries when the med-ical students were part of the great band of scholars who roared Latin songs, drank uproariously, wenched, diced, and wrote and recited Latin lyrics. A figure who is the symbol of these times is the Archpoet who died about 1165 and who has been so brilliantly re-created in our time by Miss Helen Waddell. As she says – 'He travelled light, even to immortality'. A 'rather disreputable figure, keen as a razor and lean as a hawk', he wanders over Europe with his patron's cloak 'hugged about his tatters'. After some scandal about a wench, his friends, thinking to make him respectable, pack him off to Salerno to study medicine where he remains for a time. Then he returns, burnt up with the fever of consumption, and at Pavia writes his poem, the *Confessio*, the eternal challenge against the denying of the flesh, the cry of youth in all ages, whether medical students or vagrant scholars. The poem is the greatest drinking song in the world. The Latin lines pound out their rhythm vehemently.

> Estuans intrinsecus
>   Ira vehementi . . .

> Seething over inwardly
>   With fierce indignation,
> In my bitterness of soul,

>   Hear my declaration.
> I am of one element,
>   Levity my matter,
> Like enough a withered leaf
>   For the winds to scatter.

> Yet a second charge they bring:
>   I'm forever gaming.
> Yea, the dice hath many a time
>   Stripped me to my shaming.
> What and if the body's cold,
>   If the mind is burning,
> Or the anvil hammering,
>   Rhymes and verses turning.

> Look again upon your list
>   Is the tavern on it?
> Yes, and never have I scorned,
>   Never shall I scorn it,
> Till the holy angels come,
>   And my eyes discern them,
> Singing for they dying soul,
>   Requiem aeturnam. – *Medieval Latin Lyrics*:
>   translation, Miss Waddell

In these centuries verse was the medium for medical teaching. Probably the earliest physician-poet was Floridus, who lived in France in the ninth century and wrote a lengthy collection of hexameters about the medical virtues of plants. The most famous poem of this type is the *Regimen Sanitatis* written at the medical school of Salerno about 1101, its author probably one John of Milan. This work was addressed to the lay public, was one of the earlier printed books in 1480, and has passed through over one hundred editions since then. As recently as 1922 an edition of Sir John Harington's English version was published in London.

This practice of using alliterative rhyming verse, particularly for works on domestic medicine was, of course, merely the result of classical tradition. The writing of verse by physicians, mostly epigrams and didactic epics, was common during Greek and Roman times. Nikandros of Kolophon (*circa* 133 BC), the son of a priest of Apollo, and himself a priest-physician wrote two works of poetry of considerable length dealing with bites of noxious beasts, antidotes and the virtues of herbs. Macer, in the third century AD, wrote a *materia medica* in verse which was later commended by Linacre to his pupils. These are merely pedestrian examples of the practice which reached its highest expression in the work of the Roman poet, Lucretius (85–55 BC), whose philosophical poem *De Rerum Natura* is one of the great poems of the world. The only other didactic medical poem which we need consider is the poem *Syphilidis sive de Morbo Gallico tres libri*, published at Venice in 1530 and translated into English in 1686. Osler describes it as 'the most successful medical poem ever written', presumably because it gave us the name of a disease. Its author, Girolamo Fracastoro (1483–1553), was born at Verona, became professor of logic at Padua, and afterwards practised medicine with great success. Like so many of his contemporaries he was an accomplished scholar, and was proficient in astronomy, natural philosophy, and poetry.

In search of our physician-poets we may pass at once to the sixteenth century. Ambroise Paré, a mighty figure in medical annals, wrote sonnets, and short verses appear in his various works, but he can hardly be ranked as a serious poet. In England there was an interesting group of poet-surgeons whose verse reflects the mediocrity of the time in literature. John Halle (1529–1568) published a poem in the metre of In Memoriam, entitled *The Court of Virtue Containing Many Holy or Spiritual Songs, Sonnettes, etc.* Thomas Gale (1507–1587), a prose poet whom Izaak Walton imitated, wrote *Certaine Works of Chirurgerie and Certain Works of Galen.* Thomas Vicary, the author of a work with the curious title *The Englishman's Treasure, or Treasor For Englishmen with the True Anatomye of Man's Body* (1585) wrote occasional verses. And John Read, an Elizabethan surgeon, wrote in metre *A Complaint of the Abuses of the Noble Art of Chirurgerie.*

The Golden Age of English poetry which began with Edmund Spenser's *Shepherd's Calendar* in 1579, and gave to the world the glorious, varied plenty of Elizabethan poetry finds two physicians in the long bead-roll of famous names, each of whom has given us some of the loveliest lyrics in the language. These two men are Thomas Lodge and Thomas Campion. Thomas Lodge (1558–1625), the son of Sir Thomas Lodge, Lord Mayor of London, first tried his hand at law, then for a time was soldier, literary man, and later freebooter in the Spanish Main and the Brazils. He finally turned to medicine and graduated from Avignon and Oxford. He began practice in Warwick Lane, London, was successful as a physician, and continued to write. On May 11, 1604, he was examined at the Royal College of Physician with a group of candidates which included Matthew Gwinne, Raphael Thorius, and the great William Harvey. He failed on that occasion but was successful in 1609. The first two men mentioned in the above group are worthy of some slight degree of immortality as they celebrated in verse the delights of tobacco in the early years after its introduction into England and were therefore among the first to establish for the profession of medicine that devotion to the ambrosial weed which has finely characterized it down the centuries. Thorius wrote the *Hymnus Tobaci*, while Gwinne, also a lesser poet, argued in its favour, in spite of the royal prejudice against it, at a medical disputation at Oxford for the edification, if not conversion, of James I in 1605. Lodge, in his practice of medicine, was somewhat of an authority on the plague, from which he died in 1625, nine years after the death of his greatest contemporary, William Shakespeare. It is Lodge's most famous work, *Roselynde, Euphues Golden Legacie*, that provided Shakespeare with his material for *As You Like It.* Lodge's chief volume of verse was *Phyllis* (1593), which contained some forty sonnets and lyrics and a long narrative poem. He is remembered by his little songs and madrigals, two or three of which, such as "Rosalind's Madrigal", still find a place in every anthology of English verse. His lyrics have the limped beauty characteristic of all the songs of the time, chastened at times by the poignancy of the uncertainty of life, for *carpe diem* was the theme of men living in a time when even the highest or most brilliant were apt to meet death on the scaffold. So we find Lodge writing –

> Pluck the fruit and taste the pleasure
>   Youthfull lordlings of delight;
> Whilst occasion gives you seizure,
>   Feed your fancies and your sight:
> After death, when you are gone,
>   Joy and pleasure is there none.
>   *From Robert, Second Duke of*
>   *Normandy*, 1591

Master Thomas Campion (? – 1619), poet, musician, and Doctor of Medicine (or 'doctor in phisicke' as he was styled) was born about the middle of the sixteenth century, the precise date and place being unknown. Like Lodge, he was first of all a student of law in London, later turning to medicine and graduating from Cambridge. He had a most successful practice in London, and was a cultured, urbane man, with a wide circle of friends. His first book was a collection of Latin epigrams. He later wrote masques for presentation at court which are among the finest of their kind, a volume of songs on the death of Prince Henry, and four Books of Airs containing songs and lyrics, many of which were set to music by Campion himself. Campion has provided us with one of the strangest and most delightful surprises in English literature. His work was entirely forgotten until about forty-five years ago, when Mr. A. H. Bullen rescued it from oblivion, and since that time Campion's fame has grown steadily. His lyrics are perfect and exquisite examples of their kind, completely satisfying the relationship between music and poetry. To fully appreciate the beauty of his words, one must hear them sung to their music. Probably the best known of his songs is the one beginning 'There is a garden in her face,/Where roses and sweet lilies grow'. In another of his songs there occurs one of the most beautiful lines in our language. It is the last line of this stanza:

> Shall I come, Sweet Love, to thee,
> When the evening beams are set?
> Shall I not excluded be?
> Will you find no feigned let?
> Let me not, for pity, more
> Tell the long hours at your door.

One of his sonnets, in its astringent dramatic quality, has a curiously modern flavor. It is addressed to a coquette:

> When thou must home to shades of underground,
>   And there arrived, a new admired guest,
> The beauteous spirits do engirt thee round,
>   White Iope, blithe Helen and the rest,
> To hear the stories of thy finished love
> From that smooth tongue, whose music hell can move:
>   Then wilt though speak of banqueting delights,
> Of masks and revels which sweet youth did make,
>   Of tourneys and great challenges of knights,

And all these triumphs for thy beauty's sake.
  When thou hast told these honours done to thee,
Then tell, O! tell, how thou didst murder me.

Poems expressing religious aspiration are seldom more than mere verse, but one such of Campion's beautifully unites expression and sentiment. It is included in Lewis Hind's anthology of the one hundred best poems in our language:

Never weather-beaten sail more willing bent to shore,
  Never tired pilgrim's limbs affected slumber more,
Than my weary spring now longs to fly out of my troubled breast.
  O, come quickly, sweetest Lord, and take my soul to rest.

Ever blooming are the joys of Heaven's high Paradise.
  Cold age deafs not there our ears, nor vapour dims our eyes,
Glory there the sun outshines, whose beams the blessed only see.
  O! Come quickly, glorious Lord, and raise my sprite to Thee.

Thomas Campion is certainly of the select few among the great poet-physicians.

Abraham Cowley (1618–1667), a native of London, scholar of Trinity College, Cambridge, and later of Oxford, spent his earlier years in the Royalist cause, living for a time in France as secretary to the exiled Queen Henrietta Maria. He was created in 1657 a Doctor of Medicine at Oxford by the Archbishop of Canterbury, by virtue of an ancient right which this office still possesses. He applied for the mastership of the Savoy hospital, but this was not granted. Finally, after the Restoration, a competence was provided for him by the Earl of St. Albans and the Duke of Buckingham and he retired from public life to the country. He does not appear to have practised medicine. He was, however, an original member of the Royal Society and published a Latin poem on plants. During his lifetime he was regarded as the greatest English poet and on his death was buried in Westminster Abbey. His face quickly waned; indeed, there is a melancholy note in Cowley's writing about himself, for, while fortune treated him rudely, he never really fulfilled the promise of his youth. He had been an amazingly precocious boy, writing poetry at the age of ten, and publishing his first work when fifteen. Later he set the contemporary fashion of writing poetry, and in literary history is remembered as one of the first to establish what may be termed the modern prose style. In 1737 Pome wrote of him:

Who now reads Cowley? If he pleases yet,
  It is his moral pleases, not his wit;
Forgot his epic, nay, Pindaric art,
  But still I love the language of his heart.

The language of Cowley's heart is in his prose and there is little in his poetry that merits quotation in these days.

The next figure, Henry Vaughan (1621–1693), is one for whom poetry is deeply in debt to medicine. Vaughan, the 'Silurist', as he was called because of his native place among the Silures in the county of Brecknockshire in South Wales, was educated at Jesus College, Oxford, and was a staunch Royalist, being imprisoned for a time during the Civil War. He practised medicine in his native town and achieved a considerable reputation. His literary work was an avocation pursued for the love of writing and for the opportunity it gave him to express a singularly religious and mystical nature. During a long life he remained aloof from the turmoil of the world, and in genuine humility of aim and spirit he achieved immortality. It is of interest that he had a twin brother, Thomas, who was also a poet and a famous Rosicrucian. Both brothers have places in the Dictionary of National Biography, two twins thus achieving fame apparently being unique in history.

Vaughan's great poems are contained in the volume entitled in quaint classical fashion – *Silex Scintillans, or Sacred Poems and Private Ejaculations*. His poem *The Retreate* provided Wordsworth with some part of his inspiration for the famous *Ode on the Intimations of Immortality*. Some half dozen of his poems are the finest expression in our language of spiritual aspiration. As a writer of religious verse he is of the company of George Herbert and John Donne. If there is a question as to the finest poem ever written by an active practising physician, there is no doubt at all that the choice would be Vaughan's magnificent elegiac stanzas for departed friends beginning:

> They are all gone into the world of light!
>   And I alone sit lingering here;
> Their very memory is fair and bright,
>   And my sad thoughts doth clear.

Two other poems which gleam with the lights of magic phrases are *The World* and *Peace*. The imagery of the opening stanza of *The World* is superb:

> I saw Eternity the other night
>   Like a great Ring of pure and endless light,
> All calm, as it was bright,
>   And round beneath it, Time in hours, days, years
> Driv'n by the spheres
>   Like a vast shadow moved, in which the world
> And all her train were hurl'd . . .

Contrast this with the calm fervour of *Peace*:

> My Soul, there is a Countrie
>   Far beyond the stars,
> Where stands a winged sentrie
>   All skilfull in the wars.
> There above noise, and danger
>   Sweet peace sits crown'd with smiles,
> And one born in a Manger
>   Commands the Beauteous files . . .

The spirit of Vaughan is best expressed in the Latin inscription which he wrote to be placed on his tomb: 'An unprofitable servant, the chief of sinners I lie here. Glory be to God! Lord have mercy upon me'.

Two lesser names complete the roll of seventeenth century poet-physicians. Martin Llewellyn (1616–1682), scholar and cavalier, fought for the Royalist cause and afterwards practised in London. Later he became a Fellow of the Royal College of Physicians, and with the Restoration he was made physician to Charles II and Principal of St. Mary's Hall, Oxford. After four years he settled at High Wycombe where he practised till his death. His best-known work was *Mere Miracles*.

A number of his poems were satirical, and one of the last *Wickham Awakened*, or the *Quaker's Madrigal*, written in rhymed doggerel, was an attack on a Quaker rival who had annexed much of his practice. Francesco Redi (1626–1697) was a student of Pisa and physician to the dukes of Tuscany. In his scientific work he is regarded as the founder of comparative helminthology and did much to refute the theory of spontaneous generation. He was a distinguished poet in his day, publishing *Bacco in Toscane*, *Arianna Inferma* and other works.

With the single exception of Goldsmith, the physicians of the eighteenth century produced little poetry of worth. They were men who in the custom of the time wrote verse of a sort, much of it polished, but little memorable. They talked and drank with the wits in the coffee houses, and certain of them were members of the reigning literary circles of the time. As Sir Edmund Gosse has pointed out, these friendships forged the abiding ties between literature and medicine which have persisted to our day and have found their modern expression in the figure of the late Poet Laureate, Robert Bridges.

To use Gosse's figure, the last embargo dividing literature from medicine was broken down by Sir Samuel Garth (1659–1718), a distinguished member of the Royal College of Physicians and a Harveian and Galstonian orator. Known as the 'Kit-Kat Poet', he was a friend of the leading literary and political men of the age – Addison, Steele, Walpole, Halifax and Marlborough. Pope called him 'the best of Christians without knowing it' and Dr. Johnson, always the master of the telling phrase, said of him that no man knew his art more or his trade less. His mock-heroic poem *The Dispensary* ridiculed the apothecaries and those physicians who opposed the establishment of a dispensary where the poor could get advice from the best physicians. The poem is celebrated less for its verse than for its recognition of the claims of literature and medicine on an equality of importance. In 1700 Garth pronounced the funeral oration over John Dryden, the laureate, as the body lay in state in the hall of the Royal College and was present when it was buried in the Poets' Corner in Westminster Abbey. This oration of Garth's, it should be added, caused something of a scandal by its fulsome praises of Apollo and the classical ideals and its rather scant references to Christianity – the ever-recurring voice of the medical pagan!

Erasmus Darwin (1731–1802), grandfather of Charles Darwin, practised medicine successively at Nottingham, Lichfield and Derby. In his fiftieth year he wrote a long poem called 'The Botanic Garden'. Another of the lesser versifiers was John Armstrong (1709–1779), a Scot, and a rather splenetic gentleman, whose first poem *The Oeconomy of Love* created something of a stir, one commentator writing that 'he humned the praises of Venus in strains so warm that they dissolved away his practice'. He later atoned for this error with the didactic poem expressing, with the utmost medical decorum, *The Art of Preserving Health*.

John Wolcot (1738–1819), who wrote under the pseudonym of Peter Pindar, figured in some of the literary quarrels of the day. He had great satirical ability, but his humour at times was rough and libellous, while his verse resembled the slashing surgery of his time. In the literary battles which gave spice to this century a lone figure, attacked by both the medical and literary camps, was Sir Richard Blackmore (1653–1729), who had graduated in Arts at Oxford and in medicine at Padua, and was physician to William III and afterwards to Queen Anne. He was a prolific writer, and it was said: 'In leisure hours in epic song he deals,/Writes to the rumbling of his coach's wheels'. His poem *Satyr against Wit* brought on his head the stinging couplets of a band of literary enemies, including Dryden, Pope, Steele, and Garth. While in his own day Blackmore was praised by Dr. Johnson for his philosophical poem *The Creation*, the judgement of posterity is with Gosse, who dryly remarks that as an epic poet not even Phoebus Apollo can resuscitate him.

Another figure whose eminence in medicine far outstrips his ability in verse is Mark Akenside (1721–1770), the son of a Newcastle butcher, who graduated as Doctor of Physic at Leyden and later became physician to the Queen and a Harveian Orator. Wealth came to him suddenly through the bequest of a certain Jeremiah Dyson who gave him a house, an allowance, a chariot, and considerable advertisement. His principal work *The Pleasures of the Imagination* is a long didactic poem in blank verse. He also wrote many odes in the manner of Gray and Collins. His arrogant manner made him many enemies, and probably on this account he was satirized by Smollett in *Peregrine Pickle*.

Part II

The eighteenth century is notable in literary history for the number of poets whose work was acclaimed in their own day but who to later times seem dull to the point of dreariness. George Crabbe (1754–1832) is of this group. Byron called him 'Nature's sternest painter, yet the best'. Even Jane Austen said that she 'could fancy being Mrs. Crabbe'. But he sounded no strain to stir posterity. He was apprenticed to a village surgeon near his native place, Aldborough, in Suffolk, and later spent a year in London hospitals, during which time he was hauled before the magistrate because his landlady mistook the baby which he was dissecting for her own child who had just died. He failed to make a success of practice and later took orders. As a clergyman he was a friend of the poor and could combine medical advice with his work as a cleric. Crabble was a realist who wrote grimly of life as he saw it, and particularly stressed the sordid existence of the poor. He is an important figure in literary history, representing the reaction against the frigid conventional writing of the time and the artificial manner of verses to Phyllis and Corydon and my lady's eyebrows.

It is of the very essence of the irony of history that a man whom the arrogant Akenside and the other imperious medical men of the day frequently passed in the Fleet Street or the Strand with a pitying glance, or more probably splashed with mud from their carriages – a man, shabbily dressed, short of stature, with an ugly, pale face pitted with small-pox, long, protruding upper lip, and forehead broad and projecting – that this man should have gathered about himself a host of legends and become one of the best-loved figures in our literature. Such is the way of genius; and Oliver Goldsmith (1728–1774) is of this select company.

It is unnecessary if not quite impossible, to sketch in a few words the sprightly mixture we call Goldsmith, the open-hearted, improvident Irishman, 'the ugly duckling of the Johnsonian circle of immortals'. We may be permitted, however, to examine the reason for the M.B. which appeared after his name on an early title page. After graduating B.A. at Trinity College, Dublin and spending several advances of money from his family in an attempt to get out of Ireland, he turned up in Edinburgh where he studied medicine for a short time. He then wandered over Europe, playing on the flute, and debating at the universities for a livelihood; returned to England, where he was a druggist's assistant and set up as a physician for a time at Southwark. Coming to London, he went up for examination at the College of Surgeons in a suit of clothes which he had borrowed and which he afterwards pawned, but he was marked 'not qualifyd'. He was similarly rejected by the naval boards to whom he applied as a surgeon. In a cloud of misery and at times starvation he was in succession, school usher, proof-reader, journalist, and apothecary. His attempts at practice were as happy-go-lucky and as prodigal as his nature. The patients and the attending apothecary quarrelled with his advice and his dosages which were apparently given under the impulse of the extravagant inspiration of genius. Finally, his resolution to drop practice was fervently seconded by his friend Topham Beauclerc, who advised him, if he were resolved to kill, to concentrate on his enemies.

It would appear from a contemporary newspaper that in February, 1769, Oxford University gave him an *ad eundem* degree of Bachelor of Medicine, and it is supposed by students of his life that Goldsmith after his travels on the Continent obtained the Dublin M.B. *in absentia*, thus making this later English degree possible. This would account for his medical title which he most certainly acquired, for Goldsmith was too honest a man to claim a fictitious degree. Let it be recorded, too, as pointed out by Crane, that Auenbrugger's treatise on percussion of the chest, published in 1761, was made known in England by a review of the work which Goldsmith wrote in the same year.

In any event, such a wayward genius could contrive nothing but misfortune from the practice of medicine, which demands some limits to the exuberance of its members. And medicine, in one of the queer turns of fortune which marked all of Goldsmith's life, did exact a final toll from him. In his last illness Goldsmith, in spite of the protest of his medical attendant, William Hawes, insisted on dosing himself with large amounts of the famous James's powder, then having a great vogue. This was an antimonial preparation, and it is probable that his death was accelerated by antimony poisoning. There was certainly a stir in the press over the matter at the time. This last outrage of genius on nature was thus revenged; Goldsmith paid his 'cock to Aesculapius'. But what medicine denied him, 'the draggle-tailed Muses', as he called literature, paid him in full measure. As one of our few universal men of letters he produced a great book, *The Vicar of Wakefield*, a great play, *She Stoops to Conquer*, and poetry which is the best of its kind. The memorable couplets of *The Deserted Village* have in many instances become part of our daily speech. It is often forgotten how frequently Goldsmith is on our tongue:

"When lovely woman stoops to folly."
"A youth of labour with an age of ease."
"A man he was to all the country dear,
And passing rich with forty pounds a year."
"And fools who came to scoff remained to pray."
"And still they gazed, and still the wonder grew
That one small head could carry all he knew."
"Ill fares the land, to hastening ills a prey,
Where wealth accumulates and men decay."
"Silence gives consent."
"For he who fights and runs away
May live to fight another day."
"To husband out life's taper at the close,
And keep the flame from wasting by repose."

When Goldsmith died, the staircase of his lodging in the Temple was crowded with the weeping figures of London's derelicts and its poor whom he had helped, however blundering his medical aid. 'Goldie' he was to his friends. His monument in Westminster Abbey with the famous Latin inscription written by Dr. Johnson, says in part, 'There was no kind of writing that he did not touch, none that he touched that he did not adorn'.

While still in the company of genius it should not be forgotten that the brilliant and versatile German poet Schiller (1759–1805) qualified as a Doctor of Medicine at the age of twenty-one and practised for a time as an assistant surgeon in a grenadier regiment at a salary of eighteen florins (C\$7.50) a month. He speedily found his true vocation in literature, and left army surgery to rougher spirits.

There are other names in this century – hardly even minor poets – who may be mentioned. James Grainfer (1721–1766) depended chiefly on his pen rather than on his practice for a living. While in the West Indies he wrote a poem in four books called *The Sugar Cane*, which dealt in doubtful lyric fashion with the cultivation of that plant. It is chiefly notable for the remarkable line – 'Say, shall I sing of rats?' Dr. Johnson when reading this line thundered out a vehement 'No', to the laughter of his audience. Edward Jenner (1749–1854), of Lochwinnoch, was a famous man of letters in his day. It is pleasant to think of John Mason Good (1764–1827), translating Lucretius as he walked the London streets on his medical calls, and of John Leyden (1775–1811), in his early twenties already a master of many languages, assisting his friend Sir Walter Scott with the earlier editions of the Minstrelsy of the Scottish Border. More versatile was von Haller (1708–1777) who wrote the first great modern treatise on physiology. During the seventeen years in which he was a professor of medicine at Göttingen he conducted some 12,000 articles on almost every branch of knowledge. Osler puts in him the first rank of our medical poets.

It is possible to go on through a long list of eighteenth-century physicians who were poetasters, rough lampoonists, lively blades whose wit crackled while their rhyming couplets served the custom of the day. Through it all is expressed the intimate relation between literature and medicine which Osler and Allbutt revived in our own day. In a fanciful way Sir Edmund Gosse has suggested that this relation might be perpetuated by having a statue of the great and gentle Dr. John Arbuthnot, the author of *The History of John Bull*, with busts of Pope, Steele, Swift and Gay at the corners of the pedestal.

The roll of nineteenth-century medical poets opens with the name of the most illustrious figure in the group which we are considering – John Keats (1795–1821). In some respects, it is a Philistine presumption, almost an impertinence, for medicine to assert any claim to Keats. He is one of the immortals of our race and belongs to the world. And yet medicine in all humility may state that it cradled him. As a modern writer as put it, 'Medicine suffered a loss, but the world gained when this prodigal son strayed off into a far country'.

Keats's major works are so much a part of our common heritage that they require no comment in this paper. It is of more immediate interest to examine the way in which the poetic genius burst through the bounds which the study of medicine had placed about the young man. Keats, a spirited pugnacious lad, and a natural leader among his fellows, was left an orphan at the age of fourteen. In the following year he was apprenticed by his guardian to Mr. Hammond, a surgeon of Edmonton, in whose service he spent more than four years. The young apprentice already had a passion for literature, and during these early years completed a translation of the *Aeneid*. But it was the reading of Spenser's 'Faerie Queen', through which he ranged with delight, that awakened his genius, and his earliest compositions are in imitation of Spenser. The earliest sign that Keats had seriously committed himself to poetry occurred in February, 1815, when he impulsively handed his friend, Clarke, a sonnet entitled *Written on the day that Mr. Leigh Hunt left Prison*. He was in his nineteenth year at the time and still an apprentice. While none of these earlier efforts were precocious, in midsummer of this same year there was a sudden blaze of genius. Keats and Clarke had read a borrowed folio copy of *Chapman's Homer* far into the small hours of the morning. Keats, who left for home in a state of excitement, composed and sent back a sonnet which Clarke found on his breakfast table when he came down in the morning. It bore the title 'On First Looking into Chapman's Homer', and is one of the perfect things in our literature:

> Much have I travell'd in the realms of gold,
> And many goodly states and kingdoms seen;
> Round many Western islands have I been
> Which bards in fealty to Apollo hold.
> Oft of one wide expanse had I been told
> That deep-brow'd Homer ruled as his demesne:
> Yet did I never breathe its pure serene
> Till I heard Chapman speak out loud and bold:
> Then felt I like some watcher of the skies

When a new planet swims into his ken;
Or like stout Cortez when with eagle eyes
He stared at the Pacific – and all his men
Look'd at each other with a wild surmise –
Silent, upon a peak in Darien.

In those lines the young apprentice for the first time 'speaks out loud and bold', in accents which were to widen the boundaries of those very realms 'which bards in fealty to Apollo hold'. Poetry was already the interest of his heart.

However, he passed with credit his examination as licentiate at Apothecaries' Hall and registered at Guy's Hospital on October 1, 1815, to continue his studies. He was a diligent student, sufficiently outstanding to attract the attention of the celebrated Sir Astley Cooper, from whom he received his principal lectures. During the first winter and spring in London he lived the typical drudging life of the medical student, rooming with two fellow students in the dingy lodgings in the Borough near Guy's hospital. While here he wrote the two sonnets:

O Solitude! if I must with thee dwell
Let it not be among the jumbled heap
Of murky buildings
(the sentiment of many an obscure young student,) and
To one who has been long in city pent,
'Tis very sweet to look into the fair
And open face of heaven . . .

In the course of his first year as a student at Guy's, Keats moved to lodgings over a tallow-chandler's shop in St. Thomas's Street. Here one evening while his fellow-student Stephens was studying, Keats broke out with the announcement that he had composed a new line of poetry: 'A thing of beauty is a constant joy'. To Keats's inquiry Stephens replied that he liked the line, but it seemed wanting in some way. After an interval of silence came Keats's rejoinder: 'A thing of beauty is a joy forever'. And so there was born in the little room of a trio of medical students 'one of the imperishable lines of English poetry'.

Keats continued to do his work regularly and with considerable credit. But the poet was always elbowing aside the medical student. As he himself says, 'The other day, during the lecture, there came a sunbeam into the room, and with it a whole troop of creatures floating in the ray, and I was off with them to Oberon and fairly-land'. He worked as a dresser, but always seemed curiously apart from the work. He later told a friend – 'my last operation was the opening of a man's temporal artery. I did it with the utmost nicety, but, reflecting on what passed through my mind at the time, my dexterity seemed a miracle, and I never took up the lancet again'. He qualified with credit in July, 1816, but after a holiday at Margate returned to London resolved to write poetry, and with the ambition to be among the great. Medicine was already forgotten, and with an intensity which few poets, even the greatest, have shown, Keats gave himself up to his work as a writer.

In the following three years – three wonder-years into which he packed the sensations and achievements of a lifetime – he refers to medical practice on several occasions. In May, 1818, he writes,

Were I to study physic or rather medicine again, I feel it would not make the least difference in my Poetry; when the mind is in its infancy a Bias is in reality a Bias, but when we have acquired more strength, a Bias becomes no Bias. Every department of knowledge we see excellent and calculated towards a great whole. I am so convinced of this that I am glad at not having given away my medical books, which I shall again look over to keep alive the little I knew thitherwards . . .

And again in the course of his most famous letter, written to his brother in March, 1819: 'I have been at different times turning it in my head wither I should go to Edinburgh and study for a physician; I am afraid I should not take kindly to it; I am sure I could never take fees – and yet I should like to do so: it's not worse than writing poems and hanging them up to be fly-blown on the Review shambles'. Medical practice was never distasteful to him; he never showed for it the dislike with which so many geniuses have regarded the more work-a-day vocations. To him it was like sojourning in a far country. So (if we may correct the expression of a writer previously quoted), Keats, rather than being the prodigal son of medicine, was born to Poetry and as a lad with a sort of uneasy wonder strayed into the country of medicine, but as he became conscious of his powers returned to his own land where he received the goodly inheritance of immortality. His chief in medicine, Sir Astley Cooper, is still remembered by physicians; Keats is known to the world.

It is the destined privilege of the physician, like the Happy Warrior, 'to go in company with pain and fear and bloodshed', and to be constantly on some terms of understanding with man's ancient enemy, Death. It is not strange, therefore, that a physician should have become obsessed with the idea of Death and in his solitary quest sought even to 'uncypress' Death (as he puts it) and to make him 'the fool o' the feast.' This 'Death's jester' was Thomas Lovell Beddoes (1803–1849), whose figure is one of the curiosities of literature and biography. A man of great poetic genius whom many hailed as the successor to Keats, his life was a thwarted, sorry affair, but his achievement is that, along with Edgar Poe, he is one of the masters of the macabre in literature. He was the son of a celebrated English physician, and after leaving Oxford, went to the Continent, where he received his medical degree from the University of Würzburg. An orderly life was constantly shattered by his becoming involved in political intrigue. He finally committed suicide at the age of forty-six. His last letter is painfully revealing: 'My dear Phillips, I am food for what I am good for – worms. I have made a will here which I desire to be respected. . .. Thanks for all your kindnesses. . .. You are a good and noble man and your children must look sharp to be like you. Yours if my own, ever, T. L. B.' And the bitter joking postscript: 'I ought to have been among other things a good poet; Life was too great a bore on one peg and that a bad one'.

Beddoes bequeathed all his manuscripts to his friend, T. F. Kelsall, who in turn on his death directed that they be given to Robert Browning. The papers were contained in a large box which Browning finally allowed Sir Edmund Gosse and Mr. Dykes Campbell to explore. Gosse in 1890 published an edition of Beddoes's collected works, while apparently Campbell contented himself with transcribing all the original manuscripts. The box and its contents subsequently disappeared, but the last chapter in the story was written this year when H.W. Donner, who has had access to the Campbell copies, published the entire works of Beddoes, giving his book the title *The Browning Box*.

Beddoes's works are cast mostly in the form of the poetic drama. He is an Elizabethan dramatist of the company of Marlowe and Green, born out of season. His chief work is the play *Death's Jest Book*, upon which he laboured at interval for more than twenty years. It is the greatest dramatic variant in English on the old Dance of Death theme which has haunted painters and writers for centuries. The scenes are crowded with murder, ghosts, skulls, all cast with a strange beauty that is peculiar to Beddoes. His is the concentrated grim irony and harsh mirthless laughter of one who is preoccupied with death. The dark background of the play is lit up with an unearthly beauty by many haunting lyrics and dirges.

> The swallow by her nest,
> The soul my weary breast;
> But therefore let the rain
> On my grave
> Fall pure; for why complain?
> Since both will come again
> O'er the wave.

and:

> If thou wilt ease thine heart
> Of love and all its smart,
> Then sleep, dear, sleep;
> And not a sorrow
> Hang any tear on your eyelashes;
> Lie still and deep,
> Sad soul, until the sea-wave washes
> The rim o' the sun tomorrow,
> In eastern sky.

and again:

> We do lie beneath the grass
> In the moonlight, in the shade
> Of the yew-tree. They that pass
> Hear us not. We are afraid
> They would envy our delight,
> In our graves by glow-worm night . . ..

His lyric 'Dream Pedlary', which is in every anthology, has haunted generations of readers. 'If there were dreams to sell, what would you buy?' Beddoes failed to snare his enemy Death, but posterity has attempted to make some amends by awarding him at least a small measure of fame.

In contrast to the dark spirit of the exiled Beddoes is the figure of Oliver Wendell Holmes (1809–1894), the cheery, whimsical man of the world, scholar, essayist, novelist, poet, and physician. In his achievements in literature, he has often been called 'the American Goldsmith'. He is unique, however, in combining the career of a distinguished medical man with the avocation of letters, with such success that he is known to young and old as a writer, while few realize that he was a physician, and are quite unaware of his contributions to medical science and to the wider life of his profession. Holmes began general practice in Boston with the motto that the smallest fever would be thankfully received. He later became Professor of Anatomy at Harvard University and occupied this chair for thirty-five years. It is probably as the author of the *Autocrat of the Breakfast Table* that he will be remembered. However, his output of verse amounts to three volumes, and some poems rise above the level of well-turned craftsmanship. *Old Ironsides* stirred the country in his own day. Every schoolboy knows *The One Hoss Shay*. *The Last Leaf* is perfect of its kind.

I saw him once before
As he passed by the door;
   And again
The pavement stones resound,
As he totters o'er the ground
   With his cane.

With its concluding stanza:

And if I should live to be
The last leaf upon the tree
   In the spring,
Let them smile, as I do now,
At the old forsaken bough
   Where I cling.

The Chambered Nautilus is his greatest poem, composed, as he says, at the only time that he wrote under the urge of inspiration. Its last stanza is known to all:

Build thee more stately mansions, O my soul,
   As the swift seasons roll!
   Leave thy low-vaulted past!
Let each new temple, nobler than the last,
Shut thee from heaven with a dome more vast,
   Till though at length are free,
Leaving thine outgrown shell by life's unresting
   Sea.

Holmes's spirit and his wit are still a leaven among us.

Other names of this period which may be noticed are Edward Osler (1798–1863), the uncle of Sir William Osler, who wrote hymns and poetry; Thomas Trotter (1760–1832), a naval surgeon and author of one of the earlier treatises on scurvy; Paul Broca (1824–1880), the neurologist, who wrote poetry under the anagram name Bac Lacour; Richard von Volkmann (1830–1889), whose name is associated with ischemic contracture, and who published verse under the name of Richard Leander; and Thomas Gordon Hake (1809–1895) who retired from medicine to write poetry and who was a member of the Rosetti circle. Robert Southey (1774–1843) the poet laureate listed as a medical student for a time but failed to pursue the course.

Although only one of the 'casuals' of medicine, the name of Francis Thompson (1859–1907) must be included in any review of this kind. Among those whom we are pleased to call medical poets, Thompson stands next to Keats in sheer poetic genius and in the power to evoke the wonder of great poetry. Born in Manchester, the son of a physician, Thompson, in deference to his father's wishes, studied medicine at Owens College for six years. Failing repeatedly to pass the degree examination, he went to London to seek his fortune. There followed five years of the most terrible privation and struggle against ill-health of which the annals of genius in our race have record. Reduced to beggary and the selling of pencils in the street, sleeping in cabmen's shelters, living in the strange hell compounded of hashish and opium, Thompson sounded the very depths of human degradation. But not of human despair, for he retained a curious child-spirit and a calm, attended by the mighty spirits of his poetic imagination. As he says of Shelley, he 'fled into the tower of his own soul, and raised the drawbridge'. Finally, he was rescued by his friends, Mr. And Mrs. Wilfrid Meynell, and through their kindness continued to enjoy the care and security which he had been unable to find for himself in the world. This act of the Meynells is without parallel in literary history in its rewards, for it enriched the world with some of its greatest poetry. Mr. Wilfred Whitten (John o'London has described his friend Thompson during these years:

> A stranger figure than Thompson's was not to be seen in London. Gentle in looks, half wild in externals, his face worn by pain and the fierce reactions of laudanum, his hair and straggling beard neglected, he had yet a distinction and an aloofness of bearing that marked him in the crowd; and when he opened his lips he spoke as a gentleman and a scholar. . .. His great brown cape, which he would wear on the hottest days, his disastrous hat and his dozen neglects and make-shifts were only the insignia of our *Francis*.

He fought long against tuberculosis, and finally succumbed in a London hospital in 1907 at the age of forty-seven.

Thompson's poetical work is comprised in three slender volumes. He is a mystic, in the tradition of Vaughan, but his mysticism is illuminated by a golden radiance of phrase and imagery that at time yields lines unequalled in our language. His masterpiece *The Hound of Heaven* celebrates the age-old idea of the Divine Love that forever pursues men. It is one of the most tremendous poems ever written, and its power and imagery have been approached only by Shelley and the author of the *Book of Revelation*. The first stanza sets the glorious tempo of the poem:

> I fled him, down the nights and down the days;
> I fled him, down the arches of the years;
> I fled him, down the labyrinthine ways
> Of my own mind; and in the mist of tears
> I hid from Him, and under running laughter.
>   Up vistaed hopes I sped;
>   And shot, precipitated,
>   Adown Titanic glooms of chasmed fears,
> From those strong Feet that followed, followed after.
>   But with unhurrying chase,
>   And unperturbed pace,
>   Deliberate speed, majestic instancy,
>   They beat – and a Voice beat
>   More instant than the Feet –
> *All things betray thee, who betrayest me.*

One or two quotations from other poems must suffice:

> Nothing begins and nothing ends
> That is not paid with moan;
> For we are born in other's pain
> And perish in our own.
>   (*Daisy*)

Not where the wheeling systems darken,
And our benumbed conceiving soars! –
The drift of pinions, would we hearken,
Beats at our own clay-shuttered doors.

The angels keep their ancient places; –
Turn but a stone, and start a wing!
'Tis ye, 'tis your estranged faces,
That miss the many-splendoured thing.
                    (*In No Strange Land*)

And Thompson's prose is a previous legacy in itself. Those who would discover the infinite riches of the English language will find them displayed in the essay on Shelley. Thompson describes the imagery of Shelley's poetry in these words:

The universe is his box of toys. He dabbles his fingers in the day-fall. He is gold-dusty with tumbling amidst the stars. He makes bright mischief with the moon. The meteors nuzzle their noses in his hand. He teases into growling the kennelled thunder, and laughs at the shaking of its fiery chain. He dances in and out of the gates of heaven: its floor is littered with his broken fancies. He runs wild over the fields of ether. He chases the rolling world. He gets between the feet of the horses of the sun. He stands in the lap of patient Nature and twines her loosened tresses after a hundred wilful fashions to see how she will look nicest in his song.

Yes, one must include Thompson in our list if only for the pleasure of experiencing something of the glories and magic of language.

On an entirely different plane, and more in the nature of occasional verse, are the poems of S. Weir Mitchell (1829–1914), the distinguished neurologist, whose name is a household word in medicine. Mitchell took Holmes' advice to stick to his medical practice until he was over forty and had an established reputation before publishing any literary work. He wrote much successful fiction, based mainly on his experiences with nervous disorders.

In the field of lesser verse William Henry Drummond (1854–1907) is a master in his poetry of the French-Canadian habitant. He was born in Ireland, and in early life came to Canada with his parents. He combined medical practice in Quebec with literary work and lecturing, publishing four volumes of poetry. As the poet of a people, he possesses an original genius, and it seems certain that much of his work will live, in spite of its dialect difficulties.

One physician at least has been admitted to that select group of literary immortals whose fame rests on a single poem. On December 8, 1915, there appeared anonymously in *Punch* a little poem In Flanders Fields, which uttered the universal mood of the time, and whose lines quickly echoed round the world. The author, John McCrae (1872–1918) is now one of that vast company of gallant gentlemen who sleep in Flanders Fields. He was born at Guelph, Ontario, achieved distinction in pathology, served in the South African war, and in October, 1914, went overseas as a medical officer with the first Canadian contingent. In January, 1918, while acting as a Consulting Physician to the British Armies in the Field, he died of pneumonia. The volume of his collected poems was published in 1919, and included the beautiful memoir written by Sir Andrew Macphail, itself a notable addition to Canadian literature. All the poems are etched in greys and browns and are touched with a pensive melancholy. The metre of *In Flanders Fields* is one which McCrae had used previously. An earlier poem in the same medium and no less beautiful than the one by which he is known is *The Night Cometh*:

> Cometh the night. The wind falls low.
> The trees swing softly to and fro;
> Around the church the headstones grey
> Cluster, like children strayed away
> But found again, and folded so.
>
> No chiding look doth she bestow:
> If she is glad, they cannot know;
> If ill or well they spend their day,
> Cometh the night.
>
> Singing or sad, intent they go;
> They do not see the shadows Grow;
> 'There is yet time', they lightly say,
> 'Before our work aside we lay';
> Their task is but half-done, and lo!
> Cometh the night.

It is surely the gracious act of the divine justice of literary fame that has claimed this reticent Canadian physician for its own.

There is still another garland in the shrine of medical poetry. Robert Bridges (1844–1930) is the only medical man in the long line of the poet-laureates of England. Bridges was educated at Eton and Oxford and received his medical degree from Oxford in 1874. He continued his studies at St. Bartholomew's Hospital where he became casualty physician. Later he was assistant physician at the Children's Hospital, Great Ormond Street, and physician to the Great Northern Hospital. He gained a considerable reputation in his profession and was made a Fellow of the Royal College of Physicians. After eight years of practice, he retired to devote all his time to writing. His work includes poetic dramas, poetry, and critical essays. His first published work, a volume of lyrics was in 1873 when he was still a student of medicine. He was appointed Poet Laureate in 1913, and in 1929 received the Order of Merit. A lifetime of devotion to literature was crowned by the publication on his eighty-fifth birthday of his great philosophical poem, *The Testament of Beauty*. He must be ranked among the most learned of English poets, writing with distinction on art, music, medicine, science, history, philosophy, and literature. He was as well a classical scholar and an accomplished linguist. He died at his home at Boar's Hill, overlooking Oxford, in 1930.

In Bridges' poetry the classical and the Elizabethan traditions are most happily joined. But he is too subtle and restrained a poet ever to have a wide appeal. It is of interest, however, that since his death his fame has been slowly broadening. A master of metre, he has made music of surpassing beauty in both old and new measures. At least one of his lyrics, *Awake, my Heart, to be Loved* is one of the matchless things of its kind. For the most part his work is the result of a cultured, disciplined mind expressing the sense of beauty in experience; as Robert Lynd says, he is the poet of nine o'clock in the morning. It is worth recalling the sonnet which he wrote when he deserted medicine for poetry:

> I will be what God made me, nor protest
> Against the bent of genius in my time,
> That science of my friends robs all the best,
> While I love beauty and was born to rhyme.
> Be they our mighty men, and let me dwell
> In shadow among the mighty shades of old,
> With love's forsaken palace for my cell;
> Whence I look forth and all the world behold,
> And say, These better days in best things worse,
> This bastardy of time's magnificence,
> Will mend in fashion and throw off the curse,
> To crown new love with higher excellence,
> Curs'd tho I be to live my life alone,
> My toil is for man's joy, his joy my own.

Bridges, the metrist, is seen in this delightful triolet:

> All women born are so perverse
> No man need boast their love possessing.
> If nought seem better, nothing's worse:
> All women born are so perverse.
> From Adam's wife, that proved a curse
> Though God had made her for a blessing.
> All women born are so perverse
> No man need boast their love possessing.

Our own generation has added a host of medical poets, some distinguished, others less well known. This is a fact worth noting in an age reputed to be poor in poets. Sir Arthur Conan Doyle (*Songs of Action* 1898); Sir Ronald Ross (1857–1932), famous for his work on malaria; Havelock Ellis; Sir Donald MacAlister, whose *Echoes* (1913) was an amazing *tour de force* in poetical translation; Oliver St. John Gogarty, the laryngologist (*Offering of Swans* 1923); Dan McKenzie, with his poems in Scots vernacular; Sir Rickman Godlee; Henry Head (*Destroyers*); Sir Charles Sherrington (Assaying of Brabantius and Other Verse 1925); Francis Brett Young, who is also famous as a novelist.

In these years of the floodtide of science, when we are apt to measure accomplishments by their immediate practical value, it is well to remind ourselves that a great line of poetry is probably the greatest of human achievements. Certainly, it is the surest way to avoid the iniquity of the poppy of oblivion. For men must always return to poetry, if only to express or to realize their nobler moments. It is the invisible portion of man's literary inheritance in which current shows find no entrance.

It is only natural that the one group of men – the physicians – who know 'upon what tender filaments' the fabric of life hangs, and whose pursuits lead them to listen to 'The still, sad music of humanity', should have chosen to record something of their experience in the only fitting and durable medium – poetry. And it is pleasant thus to think of medicine's contributions to the wealth of Parnassus. Lodge, with his singing beauty; Campion, now lying in Fleet Street Church in the heart of London; Vaughan's mystic wonder; the stern realism of Crabbe; the humanity of Goldsmith; Keats faring for all time in 'the realm of gold'; Beddoes splendidly, if forlornly, mocking Death; the witty Holmes, holding untouched by worldly fame and college drudgery the beauty which is the heart of poetry; Thompson, whose verse is like 'a fire of lights before an altar'; McCrae who was always going to the wars, and who found there his trysting-pace with destiny; Bridges quietly pursuing his quest of beauty through a world grown weary with war and change. Of poetry here is God's plenty, and worthy of record. It is part of the great tradition of medicine.

5

MEDICINE AS POETRY

John Launer

Transcribed from the original article in the *Postgraduate Medical Journal* and reproduced here with permission from the publisher *British Medical Journal*.

Launer J. *Postgraduate Medical Journal*. 2014; 90: 302.

Before I studied medicine, I did an English degree. It was at a time when cultural studies had not been invented and close reading of literary texts was still in fashion. There were a few books on this topic considered to be classics, and one of them was by a writer called William Empson (1930). It had the title 'Seven Types of Ambiguity'. Empson was something of a legend because he had come up to Cambridge to study mathematics in the 1920s but changed to English literature, wrote the book aged 21 while still an undergraduate, and was then expelled without a degree after a servant found condoms in his college room. He subsequently became a scholar of Chinese literature and a poet of distinction in his own right, while leading a colourful personal life. The reason his book became a classic was because of the way he argued that great poetry depended not just on its capacity to express complex meaning but to convey several different meanings at the same time.

The seven types of ambiguity that Empson described in his book are not exhaustive. Instead, they represent points along a scale. At one end of this scale are straightforward devices like the use of metaphor, which is almost universal in poetry, and simply calls to mind an interesting comparison (for example, 'I wandered lonely as a cloud'). At the other end of the scale, there is the kind of writing that leaves readers having to make up their own minds entirely about what the author really means. The best-known example of this is probably a novel by Henry James called 'The Turn of the Screw', where a children's governess describes events that might be either real or imagined, and the author never resolves this uncertainty. In between these two extremes, Empson describes a range of other types of ambiguity. These include the striking use of opposites, word play, revealing slips of the pen, meanings that seem to have emerged in the writer's own mind during the process of writing, and unclear expressions that leave the reader to fill in the gaps.

Since changing to medicine, I have always taken an interest in the use of language in the consultation. However, I had more or less forgotten about William Empson and his book until

DOI: 10.4324/9781003341796-9

I recently came across a reference to it in an unexpected context – an essay on medical ethics, by the Australian physician Paul Komesaroff (2005). In contrast to almost everything ever written about communication skills, Komesaroff argues that ambiguity in medical conversations can be a valuable source of expanded understanding and new meanings. While scientists usually seek certainty, clarity, and the elimination of divergent meaning, he suggests, clinical communication often requires 'the deliberate preservation of uncertainty'. Drawing on Empson and others, including the philosopher Emmanuel Levinas, Komesaroff puts the case for respecting ambiguity in our use of language and developing its use. 'We rely on ambiguity', he writes, 'when we need to express new meanings, when we wish to give voice to new or difficult ideas: for example, when we are trying to discern the goals of treatment or to clarify an emotional response'.

Nature of language

Komesaroff is not arguing in favour of muddled expression and miscommunication. Instead, he sets out a more profound and sophisticated view of the nature of language than the one that dominates medical thinking, where one word or phrase is generally believed to represent only a single thing or idea. He points out how all effective communication must start with a suspension of presuppositions, and a search for a way 'to break through the curtain of mutual unintelligibility'. This means opening oneself to 'suggestiveness and allusiveness'. It involves the careful, tentative use of 'the same devices, rhetorical forms, figures and tropes generally eschewed by philosophers and scientists, but embraced by poets and creative writers'. Speech, he reminds us, 'is not a solitary or impersonal exercise or a thought, it is not a process of mediation among contested propositions; it is a shared adventure of creation and discovery'.

Reading the article by Komesaroff and recalling the book by Empson after all these years, has brought to mind some occasions in clinical practice when my interactions with patients succeeded not because of medical knowledge, but through subtle exchanges of language, of the kind that both writers are describing. For example, I remember a patient who came in saying: 'There are three things I want to see you about'. Something about her emphasis on the word 'three' led me to ask immediately: 'What's the fourth?' She told me. It was the most important problem on her mind, and we never needed to return to the others. Another patient, irate at something I had said to challenge him, called me a 'fat lot of use' and stormed out of the room. His comment drew attention to the fact I was overweight at the time, but it turned out to be accurate in other ways as well. Two weeks later, he returned to say he had thought about what I said and decided it was true and useful. More recently, a patient came to see me with a chronic skin condition, saying she felt like Job in the Bible, who was afflicted with incurable boils. I asked why she chose that comparison, and she listed a catalogue of disasters in her life recently, including the loss of her job and home. We were then able to discuss how the Book of Job ends, with its hero restored to health and prosperity, and how 'the Lord blessed the latter end of Job more than his beginning'.

Such consultations do not take place every day – although elements of them may be present more often than we suspect. As Komesaroff suggests, they can happen at critical moments, or when the mismatch between the discourse brought by the patient and the standard one offered by doctors is so great that we are compelled to explore radical alternatives. I never kept a diary of such exchanges over the years, but now wish I had done so. I would certainly encourage students and trainees to look out for the times they manage to transcend the banal formulas of everyday medical conversations, and find themselves moving into similes, metaphors, allusions, puns, humour, paradox, or other imaginative forms of speech. If they did so, they would discover that medicine can be poetic, in the true meaning of the word.

References

Empson W. 1930. *Seven Types of Ambiguity*. London: Chatto and Windus.

Komesaroff P. Uses and Misuses of Ambiguity: Uses of Ambiguity. *Internal Medicine Journal*. 2005; 35: 632–33.

6

WHAT CAN MEDICINE DO FOR POETRY?

Poetry's incursions in the first year of the *Canadian Medical Association Journal*

Shane Neilson

With W.B. Yeats in mind ('Irish Poets, learn your trade/sing that which is well made') when delivering a talk that challenged the instrumentalist ethic surrounding poetry pedagogy in medical education, I was asked a question I've never considered before by human geographer and health humanities researcher (and contributor to this book) Sarah de Leeuw: 'The benefits of poetry for medicine have often been pointed out, but what can medicine do for poetry in the context of interdisciplinarity?' This article is an initial response to that question. I begin by sketching the prevailing instrumentalist ethic in medical education to properly frame my inquiry. I then conduct a rhetorical analysis on the question itself, rephrasing and remixing it such that it is reconsidered in a dichotomized fashion. A more complex analysis of bidirectional flows between poetry and medicine ensues such that the final movement of the article, a real-world analysis of the appearance of poetry in the first year of the *Canadian Medical Association Journal* (*CMAJ*), can have some informing theoretical scaffolding. We will find that medicine *can* do something for poetry – it can supply its metaphor hoard from clinical practice, offering poetry a greater capacity for meaningful and material embodiment, thereby increasing its imaginative range and expanding the representational palette for life (Bleakley and Neilson 2021). Yet in this very fact is the inextricability of representation from experience and the problematization of dichotomy itself. But more, as practices concerned with intensities, medicine and poetry illuminate quality of life itself beyond instrumental frames, meaning that they support one another in providing value to life independent of direct application or use. In such valuations, in other words, they find their use.

Instrumentalism and poetry in medical education

Instrumentalism and functionalism are friends to medicine but bugbears for poetry and the poetic imagination. Tero Autio (2009) describes instrumentalization as a 'method-driven, "evidence-based" orientation' that is governed by 'economic' and suffers from 'managerial stress . . . in the name of globalization'. This is embedded in a tendency 'towards colonization and standardization of all spheres of human action instead of heterogeneity, difference and diversity'

DOI: 10.4324/9781003341796-10

(*ibid.*). This sobering critique suggests that we must look closely at why medicine is so enamoured with the instrumental and whether this is a dead weight for a progressive medicine and medical education (Bleakley 2023). Poetry in particular brings a deeper appreciation for the value of language and metaphor in medicine that may not improve clinical practice (the instrumental promise) but certainly can enrich the culture of medicine. But again, what does medicine afford poetry beyond subject matter? To gain sight of this, we must first clear the dead wood of instrumentalism.

In education, as pedagogies flatten under neoliberalism, they become fit for specific and limited uses designed to maximize efficiency with a loss of heterogeneity. Learning is reduced to seeking the right answer rather than the context of the question and the factors governing what answers are permitted. Even creative writing – supposedly an open-ended, imaginative activity that depends on as much mystery as skill – bends towards the will of purpose. Within the health humanities, the popular purposes are therapeutic: the prevention and alleviation of burnout and the fostering of resilience. Yet medicine does not perceive means–ends instrumentalism as a tool in and of itself applied by neoliberal logics; it does not see instrumentalism as a logic but rather as the way things are done, as a normative ethic that invisibly governs everything taught and learned. If medicine did see instrumentalism, then its usefulness might suddenly be harnessed differently.

But it doesn't. The CanMEDs framework, for example, is quite obviously in alignment with Autio's description of instrumentalism. What does it mean to say that '(a) competent physician seamlessly integrates the competencies of all seven CanMEDS Roles' (medical expert, as integrator of: health advocate, leader, professional, communicator, collaborator, and scholar)? 'Integrating competencies' rings of engineering and closed systems, not of the uncertainties of medicine's fluid, complex, chaotic, and often messy realities. So too is Charlotte Blease's (2016) apologia 'In defence of utility: the medical humanities', which extensively lists positive, instrumentally obtained outcomes as provided via literature review, including (again) 'counteracting burnout' but also creating a 'different intellectual culture within medicine', 'improvements in decision-making', and fostering 'improvements in doctor-patient interactions by enhancing awareness of patienthood'. All of these – at first sight empty rhetorical descriptors employing labels in a supposedly explanatory manner – are all-too-familiar to anyone working in the health humanities.

Making a lively counterargument, Blease (*ibid.*) maintains that a 'wholly instrumentalist rationale for [the Humanities'] role' in medical education is best. She makes this argument through collapsing the familiar Hegelian 'use vs intrinsic value' dichotomy, arguing that these can be identified: what is of use also has intrinsic value. Well, this is fine, but it doesn't address the issue of 'quality'. A doctor may find that studying visual art somewhat improves her visual diagnostic capabilities (utility), but this is not of particular use if her diagnostic capabilities are poor or lack quality. More, does it show in a deep appreciation of colour saturation in a Mark Rothko painting?

In the specific case of poetry, a notoriously useless product and practice that strenuously avoids being used to 'improve' anything, it is hard to imagine such a 'wholly instrumentalist rationale' that isn't ridiculous. Poetry rightly shuns the functional in embracing complex aesthetic challenges. Indeed, stymying the practical is the most practical thing that poetry does. Moreover, the poetry product that has been generated in the health humanities using instrumentalist rationales has often resulted in aesthetically compromised art, or plain bad poetry. But my concern here is, what is poetry getting out of the deal? Does poetry even need medicine at all or is it a dead weight? What's wrong with thinking of this 'deal' this way? Might medicine, in an instrumental mood, be bruising rather than using poetry?

Analyzing the question

It is important to think of Sarah de Leeuw's inciting question in more general terms because in this way it connects with a larger artistic world, a non-narrativistic one in which poetry is but one player. How can we sidestep the grip of the functional on this conversation to embrace other values such as the ethical and aesthetic? Breaking down the question in terms that biomedically oriented practitioners and Hegelians might appreciate, some can look at it as a combination of the following:

What does X do for Y?

and

What can X give Y?

The variables can be defined as follows:

X is a non-representational or illustrative art or genre or creative discipline,

and

Y is an occupation or practice that is not artistic, strictly speaking.

With the terms so defined, an answer to the question *What can medicine do for poetry?* can only come into view if poetry is first considered as selfish, or a seriously malfunctioning instrument.

Can medicine do anything for poetry other than assist poetry to do what poetry is itself for, which is for a great number of things that don't have, in the main, a practical end? Poetry is less a form of knowledge production and more a means to that production, a way of understanding the world and the provider or sponsor of relationality, a means to both show how x is like y and how it is not like y and how x is both like and not like y. This is, of course, the basis of metaphor. Poetry affords masterclasses in metaphor.

Modern scholars, starting with Nietzsche (1967) and including Derrida (1982), Ricoeur (1993), and Lakoff and Johnson (2003) insist that there is no possible cognitive frame from which to operate outside of metaphor. Metaphor is how we perceive and understand the world. If this is so, then poetry is the House of our common Dwelling. If poetry can be conceived of as being itself instrumentalist, then metaphor must be its chief instrument. But in the Derridean manner, that instrument is anti-instrumental: advertising the aporia of, or becoming the surplus to, instrumentalism. Poetry then is not the means to an end but is the end in the means, as embodied process: Becoming rather than Being and the very air that we breathe.

Note the use of small case in the preceding paragraph's formulation of x and y. Let us, then, consider the capital X of the previous section. How might poetry, X, be selfish? Meaning, how might X be for X?

When the question is phrased this way, any possible answer seems lifeless. If X is for X, if poetry is only for poetry, then – what? Does this leave poetry only for conversation and companionship with other poetry? How would this possibly benefit medicine as it searches for solutions? Is it only for some ineffable refinement of the language which could never, of course, be arrived at without a source, a consciousness, a further world that had to have informed it, an author, a subjectivity – even, daresay, a medical imagination? The world intruded to make the poem some-how, in some way; so, poetry is not a closed system. Rather it is open, adaptive, and complex as the process of Becoming collapsed to an acute intensity and encapsulating quality. Breath. Once, we openly called this Beauty, Grace, and Love. Now, we are mocked for this by functionalists.

Moreover, if X is for X, then who gets to say X is even X at all, the thing we know as X; and who gets to say X is only for X? I shall try to answer these questions. But to begin, we must start with the X variable, with a definition of what 'poetry' even is, which is a notoriously poetic thing to try to attempt, an ouroboros of a definitionary process. Acknowledging the futility here, I try to meet the idea of poetry as for itself. If we think of it as a discipline composed of people currently practising it as well as past practitioners, the sum of writing in the discipline, then we can begin to think of what it might mean if poetry was 'for itself' in that poetry would be for those who love it to play with it, to grow in it, to use it for their own edification and enlightenment, for them to bet-ter create relationality in the world. This is the chief meaning of the term when one says: 'poetry is for itself'. In short, poetry is for the creation and identification of that which is beautiful in the language as it somehow coheres as poetry, tautology notwithstanding.

There is no pure poetry plane of X is X as I've argued already. Poetry is in the world and of the world. Art-for-art's-sake – X is for X only – fails as a singular rationale because art should not only be for its sake, centring aesthetics. Art cannot only be aesthetic. This failure is actually a success, a product of the reality of being a material thing.

Perhaps, again, we would agree that poetry is for the creation of beautiful things and the inef-fable sense of being in the proximity of a truth. Poetry is surely for the creation and curation of metaphors, for the celebration of language in its compact forms. What then of medicine? Is medi-cine for the creation of beautiful things and the ineffable sense of being in the proximity of a truth? No. Taking the statement at face value, on its surface, the prospect seems absurd. One can play language games and speak of diagnostic truth, but this is a strain. Medicine is for the prevention, identification, and treatment of illness if one thinks biomedically; thinking more holistically, medi-cine is for the creation of balance for individuals and populations such that they are in homeostasis with their environments. Poetry has more in common with the non-biomedical definition but not so much that an immediate homology leaps out.

Consider how poetry is for other things so that it can be for itself. In other words, how X gives Y something in reciprocity, meaning X does something for Y such that X benefits in that doing. The number of possible Ys here boggle the mind. Consider that X is for rest; incitement of the imagi-nation; the scoring of passions and the intensification of life; the full expression of languages; a refinement of sense and sensibility while also existing as a ruin of past greatness and atrocity, of low bodily function and carnality. What of the poet in the prophetic vein, the *poet vates*, who brings the visionary mode to revolutionize our conceptual frameworks? In a consideration of the poet Geoffrey Hill, Von Koppenfels (2001) argues that poetry is for a 'rendering of accounts, act[s] of memory both private and public, and an attempt to come to terms with one's own times'. Poetry attempts to be not just a history of the present but also a history of the near-future.

To render an account might be to call to account as much as it is also to define a relationship between account holders; to perform an act of memory is to define oneself and one's public in terms of one another; to attempt to come to terms with one's own times is a possible reconcili-ation or destruction, depending on the terms, but it is certainly an action. This is poetry making something happen, of course; and in making this something happen, poetry ceases to be only for X. It gives itself to Y, and in so doing, it acquires a purpose, imbuing it with a charge or life for it is addressing life itself, life which could not be conceived of outside of metaphor, outside of itself. Life is brought in to infuse poetry, to revivify it.

Since the fact has been established that poetry's X is not the same as medicine's Y, de Leeuw's question can finally be directly answered. The Y of medicine offers the X of poetry its own Y-repository of knowledge and its inherent Y-nature of *also* being structured by metaphor as all scientific disciplines are, and as all human experience is, meaning that there is a compatibility at the level of language. Medicine offers medical discourse to add to poetry's repertoire to create more poetry and the resultant broadened or sharpened understanding that this augmentation/supplementation can bring. If poetry is breath, then medicine is a scaffold allowing us to build and maintain breath, again beyond mere 'subject matter'. Medicine, as clinical practice, gives *topos* or place to poetry. It is here specifically: in this placing of a central line, that comforting word to a frightened child, this swing of the orthopaedic hammer. Furthermore, by offering its particular kind of topos – and here I give instrumentality its necessary due – medicine offers a model of intense devotion and skill-building, of dedicated practice, that could surely be emulated by poets only lightly familiar with their craft.

In summary, medicine offers two things to poetry. The first is medical discourse and activity with which to make different kinds of poetry; the second is a living example of the grotesque ends of a tyrannical instrumentality. To argue this point more broadly, returning to the more general concept of non-representational art as X and science-based profession/institution Y: to say that X (art) and Y (science-based profession/institution) will be brought forward in terms of what Y can do for X is always to come up against a fundamental misunderstanding or divide in X (the difference coming in what one believes X to be and what it is for): Is X for itself? Is X for X's sake? Or is X for something other than itself? Is X for work in the world? Or is X for itself and also work in the world? If the answer is yes to this duality, then what is Y to help X with? Is Y to assist X with X-ness or with its horizon of instrumental outcomes? Or both?

The overarching answer is, Y offers the world to X, just as X offers the world to Y, since both are of the world. How they differ is in their worldviews. These must accommodate rather than assimilate. What can be more artistic or X-like than *bios*?

Moving out into the world

Why this archive

The archive chosen to juxtapose the previous thought with, as well as to apply the previous thought to, is the entire *CMAJ*'s issuances in 1911, the first year of its existence. This archive was selected for good reasons. The author of this paper is both a Canadian physician and a scholar of Canadian literature. This paper is the first in a planned series drawing on this archive. The *CMAJ*'s beginning boundary precedes the development of literary modernism in Canada, identified as beginning in 1914 with the publication of Arthur Stringer's Open Water (Norris 1982). Thus, starting with *CMAJ* in 1911 provides an ideal publishing parallel with a period of Canadian literature that showed the most change over its course. The first editor of the *CMAJ* was Dr Andrew MacPhail (1916), a poet and poetry anthologist himself. Finally, because the current article represents only a preliminary study, the fact that the evolution of the journal to its contemporary state from the 1990s onward, in which it publishes poetry with frequency, means that there is a terminal payload to analyse in future studies. The other possible archives for study in the Canadian zone would be those of the *Montreal Medical Journal* as well as the *Maritime Medical News*, both of which folded into the *CMAJ* in 1911. McPhail himself edited the *Montreal Medical Journal* and assumed the editorship of the merged publication. Yet too large an archive makes for too unmanageable and diffuse a starting analysis. Thus the 'Canadian' iteration of the national medical journal was decided upon.

Method

Unfortunately, the archive is not searchable as full text (as digitized by PubMed), making it quite accessible but laborious for review since shortcuts aren't possible. I read all 12 issues of Volume 1 to find instances of (a) whole poems and (b) quotations/excerpts from poetry in both scientific articles and editorial content. The reading process was granular, for to find poetry quoted at the level of a line, one has to read each line in every article. Most of the scientific articles were without references, meaning that one couldn't easily skip to the back of an article as a shortcut; none of the many editorial contributions referenced anything. Nor was there a dedicated section in the first year to what one would recognize today as a health humanities section common amongst contemporary medical journals. Poetry had to be actively read for. One perilous shortcut was available, however: pages *could* be scanned for verse set off from regular prose text, yet in this first year, the manifestations of poetry could be so subtle that each line had to be read carefully in case a line was quoted and thereby missed. In addition, small quotations from other publications might have occurred to fill space in the journal, so every page had to be carefully read for its own content as well as for this other content without metadata to ensure nothing was missed. I read the archive in a Foucauldian manner, as a 'history of the present'. What were the conditions of possibility for the emergence of the very idea of 'what can medicine offer poetry' in the contemporary world?

Results

The very first appearance of poetry occurred in G.E. Armstrong's (1911) 'CANADIAN MEDICAL ASSOCIATION: President's Address':

> I feel that the Canadian Medical Association, if it would fulfil the duties of a national association, should organize and enlist the services of some of our young and enthusiastic members in this matter, and demonstrate to municipalities and the state that money expended in providing the so-called working classes with better houses, on wider and better lighted streets, would be more than recouped in a lessened expenditure in courts, prisons, asylums, and hospitals: 'the means to do ill deeds make ill deeds done'. In this way we can best aid the churches and the temperance and moral reformers. In the words of Robert Burns:
>
>
>
> 'To make a happy fireside chime
> For weans and wife,
> That is the pathos and sublime
> Of human life'.
>
>
>
> In Montreal, Professor Adami and his associates are doing splendid work in directing the public mind to these questions . . .

Armstrong is quoting from Robert Burns' 'Epistle to Dr. Blacklock' (Burns n.d.), albeit badly, for there are many errors in his transcription; the relevant lines are as follows:

To make a happy fireside clime
To weans and wife
That's the true pathos and sublime
Of human life.

Here, medicine is not subject matter, object of contemplation. Rather medicine is instigator of a natural language of care that draws on poetry. Here too is the highly contemporary notion of public health operating to challenge inequity with the payback of lessening pressure on acute care. This is prescient in light of the Covid pandemic in particular. Medicine shapes poetry as the prescription of 'a happy fireside clime' whose absence leads to suffering. Perhaps the transcription was done from a variation, or perhaps the bit of poetry appears quoted from memory, in which the verse has a more intense living life in its human vessel. Even so, this particular manifestation of poetry is decorative, used to accentuate a rhetorical point. Armstrong's published address is not a scientific article, making poetry's appearance in this context all the more expected. In the same issue, however, a complementary address by A. Primrose (1911), 'Address in Surgery', outdoes Armstrong's single use with two separate usages:

> . . . seldom able to produce, for few medical men in active practice have the leisure to sift and weigh the facts and arguments of such a discussion; yet, if they lose firm faith in the guiding principle of the treatment, the attainment of a full measure of success becomes with them a matter of impossibility. 'Felix qui potuit rerum cognoscere causas' was never more applicable than here'. This was written by Lister in 1871 when, as was afterwards shown, he was only on the threshold of that long period of years during which he was compelled to continue the fight for principles that finally became universally accepted.

Primrose continues,

> In the address to which I have referred, Lister gives most convincing proof of the correctness of his views, and relates the remarkable results obtained by him in his wards in the Glasgow Infirmary. He also cites the experiences of others, chiefly on the continent, who had followed his methods, and who had succeeded by these means in abolishing pyaemia in hospital practice. He finally concludes his paper by saying: 'After statements of this conclusive character have been published regarding what is generally admitted to be the most urgent medical question of the day, when I consider the apathy with which they have been received in many quarters, I cannot avoid being reminded of the language of Macbeth –
>
> > 'Can such things be,
> > And overcome us like a summer's cloud,
> > Without our special wonder?'

Here, Lister bemoans the slow uptake of his ground-breaking work on infection control in surgery. Note the appearance of Virgil, *felix qui potuit rerum cognoscere causas* (literally, 'a person who understands the causation of things is happy'), taken from verse 490 of Book 2 of the *Georgics*, though this use is really a quotation from Lister who used the phrase himself; poetry's second appearance comes with the snippet from Shakespeare's *Macbeth*. Lister's original usage of the Virgil and Primrose's use of Macbeth are, once more, rhetorical devices reliant on drawing analogy to canonical works in order to intensify the connections drawn and add a sense of urgency to the expression. Medicine offers poetry striking illustrative examples of poetry's wisdom. Virgil and Shakespeare both caution against the clouding over of curiosity, as neglect of seeking causes. Lister bemoans the apathy of medicine in not being more energetically curious about infection control (which patently saves lives). Poetry is the aphoristic wise old head given employment by medical curiosity and invention. And we see how poetry, these brief glimpses, come packed with 'special wonder' or curiosity and awe, in Shakespeare's description. Medicine gives poetry a reason to show off its metaphor horde ('a summer's cloud') and its shift of gear from linear, one-paced description to rhythmic living (the iambic pentameter of 'And overcome us like a summer's cloud').

In summary, the initial appearances of poetry come in issue 7 of the journal. All occur in published *oratoria* that are not scientific content and are not technically editorial content either but are rather promotional material for the sponsoring Canadian Medical Association. In one case, there is misquotation. All instances are illustrative, rhetorical devices used amidst a larger argumentative frame, which is how poetry is used in regular conversation and typical essays.

The first appearance of poetry in the editorial content comes in the ninth issue on p. 889 in a piece called, simply, 'Editorial' (n.d.):

In the freer profession of medicine, all are equal because all are free. In a profession composed largely of civil servants, there will soon be a clearage, and the salaried officials will be forced into a subsidiary position, which is not favourable to an alert and open mind.

If the Government, or its agents, accept and distribute funds which have been levied for the care of the sick, they must appoint their own physicians and other officials. These can only be drawn from two classes, from those who have failed in free practice, or from those:

who either fear their fate too much,
Or whose desert is small,
Who will not put it to the test,
To win or lose it all.

This is a misquotation of 'My Dear and Only Love' by James Graham (n.d.), Marquis of Montrose, easily checked against this version on the Poetry Foundation website:

He either fears his fate too much,
Or his deserts are small,
That puts it not unto the touch
To win or lose it all.

Medicine's democratic pledge to treat all patients without discrimination at the point of suffering is a quasi-democracy that may or may not suit the political leanings of the individual doctor. However, it is a professional duty to act into this democratic gesture. In turn, this activity of provision of care must be decided upon by the doctors themselves and not by bureaucrats in government. The warning is that the small-minded government might appoint small-minded physicians in its image who will not take necessary risks. Is this not an ongoing conundrum of medicine in an era of patient safety where regulation denies risk? Medicine gives to poetry an illustrative specific case for poetry's generalization.

The next appearance of poetry in the journal – a very dense one – is again in an editorial, this time in what is essentially a medical eulogy for a Dr James Ross:

A life so full of interest and occupation, of opportunity and accomplishment . . . was nevertheless laid down with a philosophic calm and resigned submission which does credit to our calling and attests the value of our training in opposing 'free hearts, free foreheads' 'to the sunshine and the shadow', and in meeting the last stroke of fate with equanimity. All honour to James F.W. Ross for his example, 'living and dying'.

We take our leave of him, husband, father, brother, friend, and confrère, in the old, time-honoured, simple words:

> *Accipe fraterno multum manantia fletu*
> *Atque in perpetuum, frater, ave atque vale, -*

unmatched and immortal words which have borne the burden of the many sorrows of many generations in many climes and express the grief of all, but have a special meaning for each one who uses them, whether it be the overwhelming despair 'of the poet's hopeless woe', as once in 'olive silvery sirmio', or the buoyant resignation of St. Monica's last prayer for 'Faith in God and union there;' and so once more, with disregard of scansion, *Vale, Frater, Atque, Ave!*

Unpacking the appearances instance by instance: 'free hearts, free foreheads' comes from line 49 of Tennyson's "Ulysses"; 'to the sunshine and the shadow' is likely a misquotation of line 48, which should read 'the thunder and the sunshine, and opposed.' 'Living and dying' likely refers to the drama of the poem and is not a direct quotation. The set-off Latin comes from Catullus and has been translated by James Green to *'as a sorrowful tribute in funeral rites,/and forevermore, brother, hail and farewell!'* (Catullus n.d.).

Clearly an elegy is an entirely familiar place for poetry to appear; poetry's alighting here is entirely conventional as it occurs in a medical journal, and yet, how exactly this maps onto von Koppenfels' identification as poetry as a 'rendering of accounts' and an 'act of memory both private and public'. In this particular use, we are in the vicinity of something different from only rhetorical flourish or emphasis; we are also in the realm of memorializing life. And yet there is a sense of poetry being for itself here, being in conversation with itself, for the remaining poetry sightings – 'of the poet's hopeless woe' and 'Vale, Frater, Atque, Ave!' – come from Tennyson's 'Frater Ave Atqe Vale', although Tennyson's title was taken from a poem Catullus addressed to his dead brother. What medicine offers poetry here is conversational eloquence and ease with the subject of death. This might be everyday for medicine but nevertheless remains visceral and poignant, especially in physicians remembering physicians. Medicine brings the body to the poem that necessarily remains an abstraction. Isn't medicine theorizable as the living profession of eulogy?

In the very first year of the *CMAJ*, then, poetry had a public life as well as a life in conversation with itself so as to create a different public life. As for the scientific articles, no poetry quotations could be found as epigraph or in their bodies, which is as expected, though on p. 15 of the first issue, quotation was made of a literary text, in this case a bit of Reverend Sydney Smith, within A.B. Macallum's (1911) 'The Ancient Foundations of Heredity' – what constitutes a scientific article for that time:

> Can the economist, the philanthropist, or the statesman, or all three combined, add by thinking on their behalf one cubit to the intellectual stature of a family of mental degeneration? In the words of Sidney Smith, 'You might as well try to poultice away the humps of a camel'.

The lack of editorial fastidiousness continues when it comes to quotation, for the proper spelling of the first name occurs with a y and not an i. Also in this first issue on p. 24 is an excerpt of Lewis Carroll that appears in Thomas (brother of John) McCrae's (1911) 'Rheumatism and So-Called Chronic Rheumatism':

. . . that a number of conditions are grouped together as rheumatism, which have no other feature in common than the occurrence of pain.

That you will agree with me entirely, I do not expect, but I ask that you consider the matter and reconsider the diagnosis of 'chronic rheumatism' when next it comes to your lips. I believe that it would be a gain if the use of the term 'rheumatism' could be given up. It is not necessary.

My paper, perhaps, recalls to you a quote from 'Alice in Wonderland'.

'Have some wine' the March Hare said in an encouraging tone.

Alice looked all round the table, but there was nothing on it but tea. 'I don't see any wine', she remarked.

'There isn't any', said the March Hare.

'Then it wasn't very civil of you to offer it', said Alice angrily.

Perhaps you will consider it not very civil of me to read a paper on what, in my opinion, does not really exist. However that may be, I hope these remarks may suggest some consideration on the subject of the next diagnosis of 'chronic rheumatism'.

Physicians of the day would be expected to have a broad liberal education and to draw on this to apply to medicine. There would be a readiness and willingness to cast light on a medical issue through a literary analogy, but this can be turned on its head, mirroring the March Hare's tactic. Medicine can illuminate literature (rather than the usual reading that literature can illuminate medicine). In the example above, the medical mindset of clinical reasoning is tuned back on Alice in her Wonderland. How does one diagnose a disease that doesn't exist? Or rather, that exists as a layperson's term ('rheumatism' loosely used describes rheumatoid arthritis that includes a spectrum – over 100 – of muscle, joint, and bone disorders). The medical conundrum (the unicorn diagnosis for a single condition that doesn't exist) surely offers a wonderful illumination of Lewis Carroll's poetic prose.

We might note that, like the Macallum, the McCrae is more of a review article than an actual scientific investigation. Indeed, the truly 'scientific' articles, such as case reports, pathological investigations, and the like, would feature no literary quotations.

Conclusions

The first year of the *CMAJ* featured several appearances of poetry. Though most were purely rhetorical in nature, designed to emphasize and punctuate an argument, all were quotations from famous poets/writers (Virgil, Shakespeare, Tennyson, Catullus, Burns, and Carroll). Though distinctions can be made between rhetorical emphasis, elegiac deployment, and poetry in celebration of its own knowledge-making and connection-building, the appearances lead to a series of simple observations. Medicine does indeed give something to poetry beyond seeking an instrumental return gift: medicine gives body to disembodied words; context to abstractions; specifics to generalisms; a certain ease with death; and an expertise in democratic habits learned from treating all patients equally. This is quite a yield from the flow of the medical imagination into the poetic imagination.

All of this seems to be riding on the coattails of instrumentalism. Is this a bad thing? Not necessarily: it just feels uncomfortable. How to make a clean break? Oddly perhaps, by totally aligning medicine and poetry, as though they were hewn from the same timber, albeit crooked. Medicine and poetry are embroiled in life itself but a life that is intensified. Poetry is present; poetry has a life in the *CMAJ* (as an illustrative example) because it is part of life as much as medicine is part of life; poetry has its public in the readership of the journal, and it is leaned on to do work in the journal, be it to advance an argument or to memorialize the dead. And if one considered the matter from a reverse flow, in terms of what poetry gets out of this arrangement, the answer is this: poetry has a living life in a community as well, where it is seen (with respect to the Catullus–Tennyson connection) to be taking care of itself, memorializing itself. It is as if instrumentalism has made us so tense that we have figured medicine and poetry separately out of shared ground. We can surely ease our grip and allow tense figures to relax back into common ground that is also the metaphor horde. Not yet does poetry have what I suspect it will obtain in the coming years, a refreshment of its metaphoric repertoire.

For further study

The remainder of the journal needs to be searched through in order to discover different deployments of poetry. In particular, the first poem published by the *CMAJ* by a Canadian author or otherwise needs to be identified. A historical arc should be sketched such that the conditions for poetry are identified in the journal, suggesting different uses dependent upon era.

References

Armstrong GE. CANADIAN MEDICAL ASSOCIATION: President's Address. *Canadian Medical Association Journal.* 1911; 1 (7): 591–600.

Autio T. 2009. From Gnosticism to Globalization: Rationality, Trans-Atlantic Curriculum Discourse, and the Problem of Instrumentalism. In: B Baker (ed.) *New Curriculum History.* Leiden, NL: Brill, 69–95.

Bleakley A. 2023. *Medical Humanities: Ethics, Aesthetics, Politics.* London: Routledge.

Bleakley A, Neilson S. 2021. *Poetry in the Clinic: Towards a Lyrical Medicine.* Abingdon: Routledge.

Blease C. In Defence of Utility: The Medical Humanities and Medical Education. *Medical Humanities.* 2016; 42: 103–8.

Burns R. n.d. Epistle to Dr. Blacklock. *Robertburns.org.* Available at: www.robertburns.org/works/293.shtml. Last accessed: 20/7/2023.

Catullus. n.d. *A Fraternal Farewell.* Available at: https://classicalanthology.theclassicslibrary.com/2019/05/27/catullus-101-a-fraternal-farewell/. Last accessed: 20/7/2023.

Derrida J. 1982. White Mythology, Metaphor in the Text of Philosophy. In: A Bass (trans.) *Margins of Philosophy.* Chicago, IL: University of Chicago Press.

'Editorial'. n.d. *Canadian Medical Association Journal.* 1911; 1: 883–90, 1196–210.

Graham J. n.d. Marquis of Montrose. 'My Dear and Only Love.' *Poetry Foundation.* Available at: www.poetryfoundation.org/poems/44296/my-dear-and-only-love. Last accessed: 20/7/2023.

Lakoff G, Johnson M. 2003. *Metaphors We Live by.* Chicago, IL: University of Chicago Press.

Macallum AB. The Ancient Foundations of Heredity. *Canadian Medical Association Journal.* 1911; 1: 3–17.

MacPhail A. 1916. *The Book of Sorrows.* Oxford: Oxford University Press.

McCrae T. Rheumatism and So-Called Chronic Rheumatism. *Canadian Medical Association Journal.* 1911; 1: 23–32.

Nietzsche F. 1967. *The Birth of Tragedy and the Case of Wagner* (W Kaufman, trans.). New York, NY: Vintage.

Norris K. 1982. The Beginnings of Canadian Modernism. *Canadian Poetry;* 11: 56–66.

Primrose A. Address in Surgery. *Canadian Medical Association Journal.* 1911; 1: 601–16.

Ricoeur P. 1993. *The Rule of Metaphor.* Toronto: University of Toronto.

Royal College of Physicians and Surgeons of Canada Website. *CanMEDS: Better Standards, Better Physicians, Better Care.* Available at: www.royalcollege.ca/rcsite/canmeds/canmeds-framework-e. Last accessed: 20/7/2023.

Von Koppenfels W. 2001. A Sad and Angry Consolation: Violence, Mourning and Memory. The Late Poetry of Ted Hughes and Geoffrey Hill. In: U Broich, S Bassnett (eds.) *Britain at the Turn of the Twenty-First Century.* Leiden, Netherlands: Brill.

7

POETRY AND MEDICINE

Audrey Shafer

Reprinted from *Anesthesiology Clinics*. 2022; 40: 359–72, with permission from Elsevier.
   Note: American spellings have been replaced by UK spellings following the standard format throughout this book. The exception here is the retention of North American technical terms related to anaesthetics: anesthesiology, anesthesiologist, anesthesia.

Introduction

Poetry is in us, of us, and around us. Poetry is a way of meaning-making in a complicated, confusing world, which includes not only loss, terror, and hatred but also joy, gratitude, and love. The historical roots of poetry predate writing; intergenerational knowledge transfer included bards who memorized verse. For many centuries, poetry has imbued the writings and oral traditions of religions around the world. Our exposure to poetry starts when we are young: we are taught poems in nursery rhymes and children's songs. We ask in a slant rhyme at the end of the alphabet song: 'Now I know my ABC's/Tell me what you think of me'. However, we may lose our comfort with poetry as we progress through education. Poetry itself can feel confusing, and the effort to live with a poem, to mull it over, and accept its ambiguities can feel burdensome, as well as tangential to life. Poetry put to music, in the form of lyrics from musical theatre to popular music to rap, may become the only poetry the public feels has worth.

   Poetry is often put in opposition to prose as a form of literature, but in actuality these two forms, which manifest in a diversity of ways, overlap. What is usually true of poetry, however, is that summarizing a poem so eviscerates the poem that a brief synopsis is meaningless. For example, parse Robert Frost's (1915) much quoted poem, 'The Road Not Taken', to 'choices in life's journey matter', and we have not experienced the poem itself at all. We have not walked in that 'yellow wood', have not felt the rhythms of the words, the breaths, the spaces. In other words, a poem, whether a couplet, sonnet, free form, epic, or anything in-between, needs to be fully read, experienced, and hopefully heard, either aloud or in the mind's ear.

   Poetry as incantation has a long history in healing, such as in shamanistic rituals. Such uses continue in tempered, more nuanced ways. Poetry is frequently invoked at gatherings to celebrate or mourn passages in life and death. Poetry creates community within such gatherings, and enables

DOI: 10.4324/9781003341796-11

those present to access emotions – and, importantly, first gives permission to access such feelings. Think of the funeral scene in *Four Weddings and a Funeral* (1994),[1] where the bereaved Matthew recites the poem, 'Funeral Blues' by WH Auden (1936), as an elegy for his dead partner and lover, Gareth. The poem creates a shared experience of grief and loss and provides an avenue for collective and individual healing.

An outstanding way to start or continue an exploration of how to approach and live in a poem is through the podcast, *Poetry Unbound*, by poet, theologian, and educator, Pádraig Ó Tuama (2022). Each episode focuses on one poem, read twice within the space of ten minutes, with an intervening dive into the poem, its poetics, the poet's life, and the ways in which the poem affects the host. The podcast, itself personal and universal, hence captures that which makes a poem both individual and revelatory of truths.

The value of poetry in medicine is demonstrated in the multiple medical journals that accept and publish poetry and the growing number of literary medicine contests that include poetry, or exclusively focus on poetry. For example, poems can be found in sections of the *Journal of the American Medical Association, The Lancet, Annals of Internal Medicine*, and *New England Journal of Medicine*. Medical specialty journals that include poetry include two major journals in anesthesiology: *Anesthesia and Analgesia* and *Anesthesiology*.[2,3] Medical (or health) humanities, the academic discipline devoted to the intersections of the arts, humanities, and medicine, includes poetry readings at national conferences as well as the publication of poems in scholarly journals, for example, *Journal of Medical Humanities*. Medical literary journals, such as *The Pegasus Review, The Intima, Pulse: Voices from the Heart of Medicine, Literary AMWA* (American Medical Women's Association), and *Bellevue Literary Review* include poetry. Volumes or anthologies of literary writing can include poetry related to medicine or can be exclusively composed of such poetry (Belli and Coulehan 1998). The extensive online resource chronicling literature, film, and arts related to medicine presented in the New York University Literature Arts Medicine Database includes 745 annotations of poetry.[4] Medical literary contests, such as the Paul Kalanithi Writing Award and the Irvin D. Yalom Literary Award (for students and trainees only) accept poetry entries.[5,6] Poetry contests on topics related to medicine and the human condition include those open to practitioners and the public, such as the Hippocrates Initiative for Poetry and Medicine,[7] and those exclusively for medical students, such as the William Carlos Williams Poetry Competition for Medical Students.[8]

There are growing numbers of physician-poets publishing in the aforementioned venues or compiling chapbooks or poetry collections. Historically, the most famous physician-poets include William Carlos Williams and John Keats. Williams, a family doctor and paediatrician born in 1883, practiced in New Jersey. Part of both the modernist and the early imagist movements in poetry, Williams (1984) also wrote prose, including short stories and an autobiography. Although his stories tended to deal more directly with medicine and practice, occasional poems, such as 'The Last Words of My English Grandmother' (1924) did as well.

John Keats, born in 1795 in London, attended medical school, did surgery apprenticeships and received his apothecary license (for pharmacy, medicine, and surgery). However, he abandoned medicine and surgery to become a poet and died at age 25 years of tuberculosis. In his short career he wrote poems that have lasted in the Western poetry canon, which, like 'Ode to a Nightingale' (1819), contain multiple references to the pharmaceutical and medical knowledge he had acquired in his studies. There are also several physician-writers, such as Sir Arthur Conan Doyle, who wrote poetry but who remain far more known for their prose writing. Two contemporary physician-poets, Rafael Campo and Audrey Shafer, are featured in the documentary, *Why Doctors Write*, by filmmaker Ken Browne.[9]

This article explores some of the multiple relationships between poetry and medicine. The word 'healing' is used in a broad, inclusive way, and no claim is made that poetry itself has direct curative powers. We will explore the following:

- How illness, health, and medicine are portrayed in poems, including how poetry enables us to understand the human condition in new or deeper ways.
- How poetry and anesthesiology, in particular, are related.
- How poetry and writing poetry can enhance our understanding of well-being.

This article will not provide an exhaustive overview of these topics, but rather will sample poems illustrative of such concepts and provide highlights for further contemplation.

Portrayal of illness, health, and medicine in poetry

Humans are embodied and mortal. For centuries, we have struggled to understand these truths through words. Philosopher Martha Nussbaum (1990) notes: 'We have never lived enough. Our experience is, without fiction, too confined and too parochial. Literature extends it, making us reflect and feel about what might otherwise be too distant for feeling'. Poetry extends our understanding of the world, both across time and distance.

There are many poems that illustrate the powerful, subtle, lyrical, and heart-breaking ways in which poets explore what it means to be human, to be mortal, to be ill, to care for another that is ill, to mourn, to become and be a physician or health care worker, and to experience or witness suffering. Poems, in their crystalline, spare, allusive, and expansive ways, enable us to hold a moment in hand. To both stop and explode time. Table 7.1 lists a sampling of poems currently online that can start the reader on this journey.

Table 7.1 Sample poems.

Poet	Title	Online source
bearheart, b: william	When I Was In Las Vegas And Saw A Warhol Painting Of Geronimo	https://muse.jhu.edu/article/548715
Brooks, Gwendolyn	We Real Cool	https://www.poetryfoundation.org/ poetrymagazine/poems/28112/ we-real- cool
Campo, Rafael	The Chart	https://www.poetryfoundation.org/ poetrymagazine/poems/57745/the- chart
Carver, Raymond	What the Doctor Said	https://utmedhumanities. wordpress.com/2014/10/12/ what-the-doctor-said- raymond-carver/
Clifton, Lucille	Dialysis	https://utmedhumanities.wordpress. com/2014/10/12/dialysis-lucille-clifton-2/
Coulehan, Jack	On Reading Walt Whitman's 'The Wound Dresser'	https://jackcoulehan.com/
Derricote, Toi	Pantoum for the Broken	https://wisepoets.com/2021/08/21/ toi- derricotte-pantoum-for-the-broken/
Dove, Rita	Old Folks Home, Jerusalem	https://www.poetryfoundation.org/ poetrymagazine/browse? contentId536267

(Continued)

Table 7.1 (Continued)

Poet	Title	Online source
Hall, Donald	The Ship Pounding	https://www.ncbi.nlm.nih.gov/pmc/articles/PMC2839325/
Harper, Michael S.	Nightmare Begins Responsibility	https://www.poetryfoundation.org/poems/42829/nightmare-begins- responsibility
Hoagland, Tony	Emigration	https://journals.lww.com/academicmedicine/fulltext/2000/11000/emigration.19.aspx
Howe, Marie	What the Living Do	https://poets.org/poem/what-living-do
Kenyon, Jane	The Sick Wife	https://www.ncbi.nlm.nih.gov/pmc/articles/PMC2839325/
Lee, Li-Young	Persimmons	https://www.poetryfoundation.org/poems/43011/persimmons
Neruda, Pablo	The Dictators	https://www.poetryfoundation.org/poetrymagazine/browse? contentId525873
Plath, Sylvia	Tulips	https://www.poetryfoundation.org/poems/49013/tulips-56d22ab68fdd0
Rilke, Ranier Maria	Washing the Corpse	https://poems.com/poem/washing-the- corpse/
Shafer, Audrey	Falling Fifth: The Neurosurgery Patient and the Anesthesiologist	https://pulsevoices.org/index.php/poems/falling-fifth-the-neurosurgery-patient- and-the-anesthesiologist
Vuong, Ocean	Seventh Circle of Earth	https://poetryschool.com/how-i-did-it/i-forward-first-collection-special-ocean-vuong-seventh-circle-earth/
Whitman, Walt	The Wound-Dresser	https://www.poetryfoundation.org/poems/53027/the-wound-dresser
Young, C. Dale	Corpus Medicum	https://www.poetryfoundation.org/poetrymagazine/browse? volume5187&issue52&page530

(Note: some of the poems contain strong imagery, and are on difficult topics, which can be triggering for some readers).

Three poems that explore these critical themes are provided here: a fragment by Sappho, a poem on pain by Emily Dickinson, and a modern poem on the pandemic by Adjoa Boateng. The poems cross time and oceans, and the reader is encouraged to read them aloud, to spend time with the words, the spacing, the rhythms. Sappho, born in Lesbos in 630 BCE, is known for her poetry on love and longing, much of which is only preserved as fragments on papyrus or pottery (Figure 7.1). In poem 31, she explores the bodily manifestations of love and envy, including effects on the ribcage, tongue, skin, ears, vision, and the body as a whole. This is love-sickness manifest:

FRAGMENT 31

By Sappho, translated by Chris Childers (2016).
(For the full version see www.literarymatters.org/1-1-sappho-31/).

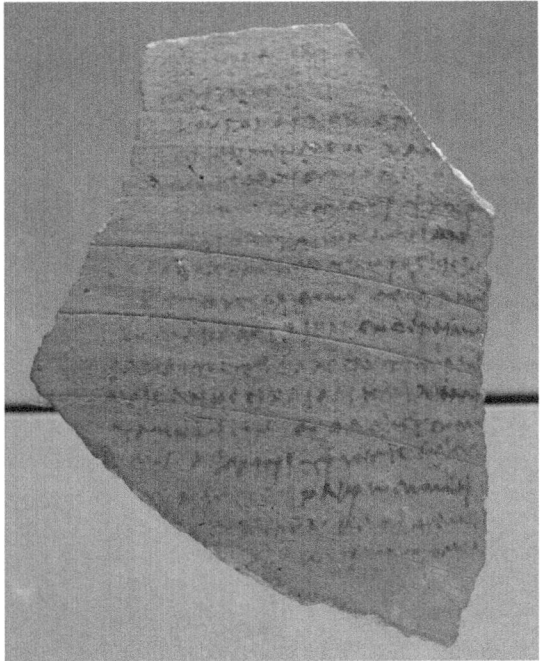

Figure 7.1   Fragment of poem by Sappho.

He seems like the gods' equal . . .
sets the heart in my ribcage fluttering; . . .
and my tongue stiffens into silence . . .
flames underneath my skin prickle and spark . . .

The poem fragment concludes:

. . . my body shakes, suddenly sallower
than summer grass, and death, I fear and feel,
is very near.

Moving centuries forward, Emily Dickinson (see 1924) addresses the experience of pain, linking the experience to timelessness and the sway pain has over us:

PAIN HAS AN ELEMENT OF BLANK

By Emily Dickinson

Pain has an element of blank;
It cannot recollect
When it began, or if there were
A day when it was not.

It has no future but itself,
Its infinite realms contain
Its past, enlightened to perceive
New periods of pain.

Pain can make us speechless, preverbal, incoherent. The questions used to elicit clinical details of the type, onset, quality, and duration of pain can feel completely inadequate when one is in the throes of pain. The erasure that pain can cause, diminishing the rest of our lives, reducing social contact, narrowing our world, is contained in the poem – pain becomes the future itself, it swallows our past, it is a void that allows for nothing else, only its return.

Suffering has both universal and highly individualistic qualities. Poetry is particularly adept at enabling such qualities to be explored. Adjoa Boateng (2021) is an anesthesiologist-intensivist who worked in critical care during the coronavirus disease 2019 (COVID-19) pandemic. Her poem, 'Grief, What Is Your Name?' launched the new section, The Human Experience, in the journal, *Anesthesia and Analgesia*:

GRIEF, WHAT IS YOUR NAME?

By Adjoa Boateng

After encountering innumerable deaths in the ICU, ushering families through the dying process virtually, grieving a life once lived, simply, amidst so much death, this piece came to life.

Today, I write to those entities my mind cannot digest.

To the novel tastes that defy even umami, the ones chewed, looking upwards, with eyes closed, to give my tastebuds a bit more bandwidth.

Today I write to you, grief.

You arrive indiscriminately, luggage brimming with both overwhelming cacophony and also deafening silence.

You disrupt conversation, causing coffee to spill over freshly pressed linen.

I weep.

What was once the fluid and graceful nature of my tongue begins to stutter through poorly concocted words or use inappropriate comedy because life sometimes, is too much to bear.

Paradigm shift.

Grief is when the life preceding no longer mirrors life thereafter.

So I pause, stare toward the muted tones around me and whisper, "Grief, what is your name?"

When we are already in mourning and there is more death, what do we call it? From where does more pain emanate when numbness prevails? How do more tears spring from a dried well? Grief, who birthed you? From whose womb were you nourished and sung lullabies? What bosom fed you emotion-scattered, over-whelming, speechless pain? How did your mother come to be? Did she adorn with delicate, yet decadent lace that lingers long after death bringing reminders of what was, via song, scripture or sermon?

I ask you, again, grief, what is your name??

Do your eyes puff with sunrise's trickling red, yellow and orange embers as you awake from a night of tear-stained weeping; a reminder that the escape of dreaming is over.

Grief, do you also wish that same sleep would rescue you back to dream, because reality is too harsh, too stinging?

Acid to an open wound?

When the tone of my mother's voice becomes less rhythmic, more monotone, less laugh-filled, more littered with pause – I want to almost say the words with her as if to blunt the stab when she breathes deeply and whispers, "I have some bad news."

But grief, I don't know you.
Not like this.

You are to come with warning, preparation, a chance to reconcile replaying voice-mails when a voice is no longer.

A chance to find old pictures when flesh travels to morgue. You are to give us opportunity to go through ritual.

We need ritual . . . or so we thought.

Your son – tragedy, robs and steals from us. So we stand, rather, we crumble, shell-shocked.

Stranger, what is your name?

Until we meet again.

But oh! Shall I never you meet again. You make the taste of my own mortality too sweet.

Boateng's poem, written and published during the COVID-19 pandemic, apostrophizes 'grief'. Grief is addressed, given attributes like lineage and the ability to carry 'luggage', and yet remains a 'stranger'. Naming is one of the ways in life and in medicine that we categorize, and hence feel, we better understand, or even control, something. That something can be a diagnosis, which may hold unknowns within it, but it can also be far more elusive: a boundless, inchoate concept. This complex poem, in which we meet the narrator's mother bearing 'bad news', conjures images of 'flesh travel[ing] to morgue' *as* we witness the narrator repeatedly attempt to understand how and why grief came to be such a dominant part of the human condition, and contextualize the pandemic within the arc of human loss and suffering.

Some of the poems examined in this section relate directly to the practice of anesthesiology, particularly because such practice includes the witnessing and alleviation of pain and suffering. The following section deals even more directly with not only how anesthesiology is portrayed in the poem but also how the act of providing an anesthetic holds poetic elements.

Poetry and anesthesiology

For the purposes of the comparison of poetry and anesthesiology, 'poetry' is used here to broadly include the genre of poetry, poetics, poetry making, and poems. Anesthesiology is also used broadly, to include providing anesthesia care (such as the practice of anesthesia, the delivery of anesthetics), the experience of general anesthesia, and the experience of the anesthesiologist or trainee.

Poetry and altered states are complex: they are both simultaneously specific and ambiguous, linear, and defiant of boundaries, well-studied entities, and incompletely defined or partially known. The dynamics of poetry are applicable to the practice of anesthesiology where both intimacy and detachment are experienced, at times, in intense and fraught ways. The reader of a poem brings their individual experience and history to the reading and thus forms a unique relationship with the poem and the poet. The patient and the anesthesiologist bring their own expectations and experiences to the discussion of an anaesthetic, and this complicated, usually quite brief, interaction can have the feel of the creation of a new relationship, a new understanding of the other.

Although vastly different in purpose and outcome, anesthesiology training and classes on poetry are both replete with new and potentially uncomfortable, overwhelming experiences, as well as providing entrées to new language, specialty-specific jargon, and rituals. Such rituals are different in tone and embodiment, but each set, such as, for poetry: reading a poem aloud before class analysis, listening for rhythms, following themes for poetry courses, or, for anesthesiology: the donning of scrubs, entering a restricted area of the hospital, preparing equipment, anticipating the pace for preoperative, intraoperative, and postoperative care, has physical, intellectual, and emotional qualia.

Exploring the properties of poetry and anesthesia, such as allusion, boundedness, porosity, disruption, voice, breath, and surprise, can illuminate both poetics and anesthesia. Figure 7.2 compares poetry and anaesthesia in three domains: form, rhythm, and purpose. For example, in the domain of form, the visual analysis of the poem as object – with its crisp hospital sheetlike border, the flush or ragged margins, the placement of title and poet's name, can be likened to a visual analysis of the anesthesia location, with the patient centre stage. Similarly, the anesthesiologist and the reader of poetry are both attuned to rhythms, disruptions in rhythms, and repetitions. However, the third domain, purpose, holds the widest divergence, because the purpose of poetry centres on interpretation and creativity, whereas the purpose of the anesthetic is caring for the individual patient.

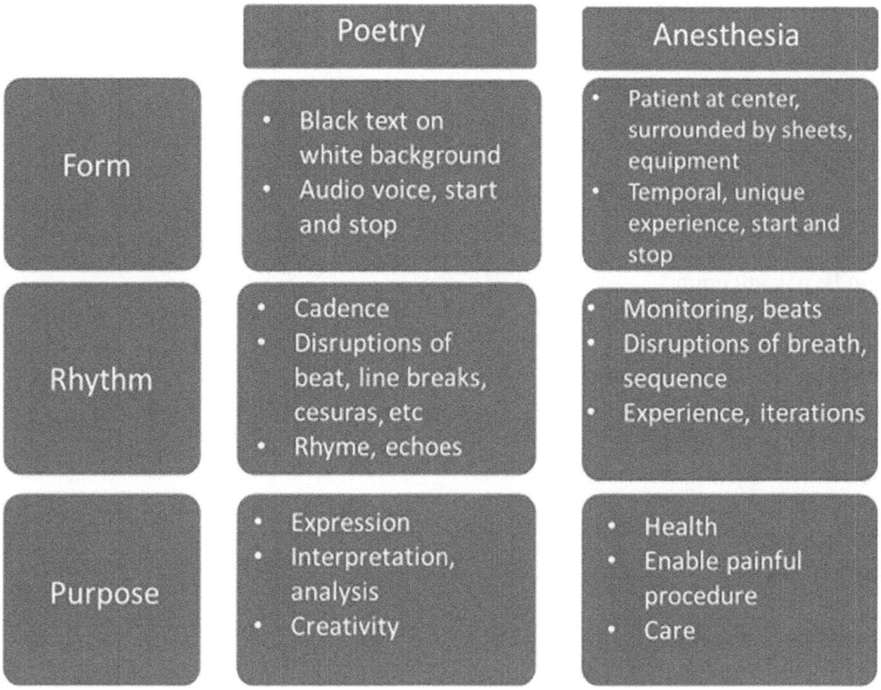

	Poetry	Anesthesia
Form	• Black text on white background • Audio voice, start and stop	• Patient at center, surrounded by sheets, equipment • Temporal, unique experience, start and stop
Rhythm	• Cadence • Disruptions of beat, line breaks, cesuras, etc • Rhyme, echoes	• Monitoring, beats • Disruptions of breath, sequence • Experience, iterations
Purpose	• Expression • Interpretation, analysis • Creativity	• Health • Enable painful procedure • Care

Figure 7.2 A comparison of poetry and anesthesia along 3 domains: form, rhythm, and purpose.

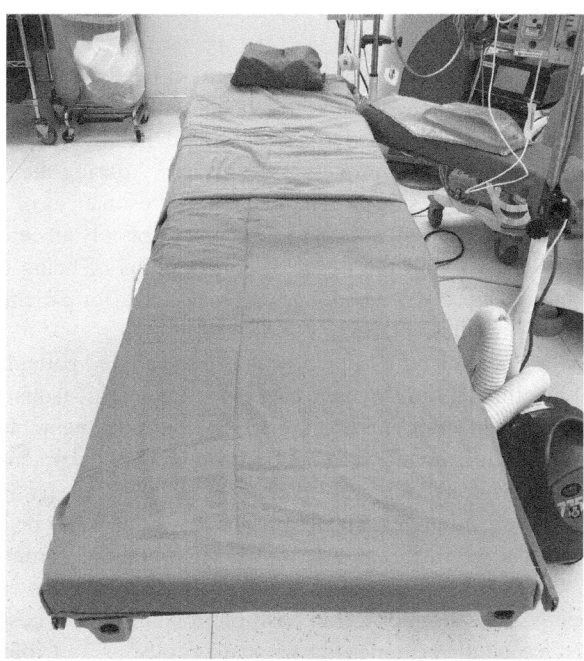

Figure 7.3 An operating room and table (photograph by Audrey Shafer).

ANESTHESIA IS A POEM

By Audrey Shafer (2019)

Begin: an arc rises
from pain, suffering, love
tendrils flow to past and future

but here, now, this matters
demands: pay attention

peaks, valleys, cadences
pauses, surprises, turns, breaths
echoes, comforts, but also
a knowledge of the abyss
a body exposed, raw

intensely intimate
layered mystery

time expands, contracts
and thus encapsulated, concludes
the end opens our eyes
light enters
look: the arc sets
just there, beyond the horizon.

The caveat of depersonalization and hence dehumanization needs to be addressed, because the patient cannot be reduced, simplified to the text of a poem without loss and distortion. In anesthesia practice, the patient is frequently alluded to – transformed metonymically to lines on the monitor, for example, or metaphorically as in a vessel for disease – during the time that the patient's personhood is hidden by general anesthesia. The metaphoric resonances of the relatively innocuous phrase, 'under anesthesia', wherein 'anesthesia' becomes not only an entity but also something one is beneath in some way, with all the negative connotations of being down (such as death, misfortune, and poor status), are explored, along with metonyms for patients and their bodies, in the article, 'Metaphor and Anesthesia' (Shafer 1995).

Although reification of the patient, particularly the incapacitated patient, is dehumanizing, to deny that patients are objectified during medical care is to forego critical analysis of the experience of illness. The risk of dehumanization increases when analogies of the nonhuman and the patient are too closely aligned, too tightly bound, leading to a distancing of the practitioner and the patient. For example, the main character of Margaret Edson's (1999) play *Wit*, Dr Vivian Bearing, whose life work was rigorous interpretation of John Donne's poetry, remarks on being ignored as a whole person while she is a patient with ovarian cancer. She attempts to confront the confusion of the physical and the metaphysical, the treatment of her as an individual versus as a vessel for anticancer therapies, while being in the disempowered position of being ill and hospitalized.

The anesthesiologist frequently becomes the advocate, protector, and voice for the patient, both before and after rendering their patient incapacitated. The reliance on close attention paid to an individual under anesthesia is a hallmark of anesthesia care. The following points summarize this comparison of poetry and anesthesiology:

- The reading and writing of poetry, as well as the practice of anesthesia demand close attention.
- Both a poem and the time frame of an anesthetic are bounded.
- Poetry and anesthesia care depend on specialized language and norms.
- Rhythms are critical to both poetry and anesthesia.
- Altered states can be attributes of both poetry and anesthesia, but the cause, purpose, and nature of those states differ.
- Critical differences between poetry and anesthesia include the life and health of an individual as the central focus in the practice of anesthesia, and the impetus to create new understanding through words in poetry.
- Comparisons of the arts and medicine can illuminate both fields, but beware of dangers such as simplification, forced equivalence, and reification.

Poetry, writing poetry, and well-being

A growing interest in the beneficial effects of the arts on health and well-being for patients and health practitioners has led to research and subsequent literature reviews. In particular, access to a variety of art interventions, including poetry, with inclusion in care ('arts on prescription') or as part of health practitioners' opportunities, has demonstrated improvement in mental health, sense of well-being, and attitudes toward the work environment (Jensen and Bonde 2018).

The experience of reading poetry can frame and illuminate one's own experiences of illness and caregiving. Furthermore, the act of writing poetry can provide a much-needed sense of perspective. Johanna Shapiro (2020), the founder of the medical humanities programme at University of California Irvine School of Medicine, writes, 'Illness in my family and myself made me feel helpless and hopeless. Writing about illness for me restored a sense of control'.

Certain subspecialties may have particular interests in how poetry impacts health care and the experiences of those involved. For example, the range of powerful emotions, including the need for solace and feelings of anger, grief, and regret, in the multi-disciplinary world of palliative care make this a particularly potent area to develop poetry and medicine workshops as opportunities for patients, families, and health care workers. Benefits ranging from breathing techniques by reciting short poems, to providing acknowledgment of difficult situations along with coping mechanisms, and community building and connection among staff have been postulated and are under study (Davies 2018).

Likewise, some illnesses can have particular symptoms or effects that benefit from the addition of poetry, and thus improve patient well-being. A preliminary study of patients with multiple sclerosis undergoing speech therapy for dysarthria found improved levels of confidence in communication when the speech pathologist was joined by a poet who included poetry in the exercises (Balchin et al. 2020). Cancer-related pain reduction through a poetry-based intervention also improved coping skills and generated a sense of hope (Arruda et al. 2016). Poetry has been found to reduce a sense of isolation felt by some patients, such as those with depression or other mental health issues; this has led to ongoing studies of the potential impact on feelings of loneliness due to social isolation resulting from the COVID-19 pandemic. Poetry may thus impact public health. Poetry, by fostering 'creative introspection', connects people to their surroundings, other people, and the world at large (Xiang and Yi 2020).

Academic and independent centres offer ways for people to connect with and write poetry. The Medicine and the Muse Program at Stanford University School of Medicine, for example, hosts a variety of programmes and collaborations. Pegasus Physician Writers[10] hold an annual poetry and music concert featuring ekphrastic poetry written by physicians and students with chamber music played by the St. Lawrence String Quartet. The Stuck@Home concert series,[11] started due to the isolation of pandemic, intermittently featured those in health care writing poetry. Stanford medical students can apply for funding to complete a poetry project through the medical scholars programme and the Biomedical Ethics and Medical Humanities Scholarly Concentration.[12] Led by writer Laurel Braitman, Director of Writing and Storytelling, students, trainees, physicians, and health professionals from around the world write and share their work through guided workshops such as retreats and the Writing Medicine programme.[13] All the programmes have generated comments on stress reduction and community building benefits (MacCormick 2020).

More research is needed on the health and well-being impacts of poetry reading and writing. In particular, studying the impacts of illness, access to health care, systemic racism, and the rigours of medical training and practice through poetry analysis, reading, and writing by a variety of patients and health care workers could illuminate how issues of diversity, equity, inclusion, and justice influence health, health care, and well-being.

Summary

Poetry and medicine interact in multiple ways, with educational and therapeutic possibilities. Because both poetry and medicine invest in understanding the human condition and forming connections, they overlap significantly in our attempts to understand life, health, mortality, and our desire to create meaning. Reading poetry related to illness, debility, death, caregiving, and medical practice can enlarge our understanding of what health care workers do, and why they do it.

Anesthesiology is, in many ways, crystallized medicine – all the elements of patient interaction and care are there, but in a heightened timeframe and within highly stylized and specialized spaces. Similarly, poetry holds all the elements of literature, and even some nonverbal arts, yet compresses them, highlighting rhythms, individual word choices, and resonances. Both anesthesiology and poetry refer to past and future, while intensely focusing attention on the present, using creative and critical thinking.

Through poetry, whether reading, sharing, or writing, we give ourselves permission to think about our roles, our lives, our interactions with others, and our relationship with the world. Thus, poetry creates a space that enables us to pause, to reflect, to recharge. Ironically, poems about difficult subjects – loss, grief, regret, pain – can improve well-being by providing connection. Poetry shows us that our individual experiences and journeys are part of the larger human experience, and hence can improve understanding and well-being.

Acknowledgements

Figure 7.1 Sappho PSI XIII 1300: 3rd–2nd century BC ostrakon from Egypt, preserving four stanzas of Sappho fr. 2 (Voigt). Now in the collection of the Laurentian Library, Florence. Photograph by Sailko. Used unchanged via license Creative Commons Attribution 3.0 Unported.

Available at: https://commons.wikimedia.org/wiki/File:Ostrakon_ PSI_XIII_1300,_II_sec._ac,_ frammento_di_un%27ode_di_saffo_sul_culto_di_afrodite.JPG Last accessed: September 3, 2021.

Emily Dickinson poem 'Pain Has an Element of Blank'. Source for quote: THE POEMS OF EMILY DICKINSON: VARIORUM EDITION, ed. Ralph W. Franklin, Cambridge, Mass.: The

Notes

1 Excerpt From *Four Weddings and a Funeral*, 1994. Available at: www.youtube.com/watch?v5DDX WclpGhcg. Last accessed: September 3, 2021.
2 Author Guidelines, *Anesthesia and Analgesia Section: The Human Experience*. Available at: https://edmgr.ovid.com/aa/accounts/ifauth.htm#thehumanexperience. Last accessed: September 4, 2021.
3 Author Guidelines, *Anesthesiology Section: Mind to Mind*. Available at: https://pubs.asahq.org/anesthesiology/pages/instructions-for-authors-paper-types#mindtomind. Last accessed: September 4, 2021.
4 *Litmed: Literature, Arts, Medicine Database, NYU Langone Health*. Available at: https://medhum.med.nyu.edu/. Last accessed: September 4, 2021.
5 Paul Kalanithi Writing Award, *Stanford Medicine and the Muse Program*. Available at: https://med.stanford.edu/medicineandthemuse/events/paul-kalanithi- essay-contest.html. Last accessed: September 4, 2021.
6 Irvin D. Yalom Literary Award, *Pegasus Physician Writers*. Available at: http://www.pegasusphysicians.com/programs-awards. Last accessed: September 4, 2021.
7 *Hippocrates Initiative for Poetry and Medicine*. Available at: http://hippocrates-poetry.org/. Last accessed: September 4, 2021.
8 W. C. Williams, *Annual Poetry Competition, Northeastern Ohio Medical University College of Medicine*. Available at: www.neomed.edu/medicine/poetry-competition/. Last accessed: September 4, 2021.
9 K. Browne, *Documentary Film, Why Doctors Write Trailer*, 2020. Available at: www.whydoctorswrite.org/. Last accessed: September 8, 2021.
10 *Pegasus Physician Writers*. Available at: www.pegasusphysicians.com/. Last accessed: September 8, 2021.
11 *Stanford Stuck@Home Concert Series*. Available at: https://med.stanford.edu/medicineandthemuse/events/stuck-home-concert-.html. Last accessed: September 8, 2021.
12 *Biomedical Ethics and Medical Humanities Medical Scholars Funded Projects*. Available at: https://med.stanford.edu/medicineandthemuse/Education/publications/projects.html. Last accessed: September 8, 2021.
13 *Reflective Writing Session for Healthcare Workers and Their Loved Ones*. Available at: www.laurelbraitman.com/writingmedicine. Last accessed: September 8, 2021.

References

Arruda MA, Garcia MA, Garcia JB. Evaluation of the Effects of Music and Poetry in Oncologic Pain Relief: A Randomized Clinical Trial. *Journal of Palliative Medicine*. 2016; 19: 943–48.
Auden WH. 1936. *Funeral Blues*. Available at: https://allpoetry.com/Funeral-Blues. Last accessed: 3/9/2021.
Balchin R, Hersh D, Grantis J, et al. Ode to Confidence: Poetry Groups for Dysarthria in Multiple Sclerosis. *International Journal of Speech and Language Pathology*. 2020; 22: 347–58.
Belli A, Coulehan J. 1998. *Blood and Bone: Poems by Physicians*. Iowa City, IA: University of Iowa Press.
Boateng A. Grief, What is Your Name? *Anesthesia and Analgesia*. 2021; 133: 289.
Childers C. 2016. Translation of Sappho 31. In: *Literary Matters: The Association of Literary Scholars, Critics and Writers*. Available at: www.literarymatters.org/1-1-sappho-31/. Last accessed: 3/9/2021.
Davies EA. Why We Need More Poetry in Palliative Care. *BMJ Supportive & Palliative Care*. 2018; 8: 266–70.
Dickinson E. 1924. Pain Has an Element of Blank. From: E Dickinson. In: *Complete Poems Part One: Life XIX*. Boston, MA: Little, Brown and Company. Available at: www.medhumchat.com/discussion guides/2019/6/18/emily-dickinson- pain-has-an-element-of-blank. Last accessed: 4/9/2021.
Edson M. 1999. *Wit*. New York, NY: Farrar, Straus & Giroux.
Frost R. 1915. *The Road Not Taken*. Available at: www.poetryfoundation.org/poems/44272/the-road-not-taken. Last accessed: 3/9/2021.
Jensen A, Bonde O. The Use of Arts Interventions for Mental Health and Wellbeing in Health Settings. *Perspectives in Public Health*. 2018; 138: 209–14.

Keats J. 1819. *Ode to a Nightingale*. Available at: www.poetryfoundation.org/poems/44479/ode-to-a-nightingale. Last accessed: 8/9/2021.

MacCormick H. 2020. How Writing Helps Medical Students and Doctors Handle Stress. *Scopeblog*. Available at: https://scopeblog.stanford.edu/2020/05/20/how-writing-helps-medical-students-and-doctors-handle-stress/. Last accessed: 8/9/2021.

Nussbaum M. 1990. *Love's Knowledge: Essays on Philosophy and Literature*. Oxford: Oxford University Press.

Shafer A. Metaphor and Anesthesia. *Anesthesiology*. 1995; 83: 1331–42.

Shafer A. 2019. Anesthesia is a Poem. Poster Presented at 'Aesthetics and Anesthetics: Boundaries and Crossings in Poetry and Anesthesia'. *International Health Humanities Consortium Conference*. Chicago, March 28.

Shapiro J. Healing Words: My Journey With Poetry and Medicine. *Families, Systems & Health*. 2020; 38: 334–37.

Tuama PÓ. 2022. Poetry Unbound: 50 Poems to Open Your World. *'On Being' Podcast Platform*. Available at: https://onbeing.org/series/poetry-unbound/. Last accessed: 6/9/2021.

Williams WC. 1924. *The Last Words of My English Grandmother*. Available at: www.poeticous.com/william-carlos-williams/the-last-words-of-my-english-grandmother. Last accessed: 6/9/2021.

Williams WC. 1984. *The Doctor Stories* (R Coles, Comp.) New York, NY: New Directions.

Xiang DH, Yi AM. A Look Back and a Path Forward: Poetry's Healing Power During the Pandemic. *Journal of Medical Humanities*. 2020; 41: 603–8.

8

A POET IN THE CLINIC

Iain Bamforth

A consultation

I thought he was the most atrociously contorted mumbler I'd ever encountered and despaired of understanding anything he might want to say to me until it hit me: he was gesticulating *inside his mouth* (the clinical term for this symptom in psychiatry is the German *Würgstimme*). Perhaps he had taken to heart Jesus's words in Matthew 15:11: 'Not that which goeth into the mouth defileth a man; but that which cometh out of the mouth, this defileth a man'.

Then again, the Gospels leave no doubt that what is brought forth from the oral cavity possesses far more creative energy and potential than words merely read from a page. It mixes with saliva, gets kneaded by a tongue and dented, and ends up as a sweetsour regurgitated pulp. Perhaps that's why garbling has always been such a venerable feature of mystical faiths, not to speak of the gabbling in tongues that is the only thing most people know about Pentecostalism. There is this arresting line in one of Gilles Deleuze's dialogues: '*Un style, c'est arriver à bégayer dans sa propre langue*' ('Style is managing to stammer in your own language').

Do me in

Volenti non fit iniuria is the common law doctrine – if you are consenting then you cannot claim harm – which stands behind acts of what has been called 'altruistic violence' and prevents a medical procedure (surgery usually but any kind of invasion of bodily integrity) from being an act of trespass to that person. When the poet Paul Valéry addressed the annual congress of French surgeons in 1938, he reminded them that they had the onerous privilege of being the only persons entitled to cut open the body of a living person and not be charged with a crime. Of course, altruistic violence has to be within the reasonable bounds of what might be expected during a medical procedure, which is why the surgeon in Birmingham who used an argon beam laser to pen his initials on the peritoneal covering of two transplanted livers was convicted of assault – although the physical harm suffered by the patients was 'no more than transient or trifling' according to the judge who sat on the case – and also lost his licence to practice medicine for several years.

 DOI: 10.4324/9781003341796-12

Thick-skinned

Type 'rhinoceritis' in a search engine and you're likely to find yourself on a website offering you cures for rhinosinusitis. *Rien à voir*. Rhinoceritis is the condition that descends on the characters in Ionescu's play *Rhinoceros* who lose their ability to think critically and start mouthing platitudes. They become infected with the need to be a herd.

Borborygmi

The French surgeon René Leriche's famous phrase about *le silence des organes* is gainsaid by a comment in Nietzsche's *Notebook* 5 (summer 1886–autumn 1887): 'people in whose body there's a constant grunting and uproar from the inner brute'. Was Nietzsche thinking of his own digestive problems, mentioned in some of his letters to friends? 'It is in moments of illness', wrote Proust, 'that we are compelled to recognise that we live not alone but chained to a creature of a different kingdom, whole worlds apart, who has no knowledge of us and by whom it is impossible to make ourselves understood: our body'.

The failing

If there isn't something wrong with you, there's something wrong with you. So runs the contemporary mantra that proves our modernity.

Depreciation

One of the revelations in Oliver Sacks's extraordinary autobiography – extraordinary if solely on account of what it reveals about his drug habits in the early 1960s – is that he was saved, after years of taking massive doses of amphetamines and being an unsuccessful researcher, by discovering when he started clinical work in a headache clinic in the Bronx in October 1966 that his patients fascinated him and that '[he] *cared* for them'. In fact, his friend Thom Gunn defined this momentous change for him in a letter written after his book *Awakenings* had appeared: 'I found you so talented, but so deficient in one quality . . . humanity, or sympathy, or something like that'. He couldn't see how his friend would have been able to overcome this deficiency: sympathy was a quality that couldn't be taught to somebody who manifestly lacked it. But Gunn freely acknowledges that this former deficiency in his friend's character has become 'the supreme organizer' of his style, and if he could see this clearly, it was because he had experienced something similar: the difference between his stylish but nihilistic early poetry and his later work is palpable. Both men experienced a growth of sympathy in their thirties. This made me realize, with a start, that my experience in Strasbourg was the opposite: it was discovering I *no longer* cared for my patients that contributed to my decision to abandon clinical practice.

Gottfried Benn was certainly not enamoured of his profession as dermatologist cum venereologist and was known to refer (in best Berlin manner) to those who called in on his practice as 'dirty urchin patients' (*Schmutzfinke von Patienten*). Now I have odd moments of peripatetic involvement with the medical problems of friends and family but no clinical practice. 'I borrow heavily from my reading, because I take my reading seriously. It is part of my total experience and I base most of my poetry on my experience' (Thom Gunn).

A cautious empiricist

John Aubrey in *Brief Lives* tells us that Thomas Hobbes 'was wont to say that he had rather have the advice, or take Physique from an experienced old Woman, that had been at many sick people's Bed-sides, than from the learnedst but unexperienced Physitian'.

Gogol and generalism

The GP and medical historian Brian Hurwitz once made the interesting point that the gatekeeper system of the British National Health Service, which is based on a capitation payment for the general practitioner established on the basis of a list of patients (for whose care the GP is paid irrespective of whether they attend the surgery), displays similarities with the former Russian landowning system: landowners could buy or sell their serfs as chattel and used the word 'soul' metonymically for counting purposes: 'fifteen hundred souls of patients'. On another level, of course, Gogol's great novel, in which his main character Chichikov describes a circle around the *guberniya* in his bizarre search to buy up some of these dead souls in order to boost his social standing, is a satire on their quality, their very deadness, which is rendered by the untranslatable Russian word *poshlost*, a kind of fatal complaisance with overtones of philistinism and cravenness, or as D.S. Mirsky defined it, 'self-satisfied inferiority, moral and spiritual'.

At the butcher's

With his trademark, casual, sometimes grotesque reductionism, Louis-Ferdinand Céline outlines the problems of securing payment in French general practice as faced by the psychiatrist Baryton in *Voyage au bout de la nuit*: 'Impossible to get a family to understand that a man, father or no, is in the end nothing more than putrefaction pending (*pourriture en suspens*). . ... A family won't stump up for putrefaction pending'. This is the same physiological scandal described by Francis Bacon in his famous interview with David Sylvester: 'Certainly we are meat, we are potential carcasses. If I go into a butcher's shop I always think it's surprising that I wasn't there instead of the animal'.

Turning tables

In the form of compassionate psychology developed by the psychologist Richard Bentall, clinicians do not ask 'What's wrong with you?' but 'What happened to you?' This turns the table of agency, but it clearly offers new possibilities for sarcastic clinicians if the speaker places the emphasis in the sentence not on 'happened' but on the last word: 'What happened to *you*?'

The service economy

The 'hideously healthy ones': a phrase used by Lou Andreas-Salomé in her memoir *Lebensrückblick*. Now we have wellbeing as government policy, with dedicated ministers and supporting data and the distinct impression, at least for me, that our societies are afflicted with an incurable desire for *goodness*. Politically speaking, it is disconcerting that although many people declare themselves prepared to take 'whatever medicine is necessary', nobody is prepared to give it them.

A mark of distinction

Cyrano de Bergerac was sensitive about his nose, which he defended with his rapier when the pen wasn't sharp enough. A large nose, he wrote, 'is the mark of a clever, courteous, affable, generous-spirited and liberal man; a small nose indicates the opposite'. All of which suggest that the large-nosed Cyrano had other legitimate claims on our attention.

I was pleased to find, while working there, that some people in the islands of the Indonesian archipelago had a similar feeling about noses: I was told that a long Western-style nose was considered particularly distinguished. The pregnant woman in one Sumatran clinic who touched my nose and then touched her belly was replicating a kind of magical thinking, or at least a mentalist presupposition that was common in Europe until the nineteenth century: that the imagination could affect the body just as effectively as the passions if its imaginings were vivid enough. The maternal imagination was thought to have special powers of projection, and I was happy to let her child have my nose.

Exthused

Coleridge was not impressed with the implications of the Authorised Version of the Greek verb *exelthousan* in Luke 8.46, which states that Jesus directly perceived the virtue (or vulgarly 'power') passing out of him when the timid woman touched the hem of his garment in the hope of a cure: it implies, he wrote in his copy of the Bible, 'that our Lord no longer possessed it, as if it had been a charm, or an amulet charged with Mesmer's fluid'.

An obit

He passed away peacefully, after a long battle against the successive encroachments of military-medical metaphors.

How a poem works

A smart literary journalist, should he or she ever be unfortunate enough to come across some of the barely competent poems which now feature in medical journals, might be tempted to call them 'sick lit'. Most of these poems fall into a subgenre that ought to be avoided at the risk of succumbing to what appears to be a toxic empathy and the naïve belief that the emotions reveal themselves unmediated in poem and prose. Purveyors of the subgenre evidently believe all writing is sanctified by experience ('it must be personal'). But 'life-poems', as they are sometimes called, often lack the editorial perspective that made the experience meaningful to the writer in the first place, however much assuagement they might have brought by having first been committed to paper.

But there are some aspects of writing that shouldn't be forgotten so blithely. There is an implicit contract between writer and reader in which 'poetry' and the 'poetic' emerge from a performance under very specific conditions. Syntax enacts compassion. Style constructs spontaneity. Depth is an effect. Should I ever to be asked to give writing classes, all my students would have to learn by heart Pessoa's great lyric poem 'Autopsicographia' on the double remove of the feelings in literature and how writing (and reciting) are intimately connected with reading (and listening):

The poet loves to put it on.
He puts it on so thick

He ends up mimicking the pain
That really cuts him up.

And those who read his poems
Feel in the printed pain
Not the two he's coping with
But one that isn't theirs.

So round and round it goes,
This little string-pull train
Referred to as the heart.
It leads the mind a game.
(My translation from the
Portuguese)

'And those who read his poems/Feel in the printed pain/Not the two he's coping with/But one that isn't theirs'. Pessoa's insight is itself is an elaboration of Shakespeare's famous line in *As You Like It* that 'the truest poetry is the most feigning'. The implication then is that when we criticize a poem for being 'contrived', what we actually mean is 'not contrived enough'. Oscar Wilde was right to remark that 'all bad poetry springs from genuine feeling' – and he didn't mean that feeling ought to be banished from good poems: it needs to be considered feeling. A wholly successful piece of literature should be so well put together as to occlude its artful nature; those tiny neural delicacies worked into the substance of the poem mean that the reader will get it in his guts. As Elizabeth Bishop said, 'Writing poetry is an unnatural act. It takes great skill to make it seem natural'.

Being a poet means more than just feeling you're a poet. You have to risk producing a work that can be ruined by a single misplaced or poorly chosen word. Furthermore, the experience of being a poet is an intermittent one: strictly speaking, the 'poet' is every bit as much a construction as the poem itself. Emily Dickinson said this very clearly when she wrote to her 'preceptor', Thomas Wentworth Higginson: 'When I state myself, as the Representative of the Verse – it does not mean – me – but a supposed person'. Her claim to imaginative freedom as the 'Rep' is the precondition to her writing the truth. Others have said the same. 'If you've written poems it means you *were* a poet', as Miroslav Holub's questioner asserts in one of his epistemologically exacting teasers. 'But now?'

Degas, that great solitary French painter, made a cynical but clarifying remark about making things that surely applies to the page too: 'A picture is something which calls for as much cunning, trickery and vice as the perpetration of a crime'.

To wit, art is engineering.

Invisible enemy

I was watching a French film from the Second World War period when I realized that the word 'microbe' was a word of great potency in France in the era of Pasteurization – comparable with the word 'germs' in English perhaps. It designated the entire realm of uncanny and invisible alien forces lying in wait to attack the human (and social) body. Jules Romains allows the eponymous 'doctor' in his play *Knock* – which is about a world poised to 'believe' in medicine – to put it to effective use when terrorizing the impressionable teacher M. Bernard: 'Do you think, doctor

. . . I may be a carrier of germs?' It has been replaced in the twenty-first century by the no less threatening but somehow pindownable 'virus', a word that had only just started its career in that era: the first electron microscopical images of the tobacco mosaic virus were produced in 1939 by Kausche, Pfankuch, and Ruska.

Camp followers

Seamus O'Mahony, in *The Ministry of Bodies* (2021), coins the word *hospitaleras* – by analogy with the Spanish word for the volunteers who assist pilgrims on the road to Santiago de Compostela – to describe women who although having no institutional recognition or post spend most of their days in hospitals, seeking the warmth in the clinical setting that their ancestors might have received by frequenting cathedrals and churches. But perhaps it is *their* presence which brings warmth to the clinics which surely stand at the bluer end of the emotional temperature scale.

A screech

One of the great doctors' names: Dr Alfred Prunesquallor, in Mervyn Peake's *Gormenghast*. An intelligent, sharp-tongued, and ultimately sympathetic character, his main defect is his maddening 'hyena laugh'.

Krebserkrankt

In *Ill Feelings*, Alice Hattrick tells the story of a woman who tried to convince her doctor that she had a crab inside her guts 'tearing at her with its claws'. Of course, there was no physical evidence of any such thing, and owing to her persistent demands on members of the medical profession, she ended up in a mental hospital. Many years later, a surgeon had to perform an emergency laparotomy on the same woman and discovered that she had a large stomach ulcer. Hattrick comments that 'there was a mass in her body – not crabs, exactly, but not nothing either. It was as if she had had too much flair for metaphor'. If it had been a cancer, there would have been a real flair for metaphor across languages, since *Krebs* is the German word for both 'cancer' and 'crab'.

Bamboozled

It sank in, as soon as he, with a smug knowingness, began to talk about 'the release of dopamine and serotonin at receptor sites' that he was spouting obscurantist jargon little different from the metaphorical overspill of 'black bile' that Robert Burton famously instanced in his *The Anatomy of Melancholy* (1621) as the source of melancholy. We might mock the seemingly quaint theories of humoral medicine, but referring to 'neuromodulators' (as if this offered an *explanation*) is just as worthy of being mocked: all that the language registers is a shift in bodily disposition as manifested in a mood that now goes under the name of 'depression' rather than 'melancholy'. The four centuries since Burton have not brought us closer to understanding the social, personal, and spiritual dimensions of this dislocated sense of experience. And it could be argued that Burton, in his elaborate reflections on melancholy and life in seventeenth-century England, was more attuned to the role played by many factors other than the humours in triggering this dislocation.

Today's prescriber of medications, most of which have been shown to be no more effective than placebos, wouldn't have that breadth of understanding and certainly wouldn't have read Burton. And the latest studies, based on proxy measurements of serotonin in the blood and fluid around the spinal cord, show no difference in levels between clinically depressed and healthy people.

Papery

'The more weight I lose, the flatter I become', said my patient. I looked at her, uncertain whether she had used the adjective 'flatter' because it made a heavily assonantal allusion to 'fatter' yet gainsaid it or because she knew that I would associate her act of personal autonomy with the writer whose 'dietary' writings we had discussed at a previous encounter, Franz Kafka, and his lifelong obsession with establishing the inverse relations between words and food.

The physical experience of refusing nourishment had brought her close to the fasting showman in Kafka's story 'A Hunger Artist'. We both knew how that that story ends:

Rediscovered in his cage after years during which his initially sensational 'fasting' act had been forgotten, the dying showman tells the circus-barker with his last breath that he simply couldn't find any food he liked (and had he found any would have eaten it with abandon just like anyone else). In the end, his remains are unceremoniously swept out of the cage, its new inhabitant an energetic young panther whose liveliness comes as a pleasurable shock to the paying viewers.

Soul-care

In the 1950s, medicine sold its soul and gained the world; it abandoned its mission to care for individual human beings and acquired many effective cures, both pharmaceutical and interventional. Nobody would seek to gainsay a cure, least of all someone who has been seriously ill or threatened by disease, but a few doctors and commentators at the time worried that medicine might neglect its traditional insight into human nature (which included knowing when *not* to treat) in favour of a blind belief in the benefits of increasing specialization and technical commitment. Doctors saw part of their traditional brief as being to help people live but also to tell them, cheerfully but firmly, when they were likely to die. There was a time, indeed, when doctors were comfortable with this helplessness, knowing their presence – and little more than that – was the remedy.

At the same time, philosophers took a special interest in what they called 'care'; by 1976, when Ivan Illich's *Medical Nemesis* exposed the medical profession as strategically self-interested and well on the road to a medico-industrial complex, notions such as 'care of the self' or even 'care of the soul' were common from Paris to Prague. Jan Patočka (1907–77) was a Czech philosopher who lived most of his life resisting the oppressive political regime in his native Czechoslovakia. Being a genuine philosopher, he was under obligation to do so, as he explained in one of his lectures, and he was certainly aware of the dangers of a technical turn in medicine and other fields, as the title of one of his lectures (to friends in his house) confirms. 'Soul-care' in Democritus, Plato, and Aristotle was, according to Patočka, a response to the loss of groundedness originally provided by myth: Oedipal wandering is the outcome of philosophical reflection and only overcome by soul-care. Democritus's is radically private, taking its bearing from the concrete world of politics but always aspiring to an extramundane form, while Aristotle's is horizontal, allowing a kind of creative play which Plato's cannot, simply because it is more alert to the actual political world.

What soul-care seems to entail is what Patočka calls solidity or endurance. By this he means an array of settled convictions that cannot be dislodged by further dialectic probing, a kind of post-analytical reintegration into the community. But can human beings have settled convictions once they have taken up thinking about their existence? Perhaps care simply means asking the right questions.

A very short history of the ego

For Blaise Pascal and the Port-Royal thinkers who popularized the word 'egoism' in the seventeenth century in order to mock it, the self is something to be despised (*le moi est haïssable*), and a good Christian would be loath to say 'I'. Pascal was the first person to turn the pronoun into a substantive ('*le* moi') in order to criticize contemporaries who insisted on drawing attention to themselves: 'moi, je fais ceci et cela . . .'. Rhetorically as much as spiritually, it was an affront. For Arthur Schopenhauer, on the other hand, self-interest is essential to every living being, traversed as it is by the blind undifferentiated force that he hypostatizes as 'will'. In Ayn Rand's philosophical egoism, exceedingly influential among living American economists, the *only* valid ethical reference is the ability to say 'I', the linchpin of the liberal world-view . . . until Christopher Lasch pointed out that this kind of egoism, under the disinhibiting impact of the 1960s, had become narcissistic, self-serving, and thoroughly agnostic about the public domain – in a word *asocial*.

The American writer Guy Davenport was even firmer about the term 'liberal' turning into its opposite. 'Not only illiberal: puritanical, narrow-minded, mean'.

Wrong again

Aristotle famously attributed the misfortunes of tragic heroes to *hamartia* (commonly referred to as 'the tragic flaw'). These misfortunes were to be assigned not to some kind of essential character defect or inherent badness but to an error of judgement, a misperception, or a bit of bad luck. Writers and critics too could err in committing various kinds of poetic errors and were able to avoid *hamartia* by the proper acquisition of *techne* or skill.

Hamartia, equally, was implicated in the aetiology of illness, which in Greek times was often attributed to a shortcoming in what the Greek called *diaita* – a word cognate to our 'diet' but with much wider scope, meaning something like regimen or lifestyle. External factors such as overexertion, contusions, vomiting, and fever were all instances of *hamartia*. The treating physician might 'err' too by administering a treatment (wrong strength or wrong rhythm) that did not correspond to the appropriate *kairos*. *Hamartia* could be due to simple ignorance (*agnoia*) but was often associated with imprudence.

Be my monster

The Centaur (horse-man) was a monster too, exhibiting the hybrid form or dislocated parts also found on the Minotaur (bull-man), Echidna (snake-woman), Pegasus (horse-bird), Sphinx (woman-lion-bird), Siren (bird-woman), griffin (lion-eagle), mermaid (woman-fish), and mandrake (plant-man).

'Monster', 'monitor', 'monument', 'monstrance', even 'demonstration': all these words are related, going back to the Latin verb *monstrare*, to show, itself a derivative of *monere*, warn, prevent, put on guard. The etymology suggests a contradictory sense of wanting to ward off a harmful or horrific portent and yet a beneficial revelation: something that should have remained hidden has surged into view and is now a part of our own phylogeny, and it may even have returned to avert a worse evil still.

Monstrum in medieval Latin was 'that which teaches'. The new biology of the nineteenth century saw the monster reach beyond the uniformity of the laws of nature and become the object of a discipline dedicated to its study – teratology – and an aesthetic category – the grotesque.

The monster became in a paradoxical manner the guarantor of the dominant order, of normality in the social and natural orders, and the monstrous not necessarily a physically unsightly figure like Victor Hugo's hunchback. One of the most frightening of all nineteenth-century creations is 'the average man' ('*l'homme moyen*'), a moral monster devised by the Belgian astronomer and statistician Adolphe Quetelet in the 1830s. The average man is an abstraction based on the mean values of any number of human activities that exhibit the pattern known as 'normal distribution' and not a person who will ever be met in ordinary social life. That hasn't stopped this fictitious grey man from having a fabulous career as a recommendable *prototype* – the celestial mechanic of the social body.

Having initially regarded his *l'homme moyen* as a fictitious entity, Quetelet later recommended him as virtue personified making his way in the world between vicious extremes, the man of moderation (some would say mediocrity) in a world in thrall to revolutions.

On coke

It is conveniently forgotten, aided of course by Freud writing it out of his *vita*, that the self-same ambitious young Viennese physician (the 'conquistador') was also a world authority on the therapeutic and recreational use of cocaine, following the publication of his monograph *Über Coca* in 1884. Perhaps not ambitious enough, since Karl Köller, a fellow intern with an interest in optical physiology whom Freud had engaged to help him with his dynamometer experiments (which measured the physical strength of subjects after the experimental administration of cocaine), also remarked on the instantaneous numbing effect of the drug on lips and tongue when swallowed in a glass of water. Köller realized that the drug might be useful in ophthalmological surgery: existing analgesics were unable to prevent the reflex blinking and twitching that made operations on the eye technically difficult for the operator and exquisitely painful for the patient. Köller promptly demonstrated the anaesthetic effect on animals and published his own findings at a congress in Heidelberg. Although Freud had mooted the suggestion that cocaine might be effective as a local anaesthetic, Köller developed the idea and ran with it, in 1888, to a lucrative ophthalmological practice in New York and many lifetime distinctions: cocaine's topical application in ophthalmological and otorhinolaryngeal surgery to provoke vasoconstriction and enhance the operative field proved to be its only uncontroversial application in twentieth-century medicine.

It seems Freud was in the habit of referring to his colleague, with whom he stayed in touch, as *Coca Köller* without reference to the cocaine- and alcohol-containing beverage that was first patented in 1886 by John Pemberton, an American pharmacist and Civil War veteran, and that later became known as Coca-Cola.

Indomitable

The poet Alexander Pope, who had Pott's disease – tuberculosis affecting the developing spine and causing severe hunchback and stunted growth – and probably hardly went a day without some degree of suffering, and wrote 'this long Disease, my Life', still found much worth celebrating in that same life, as well as many targets for his satire.

Breaking the tension

There's a moment of genial insight in Tolstoy's *Anna Karenina* when 'Kitty' (Princess Ekaterina Alexandrovna Shcherbatskaya), wife of Levin, begs her mother to take off her earrings because she thinks they're getting in the way of her contractions, in what is a long and difficult labour. This is one of the many telling details that dot Tolstoy's novels. It brought to mind one from my own life also associated with childbearing. Called to the obstetrical ward of the Broken Hill Base Hospital in the absence of the senior midwife, I discovered a mildly distressed patient pregnant with her third or fourth child whose labour pains had come on so quickly that she was already expelling the child. We helped her smartly on to the birthing chair. What I hadn't realized was that her waters hadn't broken, and a swiftly emerging distended amniotic sac exploded in my face – to the glee of the attendant midwives – as I bent down to cradle the crowning infant slippery with its custardy vernix.

'Heart of hearts'

A curious, intensified, 'noun of a noun' phrase, where the first noun serves as a modifier of its own plural. This surely goes back to the Bible translators who nativized repetitive phrases such as 'holy of holies' because Hebrew lacks the positive/comparative/superlative distinction to express adjectival degree. Other examples: 'king of kings', 'song of songs', etc.

Moderation and medicine

'*Je n'ai pas toujours pratiquer la médecine, cette merde*'. Céline has his narrator, at the start of his second novel *Mort à credit*, disavow his bonds with the profession. The generally reliable translator Ralph Manheim puts this into English as 'I haven't always been a doctor . . . crummy trade', which isn't quite what the French says, introduces an ellipsis where Céline (for once) doesn't have one, and loses the pungent force of the dismissal.

It's true that Céline's style is generally about as far as could be from the *moderato risoluto* that might be expected of a doctor. Steven Connor, quoting speculative research into ancient Indo-European root-words for treating or caring for the sick by the French linguist Emile Benveniste, suggests that the practice of medicine is associated in nearly all cultures with moderation, measure, and balance, whether in terms of magical elements (*chi*) or humours: 'The mediation of medicine involves careful reflection, as attested by the related term meditation'.

Many of his biographers mention Céline writing at top speed: 'feverishly, rabidly, anxiously', 'a delirium out of control', 'without moderation'. He might not have practised clinical medicine very successfully, but he went back to it after the war, when he was amnestied by the French government in 1951. He had very few patients. All the women he lived with, including his wife Lucette, who provided dancing lessons for middle-class schoolgirls while her increasingly shabby husband worked downstairs, remarked on his obsession with writing.

A curatorial caretaker

I made a fuss in one of my entries in my 'medical dreambook' *Scattered Limbs* about tracing the different etymologies of 'cure' and 'care' and insisting on their ontological difference too; in Foucault's last lectures at the Collège de France in February 1984 (*Le courage de la verité*), when he discusses parrhesia and Socrates's last wish for a cock to be sacrificed to Asclepius, a sentence crops up which runs them together wonderfully: 'Don't forget to make this sacrifice to the god, to the god who helps us to cure ourselves when we take care of ourselves'.

References and further reading

Andreas-Salomé L. 1974 (originally pub. 1951). *Lebensrückblick: Grundriss einiger Lebenserinnerungen*. Insel Verlag. Frankfurt am Main: Insel Verlag.
Bamforth I. 2020. *Scattered Limbs: A Medical Dreambook*. Cambridge: Galileo.
Bentall R. 2021. Richard Bentall: The Man Who Lost His Brother – Then Revolutionised Psychology. Interview with S Usborne. *The Guardian*, September 29. Available at: www.theguardian.com/society/2021/

sep/29/richard-bentall-the-doctor-who-lost-his-brother-then-revolutionised-psychology. Last accessed: 25/10/2023.

Bishop E. 2011. *Objects and Apparitions*. New York: Tibor de Nagy Gallery.

Burton R. 2001 (originally pub. 1621). *The Anatomy of Melancholy*. New York: NYRB Editions.

Canguilhem G. 1978. The Conceptions of René Leriche. In: *On the Normal and the Pathological. Studies in the History of Modern Science*. Vol. 3. Dordrecht: Springer. https://doi.org/10.1007/978-94-009-9853-7_6. Last accessed: 25/10/2023.

Céline L-F. 1971. *Death on the Instalment Plan* (R Manheim, trans.). New York: New Directions.

Céline L-F. 1985 (originally pub. 1936). *Mort à crédit*. Paris: Gallimard.

Céline L-F. 1996 (originally pub. 1932). *Voyage au bout de la nuit*. Paris: Gallimard.

Coleridge ST. 1983 (originally pub. 1817). *Biographia Literaria* (J Engell, W Jackson, eds.). Princeton: Bollingen.

Compagnon A. 2021. "Le moi est-il vraiment haïssable?" Entretien avec S Ortoli. *Philosophie Magazine*, March 25. Available at: www.philomag.com/articles/antoine-compagnon-le-moi-est-il-vraiment-haissable. Last accessed: 25/10/2023.

Connor S. 2018. Nothing Doing: The Remissions of Transmission. *A Talk at the IKKM Lab, Weimar*, June 15. Available at: https://stevenconnor.com/nothingdoing.html. Last accessed: 25/10/2023.

Davenport G. 2018. *Questioning Minds: The Letters of Guy Davenport and Hugh Kenner* (EM Burns, ed.). Washington, DC: Counterpoint.

Degas E. 1998 (originally pub. 1938). *Degas Danse Dessin* (P Valéry, ed.). Paris: Gallimard.

Deleuze G, Parnet C. 1977. *Dialogues*. Paris: Flammarion.

Dick OL. (ed.) 1999 (originally pub. 1949). *Aubrey's Brief Lives, Chiefly of Contemporaries, Set Down Between the Years 1669 and 1696*. Boston: David R Godine.

Dickinson E. 1862. *Letter to Thomas Wentworth Higginson*, July. Available at: http://archive.emilydickinson.org/correspondence/higginson/l268.html. Last accessed: 25/10/2023.

Emmerich W. 2016. *Gottfried Benn*. Hamburg: Rowohlt Verlag.

Erskine-Hill H. 2018. *Alexander Pope: Oxford Dictionary of National Biography*. Available at: www.oxforddnb.com/display/10.1093/ref:odnb/9780198614128.001.0001/odnb-9780198614128-e-22526. Last accessed: 25/10/2023.

Foucault M. 2009. *Le Courage de la vérité, tome 2: Le gouvernement de soi et des autres, 1984*. Paris: Seuil.

Freud S. 2022. *Psychonauts: Drugs and the Making of the Modern Mind* (M Jay, ed.). New Haven: Yale University Press.

Gogol NV. 1995 (originally pub. 1842). *Dead Souls*. London: Penguin.

Hattrick A. 2021. *Ill Feelings*. London: Fitzcarraldo.

Holub M. 1990. *Poems Before & After: Collected English Translations*. Newcastle upon Tyne: Bloodaxe.

Ionescu E. 1999 (originally pub. 1959). *Rhinocéros*. Paris: Gallimard.

Kafka F. 1996 (originally pub. 1922). *Die Erzählungen und andere ausgewählte Prosa*. Frankfurt am Main: S Fischer Verlag.

Mirsky DS. 1927. *A History of Russian Literature, From the Earliest Times to the Death of Dostoevsky*. London: Routledge.

Nietzsche F. 2003. *Writings from the Late Notebooks* (R Bittner, ed.). Cambridge: Cambridge UP.

O'Mahony S. 2021. *The Ministry of Bodies*. London: Apollo.

Østerud S. Hamartia in Aristotle and Greek Tragedy. *Symbolae Osloenses*. 2008 (originally pub. 1976); 51 (1): 65–80. https://doi.org/10.1080/00397677608590685

Patočka J. 1996. *Heretical Essays in the Philosophy of History* (E Kohák, trans.). Chicago: Open Court.

Peake M. 1982 (originally pub. 1950). *Gormenghast*. London: Penguin.

Pessoa F. 2006. *Poesia 1931–1935 e não datada*. Lisbon: Assírio & Alvim.

Proust M. 1999 (originally pub. 1913–1927). *Le Côté de Guermantes: À la recherche du temps perdu*. Paris: Gallimard.

Quetelet LAJ. 1989. *The Empire of Chance: How Probability Changed Science and Everyday Life* (G Gigerenzer, Z Swijtink, T Porter et al., eds.). Cambridge: Cambridge University Press.

Romains J. 2022 (originally pub. 1923). *Knock ou Le triomphe de la médecine: Comédie en trois actes*. Paris: Gallimard.

Rostand E. 1999 (originally pub. 1897). *Cyrano de Bergerac*. Paris: Gallimard.

Sacks O. 2015. *On the Move: A Life*. New York: Vintage.

Sylvester D. 2016. *Interviews With Francis Bacon*. London: Thames & Hudson.

Tolstoy L. 2003 (originally pub. 1877). *Anna Karenina*. London: Penguin.

Valéry P. 1938. *Discours aux chirurgiens*. Paris: Nouvelle Revue française.

Wikipedia. *Glossary of Psychiatry*. Available at: https://en.wikipedia.org/wiki/Glossary_of_psychiatry. Last accessed: 25/10/2023.

Wikipedia. *Holy of Holies*. Available at: https://en.wikipedia.org/wiki/Holy_of_Holies. Last accessed: 25/10/2023.

Wikipedia. *Monster*. Available at: https://en.wikipedia.org/wiki/Monster. Last accessed: 25/10/2023.

PART 3

Poiesis

Metaphor elaborates experience

9

POSITIVE NEGATIVE

Daisy G Bassen

In the Midrash, Lot's wife is called Edith

Any mammographer worth her salt
Knows down to the nanosecond
When you'll say *If men had to do this . . .*
They must learn a narrow spectrum
Of inflections, measured in the same
Millimeters they use to fit your breast
Between two panes of glass they tell
You to embrace and then hold your breath,
Hon. It's the furthest thing from a love affair,
Even though your gown is clove-pink,
And nothing must come between you
And the beloved, not even a trace of scent
Dabbed at your throat. You never remember
Her name if you get lucky.

DOI: 10.4324/9781003341796-14

Domina

There is one uterus left
Among the cadavers and it's ours now.
It's true there are more male bodies
And we never talk about why that is;
Shucked off, why we are given
These potent remnants and not others,
Because they must have understood
It was not visionary Science receiving them,
Only us in our blue scrubs, hands waxy
With gloves. The formaldehyde clings
To my covered hair, predictable funk,
Less obnoxious than you'd think.
We don't expect how hungry
It makes us, how full of lively appetites
We are. The librarian's uterus is dusky,
Like a plum, of course, like a beauty
From Solomon's Song; it was likely
She'd never been pregnant,
Though I don't call her barren.
She's our treasure trove with her complete set,
A parure of generation, her matched ovaries
Like garnet cabochons. It's hard for me
To appreciate the versatility of her womb.
I haven't been pregnant yet,
Not even a scare. I haven't found out how hard
The fundus will be, breaching the pelvic brim,
How I will carry all of you in a prison
So you don't kill me. It will be two years
Before I see a uterus born first, glossy
And taut around the baby who spills out
When we cut the smallest exit, ignoring
The cinched cervix. The baby is handed off,
Working herself up; we turn our attention
To her first swaddle, first everything, using suture
At every level to mend what's been rent.
A nurse will come in to knead the soft belly,
To force the mystery back into the unspoken depths.
I grimace, when I do it and when it is done to me.
The librarian's uterus is flattened already,
A velvet bookmark when we label it on the aluminum tray.

My abortions

We drove an hour, straight shot
On the thruway, past picturesque barns,
Milch cows, signs for public golf courses
A half-mile from the next exit.
The bare sky held no portents, clouds
Shapeless. There was no plague,
No ash, no pitchfork left smoking
Against a mile-marker, the way
The old man protesting by the on-ramp
Every Thursday would have you believe.
You were waiting for me and if Jesus
Was there, you brought him, parked
Him in the plastic chairs mass produced
For rooms like this, orderly as a library.
I never used a curette. The boxy machine
Plugged into the wall, murmuring.
The air batted about within a hollow willow,
The branches made of steel, feather-veined.
You weren't terribly far away from me
But I was careful to let the nurse
Pat your hand and lay the warmed blanket
Over you. You didn't owe me anything at all,
Not one explanation. How easy that made it.
I dealt with embryos and the blood they drew
After, without a frisson. Bodies are not tidy
As chairs, as worn blankets in folded squares.
Someone else was going to drive you home
And maybe you were going to look out
The rolled-down window or turn the station
To the country channel, wishing for Patsy Cline.
You might remember you needed a gallon of milk,
A dozen eggs. I wasn't curious. I didn't need a story
To understand an ending. We went home together
With the sun sharply gold in our eyes, unveiled,
Without bothering to say we went west.
There was no freak snow, too early, falling like ghosts.
How easy that made it. We would come back next week.

Tansy

All the little witches in my office,
Who would have burnt you up,
Soaked you like a cherry in liquor,
The larded green scum of the pond
Skimming your confit?
I hope it wouldn't have been your mother.
She's sitting beside you, reminding us both
She carried you once, she ate you
Into being. They had to cut you apart;
You're a girl, not a doll, there's always a mark.
Not the devil's print, not the scratches
Of a familiar. You used a razor, scissors,
The teeth of a spare key, hidden under a flower-pot.
Why are there so many mouths, biting,
Holding pills like the bottle they just left,
Your pink tongue the cap a child can't open?
Little witch, you would have tried to shelter
Inside a tree's bole, to shove the dryad out.
You would have sucked the ends of reeds
To put the visions in a place they could be heard.
It would have been a neighbor who denounced you,
A jealousy unnecessary. You wanted to share,
To hold her hand, to drag yourself back.

Catherine-Wheel

At 2 am, the hours before the next dose
Are four and infinite.
The darkness is also incomplete,
Stained with leached grey
From streetlights, the nursing station.
Few things are certain: the pangs,
The no, the suspicion of contempt.
You are being walled off
Like an abscess. No one
Can remember a time before demands,
When you offered yourself to the day.
If you were Einstein, maybe
You could figure out how the past
Can race away while the future
Still hugs its spool. Now
Is beyond want or need; you wish,
Wish for the dumpling heat of your cat,
An oasis, the plastic cup to rattle
With its maraca pills. The moment
Before this begins again.

Folie à deux

I knew a boy who thought he could fly.
I never met the man who knew he couldn't.
The air was not a friend, not even neutral
As Switzerland; that was the boy's mistake.
It was what the man counted on,
Not a betrayal. He'd understood the atoms
Were unsociable, that they would not rush
Together, that they were too reliable
To move so far apart he'd be held by a vacuum.
The boy hadn't imagined wings, beetle-paned
Or burning, two gashes of blue flame,
His scapulae tinder, his heels dusky
In the light; flight would come from his paddling
Hands, the helium in his lungs. His breaking voice
Would be his rudder. The man hadn't imagined
Wings or fins to beat the current of inert nitrogen,
The syrup diesel exhaust of the taxis below.
He let his suit jacket flap, a loosened hide,
Waiting, shortly, for confirmation he'd been right.

Kenoma

No one will declare you dead
In the asylum. That's what they used to call it
When medicine meant releasing the shackles,
A tin tub full of water, a canvas sail laid on top,
The air sweet off the bay, wraiths in the leaves.
Your heart stopped, your lungs collapsing,
A soaked book; they'll close your eyes
And rock back with the compressions.
Someone less necessary minds the round clock
On the wall, willing to say what time it was
When they were giving up, an asymptote
They'd never arrive at. They're all waiting
For the sounds of the siren, a way to make you leave;
You're more present now than you ever have been
In your life. The nurses didn't pay this much attention
When you were born, shrieking for your lost caul,
The endless, uremic sea. There's no verb for your state,
They pick up the pencil. They'd been willing once
To spend hours with you, unpacking
The same, same, same delusions, reassuring you
Against zombies and limbo.

Training for Death Certificate Completion

God, God, God,
Will we sit at long desks,
Will there be screens like Polyphemus's eye
Gazing back at us, incurious, encompassing
As amoebae? Will it be in triplicate,
Each third page the Holy Ghost, a fairy tale
Triumvirate to confirm you are gone:
Gone even though you lie there in front of me
Still apparently yourself because I can't see
How you continue to die, every bit of you
Coming apart, cascades stretched, snapped?

There will be an evaluation at the end,
How well you learned, any complaints
Typed, logged, filed, a bored administrator,
Mid-level pay scale, eyeing the last of the cola,
Who never says the word *coffin*
                          body
                          pyre
                          prayer

Who never says what it does to you,
Signing the certificate with your own name.

10

EMBRACING METAPHOR IN PAIN MEDICINE

Peter Stilwell and Christie Stilwell

Overview

There is a widespread assumption that medicine should be objective, using standardized terminology and plain speech to relay raw facts about disease and health (Bleakley 2017). Within this paradigm, figurative language, such as metaphor, is viewed as unnecessary and to be avoided. Yet the blind spot of this view is that medicine, science, and human languages are built on a foundation of metaphor (Lakoff and Johnson 1980; Bleakley 2017). In this chapter, we focus on the use of metaphor in clinical practice, specifically pain management. Drawing from our own and others' theoretical and empirical work, we argue that metaphor is essential, unavoidable, and potentially quite helpful. Rather than attempting to sanitize clinical practice by suppressing metaphor use, there is a need to intentionally and carefully co-construct metaphors with people living with pain to facilitate mutual understandings and enhance health-related outcomes (Neilson 2016; Bleakley 2017; Stilwell et al. 2021; Stilwell and Coninx 2021). Overall, this chapter represents a call to embrace metaphor in medicine to improve communication about the idiosyncratic complexities of pain and to avoid overly simplistic messages that may do more harm than good.

If poetry is the primary medium for innovation in metaphor, then a poetic imagination is needed to grasp the meanings of metaphor use in medicine and health care. Here, we investigate this link not only with words but also images – themselves carriers of metaphor.

First things first: what is metaphor?

Metaphor is understanding one kind of thing (or experience) in terms of another (Lakoff and Johnson 1980). Metaphor is commonly framed as figurative language used to map something more abstract or unfamiliar onto something more concrete and well-known. Consider the following: *chronic pain is a never-ending marathon.* Chronic pain is a subjective experience that is abstract and difficult to express, so it is compared to running a never-ending marathon, which may be more understood. This metaphor may be helpful to some, relaying what it is like to live with chronic pain by provoking thoughts of a gruelling marathon requiring endurance, sacrifice, suffering, and pacing. Of importance, we don't just talk with these types of metaphors, we think with them (*ibid.*).

 DOI: 10.4324/9781003341796-15

One way to get at the complex roles that metaphor plays in our lives is to consider the 'two-way traffic' between linguistic metaphors and bodily actions/experiences (*ibid.*; Kirmayer and Ramstead 2017). In the first direction, bodily states give rise to metaphors. For instance, erect or crumpled postures relate to feeling *up* or *down*, respectively. Also consider how the bodily experience of anger is mapped onto being *hot-headed* or *boiling*. In the second direction, metaphors shape bodily actions/experiences. For instance, for many years we hosted a bi-weekly community-based walking programme that also included a health information-sharing talking piece where we would translate research and best practices in ways that were appreciable for a lay audience. To relay the importance of exercise for joint health and overall wellbeing, we often used the metaphor *motion is lotion*. We were pleasantly surprised to receive feedback that this simple saying had a lasting impact on our members, prompting them to engage in regular walking and view their bodies and exercise more positively. We intentionally used this metaphor knowing that it has potential to move people, whether they realize it or not (Lakoff and Johnson 1980).

Once we acquire language, we perceive ourselves and our world, including other people, through the lens of language (Loftus 2011). Language allows us to communicate experiences but also plays a role in shaping them (Hofstadter and Sander 2013; Lupyan and Clark 2015). We subconsciously create categories through metaphor, which helps us compare and contrast the past with the present, enabling us to navigate the world and make sense of new life experiences (Hofstadter and Sander 2013). Of importance, metaphors, experiences, and actions all dynamically interact with one's culture and personal history (Kirmayer 2008). For example, in westernized cultures, dementia is viewed as a problematic condition that requires medical intervention and is metaphorically depicted as a 'return to childhood' or a zombie-like 'living death' (Hutmacher 2021). However, some First Nations cultures view dementia and the return to 'childhood' in a positive light, embedding age-related changes in a cultural understanding of the life cycle (Cornect-Benoit et al. 2020).

For readers who are more linguistically inclined, we offer a caveat before we continue. We recognize that there are many forms of figurative language such as similes, analogies, and metonymy (name of one thing is substituted for another). For simplicity, in this chapter, we follow the common practice of putting all these different forms of figurative language under the umbrella term 'metaphor'.

Metaphor in pain medicine is unavoidable!

Work on pain-related metaphor has stimulated rich discussions about pain amongst students and clinicians (Butler and Lorimer Moseley 2003; Moseley and Butler 2017; Stilwell et al. 2021). To launch discussion, we often use artwork and visual imagery representing pain-related metaphors – like the figures later in this chapter. What we regularly find is that students and clinicians do not realize how much they use and rely on metaphor. Yet in passing, we have also encountered some commentators who argue that they do not use metaphor and that patients want to be given 'straight facts' about their pain. This is not surprising given that metaphor in health care has long been debated, overlooked, and often rejected (Bleakley 2017). Further, prominent authors such as Susan Sontag pleaded that we need to remove metaphor entirely from health care as it harms patients (Sontag 1978).

While we agree that many metaphors can be unhelpful or harmful, we also recognize that metaphor is pervasive in life and cannot simply be removed. Metaphors are not just poetic or literary devices that one can choose to not use. Medical culture can try to sidestep or obscure metaphor, but no language, even the technical varieties, can prevent metaphor from surfacing (Bleakley 2017; Bleakley and Neilson 2021). Consider the following widespread metaphors that are directly or indirectly related to pain medicine: femoral *neck* fracture, *butterfly* rash in lupus, carpal *tunnel* syndrome, nerve *root* impingement, *cauda equina* (horse's tail) syndrome, visual *field* disturbance in migraine, and *phantom* limb pain. Everyone uses metaphors whether they realize it or not. Pain medicine is no exception.

Pain-related metaphors have a bi-directional purpose

Patients use metaphors to express their pain, and this information is often useful for clinical decision-making and for better appreciating the suffering the patient is experiencing (Stilwell 2020). Further, clinicians use their *own* metaphors to explain pain to patients to help them make sense of their experience (*ibid.*; Stilwell et al. 2021). This bi-directional use of metaphor is needed because pain is a complex, subjective experience that cannot be found by examining blood, brain, or other bodily tissues. Neither clinicians nor scientists can *directly* 'see' or fully understand exactly what a particular patient's pain experience is. To somewhat express *what it is like* to experience a particular pain, those affected rely on metaphor to describe their experience. For instance, a person may say their pain is *stabbing* or *burning*. They are not literally being stabbed or burned; rather these are metaphors to communicate what their experience is like.

Clinicians use these same metaphors verbally or through questionnaires to better understand the patient's situation and determine a potential diagnosis. For example, *burning* can indicate that nerves or the nervous system may be involved (i.e. neuropathic pain), which helps inform further testing or laboratory investigations. One has to look no further than the McGill Pain Questionnaire (Melzack 2005) to appreciate the rich metaphors that are used to characterize pain. For instance, pain may be described as *drilling*, *gnawing*, *wrenching*, *scalding*, *splitting*, *freezing*, *torturing*, and our personal favourites, *lancinating* and *rasping*!

Metaphors are also co-constructed between clinicians and patients. Patients often have difficulty expressing their pain, and the co-creation of metaphors with clinicians offers a way for patients to express themselves. In other words, metaphors are a communication tool that enables clinicians and patients to work together to discuss the abstract experience of pain in more tangible and concrete ways. The next sections include examples of the unfolding of metaphors in clinical practice using original data from Peter Stilwell's PhD research (Stilwell 2020).

Metaphor in action: real-time sense-making between clinicians and patients

To illustrate the use of metaphor in everyday clinical practices, in what follows we draw from our qualitative study that involved audio-recording clinician–patient interactions and subsequent individual post-appointment interviews with the patients (*ibid.*). All these patients were seeking care for their back pain from physical rehabilitation professionals. The exchange below demonstrates the use of metaphor where the patient connected with and held onto the words provided by the clinician:

Patient: *It feels like someone hit me with a hammer on my lower back.*
Clinician: *It's like bruised almost?*
Patient: *Yeah, that's exactly what it feels like, like I'm bruised.*

Later, the patient engaged in an individual interview and clearly adopted the word 'bruised' offered by the clinician when asked how they would describe their back pain:

Patient: *My lower back feels like it's bruised.*

A similar exchange occurred with another interaction; this time the clinician probed further, and the patient provided a sequence of clinically useful metaphors suggestive of allodynia (pain due to a stimulus that does not normally provoke pain):

Patient: *Ahh, it's been a rough couple of weeks.*
Clinician: *Yeah?*
Patient: *Yeah.*
Clinician: *How so?*
Patient: *Oh, just pain, you know . . . I mean it's still in the lower back, but it feels like it's kind of creeping all the way up my spine. . . . And it's like it's almost like a bruise in the sense that like just light touch sometimes like hurts a lot more than it should.*

In a post-appointment interview, another patient described their past interactions with their clinician, noting how it was helpful for them to express their experience in metaphorical terms:

Patient: *When I first met him* (the clinician)*, he asked how I felt the pain. And at first it was, 'I don't know, it's pain'. And he's like, 'Okay, well, like how did it feel?' I was like, well . . . 'it feels like someone stabbing me. Stabbing me and twisting'.*

Having that conversation with the clinician validated their language, making it easier to then use it when expressing themselves to others. Their 'stabbing and twisting' metaphors sustained beyond their clinical appointment, as this same patient went on to talk about a subsequent exchange with a work colleague which resulted in a mutual understanding:

Patient: *It was nice to feel like she* (colleague) *knew what I meant when I would describe it felt like someone was stabbing me or twisting. She could actually understand that. Not give you a weird look, like, 'What do you mean?'*

So far, we have depicted pain-related metaphors as being generally helpful. However, as we unpack below, pain medicine is rife with unhelpful metaphors as well.

Good or bad? The valence of pain-related metaphors

Like others, we take the perspective that metaphors are not *inherently* good or bad, or true or false (Loftus 2011; Gallagher and Lindgren 2015). Their valences, and whether they help or harm, ultimately depend on the meanings that are (co)constructed. A good metaphor in pain medicine will create new insights, enhance clinician-patient communication and understandings, or positively shape how a person views and experiences their body. However, many metaphors in pain medicine seem to mislead patients, create uncertainty, or result in confusion (Bleakley 2017). Unfortunately, negative meanings may persist more than positive ones (Greville-Harris and Dieppe 2015).

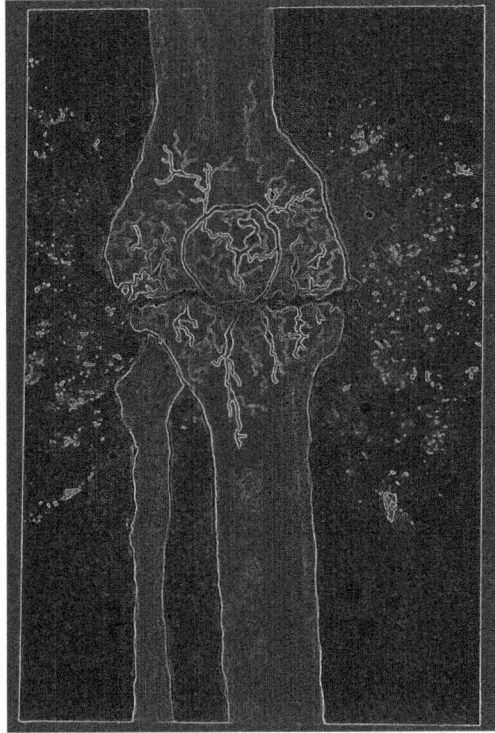

Figure 10.1　'Bone-on-bone' knee joint with no cartilage; the bones grating, cracking, fragmenting (graphite) by Christie Stilwell.

The most prominent unhelpful metaphors in pain medicine are related to the idea that the *body is a machine* (Neilson 2016; Stilwell et al. 2021). We see this frequently in verbal descriptions and medical visuals. For instance, images with clear 'pain pathways' reinforce the Cartesian impression that pain is something that simply travels from the periphery to the brain (Neilson 2016). These types of images conflate nociception and pain and endorse a linear and mechanical conceptualization of pain. Again and again, we see pain being simply equated to poor posture, *wear and tear*, or the dreaded *bone-on-bone* (Figure 10.1). The body is treated like a mechanical clock, and pain is the indicator of a broken gear that needs to be fixed (Cormack et al. 2022). This leads to the idea that a person in pain has isolated parts and linear processes that can be easily identified and fixed when they break down (i.e. find and fix the broken gear) (Stilwell and Coninx 2021).

These reductionist pain explanations conflict with contemporary understandings of pain as a *biopsychosocial* or *enactive* phenomenon wherein there is an appreciation of the whole person and how ongoing interactions in our physical and sociocultural environment *enact* or *bring forth* our personal experiences (Tabor et al. 2017; Stilwell and Harman 2019; Coninx and Stilwell 2021; Miyahara 2021).

The difference between a machine and the complex system that is the human body is not merely semantics or an academic distinction. Metaphorical understandings have real world impacts. For instance, we found in our past work (Stilwell 2020; Stilwell et al. 2021) that clinicians repeatedly use overly simplistic, mechanical metaphors that reinforced a linear conceptualization of pain and conflated nociception or injury with pain. This resulted in patients viewing their pain, or the sole source of their pain, as an injury or bodily damage rather than a multidimensional experience shaped by biopsychosocial factors. Often meanings associated with these machine-like metaphors were emotion-laden and impacted the way patients experienced their bodies and engaged in daily activities.

Further, many clinicians used metaphors that conveyed that the body needs to be *fixed*, which transmits the message that the body is *broken*. This included discussion regarding patients' muscles being *knotted*, *ropey*, and *tight*; that they lacked *core* stability or strength; and that joints or bones were misaligned or *out*. This clearly had negative impacts on patients' pain-related meanings and body image; in some cases they would blame themselves for their pain (Stilwell 2020), as one patient/clinician interaction revealed:

Patient (coming into appointment with another pain flare-up): I think I did something even more stupid.

Clinician: . . . (your) core muscles may not be firing on all cylinders. So that could be what's happening with that (flare-ups).

These types of interactions have the potential to elicit hypervigilance and limitations on movement, unnecessary bracing and worry, and a quest for a fix that does not or cannot materialize. Surveys of people living with pain repeatedly emphasize this (Setchell et al. 2017; Ray et al. 2022). For instance, people experiencing back pain often believe their bodies are like a *broken machine* and that their pain is permanent and unchangeable. Further, most of these individuals report learning these beliefs from their health professionals. Additionally, there is evidence that negative beliefs stemming from overly simplistic metaphors may impede patients' engagement with evidence-based treatment such as exercise, leading them to instead favour alternative or experimental fixes that are unlikely to be helpful in the long-term (Darlow et al. 2018; Bunzli et al. 2019).

However, our work also suggests that some anatomical and machine-like metaphors may be beneficial in the sense that they help patients better conceptualize their condition and treatment, even when the information is unidimensional and may not be fully accurate. For example, the following patient from our study appreciated their clinician's explanation of a sciatic nerve 'flossing' exercise (Stilwell 2020):

Patient: So, the exercise is easier. The flossing, the way they explained it to me made a lot of sense. . . . I'm imagining this core going through that channel. And what I'm imagining is that it actually has little bristles or something on it that it's wiping off or something. And that visualization, I can sort of feel it and it's nice. And the fact that I understood . . . or I think I understand what the flossing is doing, helps me correct myself when I'm doing it. . . . The fact that it's flossing, I can kind of visualize that motion better.

Overall, the valences of metaphors depend on their meaning, and this is unique to each individual. While basic machine-like metaphors may be helpful in certain circumstances, they are likely to do more harm than good by restricting thinking about what pain is and how it is best treated. To improve pain-related clinical outcomes, our metaphors must move beyond strictly mechanical conceptualizations of the body and pain (Neilson 2016; Stilwell et al. 2021).

Getting creative: (co)constructing multidimensional metaphors

'Metaphor is our primary linguistic medium for grasping the qualities, idiosyncrasies and expressions of dynamic, adaptive, complex systems. And, of course, metaphor as process is itself an expressive complex system' (Bleakley 2017: 5). Such a complex system is the person experiencing pain: what we have called *multidimensional metaphor* (Stilwell et al. 2021) can convey a process or experience as complex and shaped by many factors. As pain is an *emergent* experience shaped by many biopsychosocial factors (Thacker and Lorimer Moseley 2012; Stilwell and Harman 2019), multidimensional metaphors better reflect the nature of pain than do overly simplistic, machine-like metaphors that blame single pathoanatomical factors.

The most common pain-related multidimensional metaphors we see are variations of pain being compared to overflowing water from one's 'cup' or 'bathtub' (Butler and Lorimer Moseley 2003). The general idea is that pain occurs when water (representing factors related to pain) in the cup or bathtub builds up and overflows. To get at the complex idea that pain (overflow) is an emergent phenomenon (more than the sum of the parts), metaphorical layers are added to make it more concrete and understandable. For instance, we can state that every person has a different-sized cup, and it fills at different rates. This is because we have different genetic predispositions and bodies, and unique past experiences and expectations that affect the rate that our cup fills.

Further, many factors can *fill* the cup, making it more likely to overflow; this includes tissue injury, nociception, fear, worry, stress, inadequate sleep, co-morbidities, etc. In many situations, these factors do not fill the cup enough to result in an overflow (experiencing pain). That is because other factors such as pacing, distraction, analgesics, and reducing stress help to *empty* the cup, making it less likely to overflow. There are always many factors mixing, interacting, and simultaneously filling and emptying the cup. It can be unpredictable when the cup overflows, and when it does overflow, we cannot attribute it to a single factor (e.g. just a muscle or joint). Clinicians can work with patients to identify what is in their cup and which factors are modifiable and may help prevent or lessen the extent to which their personal cup overflows.

The cup/bathtub metaphor is just one example and is not expected to work for everyone. A challenge with metaphors is that there needs to be a mutual understanding of their interpretation. Therefore, each metaphor needs to be relevant to the unique person and their pain experience. This is a call for clinicians to be creative and to find ways to co-construct multidimensional metaphors with their patients. For example, some may find baking analogies useful (de Haan 2020; Cormack et al. 2022), but there are endless possibilities.

Clinical trainees are already primed for this and may be more creative than they realize. Consider all the mnemonics, funny sayings, and rhymes that are used to study and remember course materials, for example, this memorable mnemonic for brachial plexus subdivision: ***Remember To Drink Cold Beer*** for **R**oots, **T**runks, **D**ivisions, **C**ords, **B**ranches. This creativity should not be confined to anatomy. We believe that metaphor, and intentionally thinking and acting more poetically, have high potential to take the confusing and isolating experience of chronic pain and make it more expressible and understandable as well as point towards potential ways it can be treated or managed. Art pieces, like Figure 10.2, can be generated by clinicians, artists, or patients to help express understandings of pain and prompt reflection and discussion.

In the context of our interest in common musculoskeletal pain conditions, such as chronic back pain, tailored multidimensional metaphors may increase discussion and exploration of diverse treatment options that may be helpful. This includes treatment not focused solely on anatomy (e.g. cognitive therapies) while maintaining openness to other treatments that are typically perceived to be more mechanical in nature (e.g. exercise). Further, the use of multidimensional metaphor

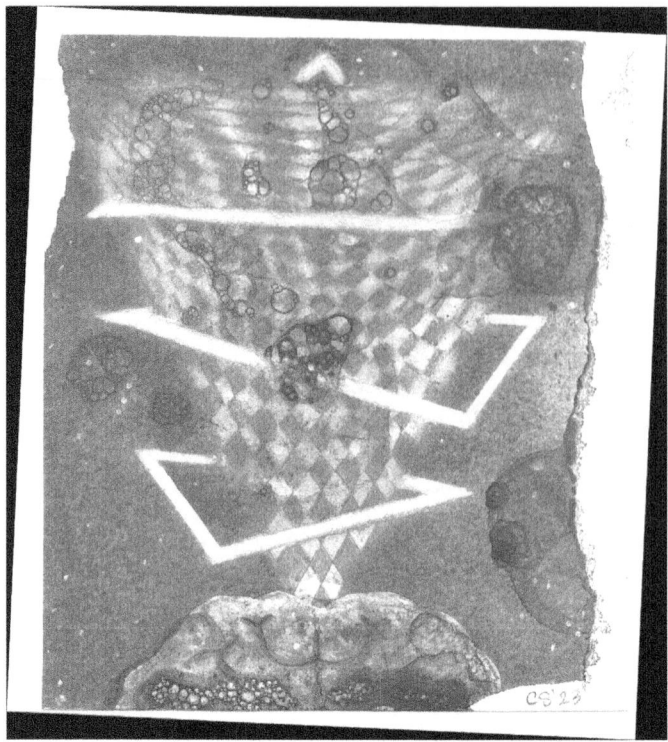

Figure 10.2 'Multidimensional metaphor mind' (graphite and soap) by Christie Stilwell.

may help patients better understand current evidence indicating that treatments such as exercise impact a variety of bodily systems and the way one engages in the world. It is not simply about flexibility, strength, or endurance (Stilwell and Harman 2017). Multidimensional metaphors may also help clinicians and patients better appreciate the role that the physical and social environments have in shaping pain experiences. This includes the important role of the clinician because 'with every utterance, the practitioner has the power to make things better or worse, and influence the outcome' (Mason and Butler 2010: 3).

Acknowledgments

Much of this chapter is based on the theoretical and qualitative research in Peter Stilwell's PhD dissertation, supervised by Dr Katherine Harman and Dr Brenda Sabo. Funding was received from Dalhousie University's Faculty of Health (internal graduate research funding and the Research Development Fund), the Canadian Chiropractic Guidelines Initiative, and a Nova Scotia Graduate Scholarship. We also thank Dr Shane Neilson and Professor Alan Bleakley for their helpful comments and suggestions.

Ethics approval

This chapter contains qualitative data from a study approved by Dalhousie University's Health Sciences Research Ethics Board (#2017–4103).

References

Bleakley A. 2017. *Thinking With Metaphors in Medicine*. Abingdon: Routledge.

Bleakley A, Neilson S. 2021. *Poetry in the Clinic*. Abingdon: Routledge.

Bunzli S, O'Brien P, Ayton D, et al. Misconceptions and the Acceptance of Evidence-Based Nonsurgical Interventions for Knee Osteoarthritis. A Qualitative Study. *Clinical Orthopaedics and Related Research*. 2019; 477: 1975–83.

Butler, DS, Lorimer Moseley G. 2003. *Explain Pain*. Adelaide: Noigroup Publications.

Coninx S, Stilwell P. Pain and the Field of Affordances: An Enactive Approach to Acute and Chronic Pain. *Synthese*. 2021; 199: 7835–63.

Cormack B, Stilwell P, Coninx S, Gibson J. The Biopsychosocial Model is Lost in Translation: From Misrepresentation to an Enactive Modernization. *Physiotherapy Theory and Practice*. 2022; 00 (00): 1–16.

Cornect-Benoit A, Pitawanakwat K, Walker J, et al. Nurturing Meaningful Intergenerational Social Engagements to Support Healthy Brain Aging for Anishinaabe Older Adults. *Canadian Journal on Aging*. 2020; 39: 263–83.

Darlow B, Brown M, Thompson B, et al. Living With Osteoarthritis is a Balancing Act: An Exploration of Patients' Beliefs about Knee Pain. *BMC Rheumatology*. 2018; 2: 15.

de Haan S. 2020. *Enactive Psychiatry*. Cambridge/New York, NY: Cambridge University Press.

Gallagher S, Lindgren R. Enactive Metaphors: Learning Through Full-Body Engagement. *Educational Psychology Review*. 2015; 27: 391–404.

Greville-Harris M, Dieppe P. Bad is More Powerful than Good: The Nocebo Response in Medical Consultations. *American Journal of Medicine*. 2015; 128: 126–29.

Hofstadter DR, Sander E. 2013. *Surfaces and Essences: Analogy as the Fuel and Fire of Thinking*. New York, NY: Basic Books.

Hutmacher F. Understanding the Self of People with Dementia. *Zeitschrift Für Gerontologie Und Geriatrie*. 2021; 54: 161–66.

Kirmayer LJ. Culture and the Metaphoric Mediation of Pain. *Transcultural Psychiatry*. 2008; 45: 318–38.

Kirmayer LJ, Ramstead MJD. 2017. Embodiment and Enactment in Cultural Psychiatry. In: C Durt, T Fuchs, C Tewes (eds.) *Embodiment, Enaction, and Culture*. Cambridge, MA: The MIT Press, 397–422.

Lakoff G, Johnson M. 1980. *Metaphors We Live By*. Chicago, IL: University of Chicago Press.

Loftus S. Pain and Its Metaphors: A Dialogical Approach. *Journal of Medical Humanities*. 2011; 32: 213–30.

Lupyan G, Clark A. Words and the World. *Current Directions in Psychological Science*. 2015; 24: 279–84.

Mason P, Butler C. 2010. *Health Behavior Change: A Guide For Practitioners* (2nd ed.). Edinburgh: Churchill Livingstone.

Melzack R. The McGill Pain Questionnaire. *Anesthesiology*. 2005; 103: 199–202.

Miyahara K. Enactive Pain and Its Sociocultural Embeddedness. *Phenomenology and the Cognitive Sciences*. 2021; 20: 871–86.

Moseley GL, Butler DS. 2017. *Explain Pain Supercharged: The Clinician's Manual*. Adelaide: Noigroup Publications.

Neilson S. Pain as Metaphor: Metaphor and Medicine. *Medical Humanities*. 2016; 42: 3–10.

Ray BM, Kovaleski A, Kelleran KJ, et al. An Exploration of Low Back Pain Beliefs in a Northern America Based General Population. *Musculoskeletal Science and Practice*. 2022; 61: 102591.

Setchell J, Costa N, Ferreira M, et al. Individuals' Explanations for Their Persistent or Recurrent Low Back Pain: A Cross-Sectional Survey. *BMC Musculoskeletal Disorders*. 2017; 18: 466.

Sontag S. 1978. *Illness as Metaphor*. New York, NY: Farrar, Straus and Giroux.

Stilwell P. 2020. Exploring Pain and Clinical Communication (PhD Dissertation). Halifax, Nova Scotia: Dalhousie University. https://dalspace.library.dal.ca/handle/10222/78346.

Stilwell P, Coninx S. 2021. A New Paradigm to Understand Pain. *Institute of Arts and Ideas (IAI)*, December 13.

Stilwell P, Harman K. Contemporary Biopsychosocial Exercise Prescription for Chronic Low Back Pain: Questioning Core Stability Programs and Considering Context. *Journal of the Canadian Chiropractic Association*. 2017; 61: 6–17.

Stilwell P, Harman K. An Enactive Approach to Pain: Beyond the Biopsychosocial Model. *Phenomenology and the Cognitive Sciences*. 2019; 18: 637–65.

Stilwell P, Stilwell C, Sabo B, Harman K. Painful Metaphors: Enactivism and Art in Qualitative Research. *Medical Humanities*. 2021; 47: 235–47.

Tabor A, Keogh E, Eccleston C. Embodied Pain – Negotiating the Boundaries of Possible Action. *Pain*. 2017; 158: 1007–11.

Thacker MA, Lorimer Moseley G. First-Person Neuroscience and the Understanding of Pain. *The Medical Journal of Australia*. 2012; 196: 410–11.

11

IS THE AUTHOR DEAD IN THE POETRY OF DISEASE?

Authorship, modern poetry, and medical language

Daniel A Romero Suarez

This article contributes to the understanding of the dynamics between poetry and disease. I will explore one of the layers that shapes poetry that is seldom considered in courses on literature and illness: I am referring to the Western tradition of modern poetry. Since this poetic language is well established in the canon, it is essential to understand how it relates to disease. The study of modern poetics is not limited to helping us to understand the flaws of medical language; it can guide us to recognize that literary texts about disease are also deficient. In other words, modern poetry keeps its own antidote within itself, preventing it from becoming a fossilizing discourse. Ultimately, poems of disease bring us closer to the tragic problem of incommunicability.

Poetry of disease, when shaped by poetic modernity, is a valuable medium for representing harrowing and chaotic experiences. Unlike a narrative or a poem that uses primarily clichéd figures of speech, there is poetic language capable of disrupting entrenched visions of health. The canon of modern poetry offers multiple depictions of pain and desolation. However, a poem is far from being a panacea for communication in medical contexts. On the contrary, modern poetics does not communicate clearly and shares with medicine one of its most harmful traits: disdain for the author. Minimizing the importance of a story's authorship may work in a literature class or when analysing X-ray plates, but when a text is written by someone who is sick, obliterating the author represents an unethical reading. Therefore, it is necessary to question contemporary notions of authorship.

Modern poetry is a language of authorial crisis that patients may use to shape extreme experiences of illness. To reach this conclusion, I first present a synthesis of the (post)structuralist debate on what was called 'death of the author'. Next, I will show how medicine has assembled a mythology of language to justify its authority. Third, I characterize modern poetics as a suitable medium for chaotic experiences of illness. Finally, the book of poems *Diario de muerte* (*Diary of Death*) by the Chilean Enrique Lihn (in 2018) will allow us to study how a terminal cancer diagnosis finds its means of expression in a poetry that constantly denies the possibility of saying something valuable and even dehumanizes the sick person. From this point of view, modern poetry shows the impossibility of communicating, leading us to a final reflection on authorship and an ethics of failure.

DOI: 10.4324/9781003341796-16

The author is dead. Long live the author!

The 1960s saw authors lose authority over their texts. Until that period, literary criticism conceived authorship as both the origin and end of the interpretative work. The authors' reality (their education, ideology, aesthetic preferences, etc.) was the starting and finishing line of exegesis; for instance, the analysis of a poem would reconstruct an episode in the sentimental education of a writer. Thus, interpretative authority was based on the critic's familiarity with the author's life experiences.

Roland Barthes' (1977) essay 'The Death of the Author' synthesizes a new way of understanding the author. Leaving behind the text–author dependency, Barthes proposes both the autonomy of the text and the fragility of authorship. He claims that 'language knows a "subject", not a "person", and this subject, empty outside of the very enunciation which defines it, suffices to make language "hold together", suffices, that is to say, to exhaust it' (*ibid.*: 145). Contrary to Romantic theories of literature, in which the author is a creator god of words, Barthes asserts that language does not have a fixed author but rather a subject that exists only in the brief moment of enunciation. Before, authorship was a primordial site – now it is only a marginal remnant of language.

Structuralism relied on the linguistic sign as a core entity capable of giving solid foundations to language and, by extension, to science and the humanities. However, critics soon discovered that the utopia of developing a metalanguage that could explain the logic of all other systems was impossible because it could not escape from the infinite deferral of meaning to another system: 'In the absence of a centre or origin, everything became discourse . . . that is to say, a system in which the central signified, the original or transcendental signified, is never absolutely present outside a system of differences' (Derrida 2002: 26). If the structuring entity of the system, or 'centre', always requires another element to secure its meaning, then it is not really a core but just another piece. If everything is discourse in the Derridean sense, language is nothing more than a chain of deferred meanings, incapable of standing on their own and always requiring recourse to another sign somewhere farther away.

The instability of language generates a centripetal force capable of absorbing and making disappear everything that surrounds it. For Barthes (1967: 145), 'the whole of the enunciation is an empty process, functioning perfectly without there being any need for it to be filled with the person of the interlocutors'. If language exists fully without its interlocutors, words float in a void. Language becomes an act that exists but is detached from consciousness, like a reflex commanded by the nervous system. Hence Barthes (*ibid.*: 146) classifies language as a performative act, living only in the instant in which it is enunciated and not dependent on the presence of the persons who pronounce or write the words.

Despite the above considerations, language did not become an infinitely acephalous entity; Barthes gives the receptor a fundamental role. The emptiness of language is unique in that rather than just absence, it is an excess of presence. Just as the rapid mixing of colours generates the colour white, giving the appearance of a lack of colour, the infinite number of meanings of a text resulting from intertextuality could lead to absolute incommunication. Only the reader can stop the dizzying wheel of signification: 'The reader is the space on which all the quotations that make up a writing are inscribed without any of them being lost; a text's unity lies not in its origin but in its destination' (*ibid.*: 148). Although readers do not fix a meaning forever because they may create new interpretations, which will continue with the postponement of signification, they do manage to keep language afloat.

Michel Foucault caught early on the problems of the erasure of the author. Foucault (1998: 211) published 'What is An Author?' two years after Barthes' essay and explained that authorship is not just the enunciative origin of language that disappears once the message is delivered:

> The author's name serves to characterize a certain mode of being of discourse. The fact that the text has an author's name, that one can say 'this was written by so-and-so' or 'so-and-so is its author', shows that this discourse is not ordinary everyday speech that merely comes and goes, not something that is immediately consumable. On the contrary, it is a speech that must be received in a certain mode and that, in a given culture, must receive a certain status.

Authorship is essential to the process of textual exegesis because it allows for establishing a classificatory horizon. Foucauldian authorship offers sufficient historical and cultural information to neutralize the contradictions generated by infinite meanings in a work and, in this way, comes to satisfy the reader's desire for coherence (*ibid.*: 215). In this perspective, authorship is a reassuring principle because it gives a clear interpretative direction. However, while the 'author' resumes presence in the text, mainly as contextual information, the flesh-and-blood author does not return.

The proposals of deconstruction have not succeeded in making the author disappear. It is undeniable that reception theory has brought the reader's subjectivity into dialogue with the text. Likewise, contemporary critical theory has reduced the author's place by giving more importance to theoretical frameworks; nonetheless, authorship has remained omnipresent in literary criticism. Texts are studied only by considering who the author is, but while leaving aside the author is always methodologically possible, in some cases the disadvantages outweigh the benefits, as with testimonial narratives. As I show below, the poetry of disease also requires the presence of its author.

A biomedical linguistic myth

Deconstruction's profound questioning resulted in a new epistemology. Now, all systems that tried to portray themselves as stable would have to be thoroughly scrutinized by critics, which would result in discovering the flaws capable of bringing down the structure: 'The newer skeptical forces deriving mostly from the French intellectual scene that asserted a new hermeneutics of suspicion, questioning the very possibility of arriving at any degree of stable knowledge' (Aryan 2020: 6–7). All major systems, then, had to come up with new ways to justify themselves. The biomedical institution subscribes to the mistrust of the school of deconstruction but in a very convenient way. On the one hand, physicians are suspicious of patients' testimonies, but on the other hand, health professionals are satisfied with their methods and do not embark on the task of deconstructing their own linear narratives about health and disease.

The birth of modern medicine required a linguistic myth of its own. Foucault (2003: xi) notes that to evaluate medical thinking, 'We must look beyond [medicine's] thematic content or its logical modalities to the region where "things" and "words" have not yet been separated, and where – at the most fundamental level of language – seeing and saying are still one'. The scientific epistemology of the nineteenth century required a particular system of signs capable of enunciating a new reality. To accomplish this objective, modern medicine resorted to a traditional view of language: the relationship between signifier and signified is totally stable; that is, what the medical institution says is the truth. This mythology was maintained even after the contributions of Barthes and Derrida.

Language is firmly tied to things in the biomedical worldview. Yet rather than linking words with abstract concepts, medicine gives fundamental importance to what we can see:

A new alliance was forged between words and things, enabling one to see and to say. Sometimes, indeed, the discourse was so completely 'naïve' that it seems to belong to a more archaic level of rationality, as if it involved a return to the clear, innocent gaze of some earlier, golden age.

(ibid.: xii)

In parallel to the poetics proposed by romanticism in the nineteenth century, biomedicine forged a linguistic worldview that implied a return to an era of greater simplicity in which what was seen corresponded to what was said; modern medicine resorted to this traditional thinking to propose, in short, that a doctor's gaze *is* language. At this point, the most important axiom of modern medicine emerges: '[t]he great myth of a pure Gaze that would be pure Language: a speaking eye' (*ibid.*: 114). The gaze-language proclaims the truth about the body, and this mythology is one of the contributing factors to biomedicine's prestige. In contrast, patients must reduce their humanity to become passive objects that facilitate the observation of the medical professional:

The patient transforms himself or herself into an object which can become the subject of clinical procedures and practice. Patients become a suitable site for clinical examination-a site which, given the correct procedures, can serve to tender certain physical functions clinically visible.

(Heath 2006: 193)

The body, in that sense, can become an obstacle to the physician's comprehensive gaze. However, medicine distrusts not only the body but primarily patients' narratives since they have not transformed their discourse following the myth of the speaking eye:

Physicians do not trust (hence, hear) the human voice . . . they in effect perceive the voice of the patient as an "unreliable narrator" of bodily events, a voice which must be bypassed as quickly as possible so that they can get around and behind it to the physical events themselves.

(Scarry 1985: 6)

Today, the physician gaze has expanded its frontiers to include all that can be observed through 'sophisticated testing and imaging such as MRI' (Bleakley and Neilson 2021: 140). In contrast, patients' personal stories are subjective and not trustworthy. The patient's language is corrupt because words and things have not maintained a relationship of correspondence as they have in the medical eye-speaker discourse – an entity that exceeds the subjectivity of a physician.

The language of modern poetry and the chaotic experiences of illness

Modern poetics pushes to the extreme the question of communicability in health care. The language of modern poetry embraces the lessons of English romanticism, French symbolism, and the avant-garde movements of the twentieth century, as seen in the work of T.S. Eliot or Sylvia Plath. These texts strongly refuse to follow the trivial norms of everyday speech or the strict parameters of scientific communication. First, poetry aspires to abandon its linguistic nature and approaches nonverbal practices such as music and visual arts (Reisz 1986: 52). Although these resources can appear in texts of diverse nature, the poetic canon preserves the most drastic and systematic cases of depragmatization and resemantization of language (*ibid.*: 54). The consequence of this rhetoric is the destabilization of meaning:

> The indeterminacy of meaning in poetry provides an experience of freedom and a release from the compulsion to signify. With its apparently gratuitous chiming and rhyming, its supplemental metrical organization and uses of lineation – in short its determination by a host of sensuous factors – lyric language works against instrumental reason, prosaic efficiency, and communicative transparency, quite independently of the thematic content of particular lyrics.
>
> (Culler 2015: 304)

Second, poetry uses semantic resources whose referents are not easily accessible. As Terry Eagleton (2008: 109) has described, poetry comes without clear contextual clues. That is, the words of a poem can interact with multiple cultural contexts that the receptor must sift through. This multiplicity makes poetry stand in opposition not only to everyday speech but also to scientific language:

> It is characteristic of poetic language that it gives us not simply the denotation of a word (what it refers to), but a whole cluster of connotations or associated meanings. It differs in this respect from legal or scientific language, which seeks to pare away surplus connotations in the name of rigorous denotation.
>
> (*ibid.*: 110)

While poetic language increases the possibilities of signification, scientific language goes in the opposite direction. If one longs for a reassuring clarity in the anguish of diagnoses, treatments, and prognoses, modern poetry would not seem to be an adequate medium. Nonetheless, this poetics has the potential to offer new ways of communicating experiences of crisis caused by illness.

Multiple authors (McEntyre 2011: 278–79; Leveen 2019: 744; Romero Suarez 2021: 310; Bleakley and Neilson 2021: 102) have noted the limitations of linear narratives in describing disease faithfully. I want to deepen the possibilities of poetic language by proposing that the tradition of modern poetry has an extensive catalogue of resources to speak of chaos, absurdity, and existential violence. The crude language of Eliot's *The Waste Land* (1922) exemplifies the poetic potential to talk about desolation. Arthur Frank (1997: 98) announced the necessity of speaking of chaotic illness without following the reassuring linearity of narrative:

> If narrative implies a sequence of events connected to each other through time, chaos stories are not narratives. When I refer below to the chaos narrative, I mean an anti-narrative of time without sequence, telling without mediation, and speaking about oneself without being fully able to reflect on oneself.

Frank suggests that we cannot control chaos. The patients' vulnerability to disease may be such that the only option for survival is to disassociate from their own body: 'The body is so degraded by an overdetermination of disease and social mistreatment that survival depends on the self's dissociation from the body, even while the body's suffering determines whatever life the person can lead' (*ibid.*: 103). Frank's proposal is in line with Jane Marston's (1986: 110) findings on how terminal patients live 'the equation of loss of body with complete loss of self'. The solution to chaos would be an escape through the alienation of the body. By turning the body into an unfamiliar entity, at least the self can be saved.

If disassociation is a resource for patients, then we require anti-narratives that can enunciate those experiences. As Hugo Friedrich (1979: 4) explains it, modern poetry is radically removed from reality and therefore could be a suitable medium for disassociation:

> Whenever a modern poem touches on realities – of objects or people – its treatment is nondescriptive, omitting the warmth of familiar seeing and feeling. It makes those realities seem unfamiliar, estranges and deforms them. The poem is not to be measured against what is ordinarily accepted as reality. . . . Reality departs from the spatial, temporal, material, and psychological order of things, transcending those distinctions which are necessary to a normal orientation in the world.

Modern poetry distorts the world. When reality is secondary, poetry can even disregard the 'personal "I" of the poet' who does not participate in his poem as a private individual (*ibid.*: 5). Now, the images created by a fervent imagination are the centre. If reality and the author are trivial, poetic language can support the disassociation that, according to Frank, can save the self.

Reassuring narratives are summarized in the well-intentioned wishes that 'it will get better' because people assume that a narrative scheme implies future improvement. The trust in linear progression is such that Frank (1997: 55) asserts: 'the conventional expectation of any narrative, held alike by listeners and storytellers, is for a past that leads into a present that sets in place a foreseeable future', where a stable timeline is a socioeconomic privilege. Moreover, the sick body in the present does not have the capacity to abstract time as reason can. When a patient does not seek narratives of control, modern poetry can offer a rhetorical repertoire that validates non-encouraging emotions: 'Who could unravel these intermeshed images; who could find a calm sense in them? Their meaning resides in the chaos itself' (Friedrich 1979: 45). In the search for an anti-narrative that hosts chaotic experiences of illness, the tradition of modern poetry has rhetorical and existential tools that can help patients express themselves.

What do we do with authorship when a patient writes a poem?

Barthes emphasizes that the process of enunciation functions without its interlocutors. In the attempt to turn linguistics into a science, structuralism pushed the idea that language is data. This proposal gave theoretical support to the modern poetry and biomedical practices of dismissing the authorial figure. However, these two languages fail for one fundamental reason: the patient wants to be heard. With few exceptions, a person approaches a medical figure with the intention of seeking wellness. An ethical approach to the stories or poems of the sick entails rethinking our way of approaching the texts so that the presence of the author is relevant.

Frank (1997: 2) describes the longing for a new communication system for illness. An emphasis on the difference between telling a story *about* illness or *through* a wounded body helps Frank propose that stories about illness have the dangerous potential to turn health issues into just a subject. In the case of poetry, criticism has established the importance of recognizing literary devices to guide our reading, which could turn texts into just a reworking of poetic familiar themes such as death or mourning. While this operation ties a particular experience to previous metaphors, which can create a sense of community, this expansion results in the partial oblivion of the individual wounded body.

Medical humanities curricula can fall into the contradiction of giving space to patients' narratives through a theoretical framework that denies the importance of such experiences. Affording similarity to how the quest for certainty and proven facts causes physicians to put patients' voices in the background (Andrews 2015: 15), contemporary theory can transform pain and illness into texts that teach interesting things but nothing more. In contrast, understanding poetry as a reading experience can open the way for an inclusive approach. Angela Andrews (*ibid.*: 19) has categorized this method as follows:

> A poetic understanding gives agency to the living, breathing person as a part of the medical encounter, because poetry is concerned with being in the world, as expressed through voice – where substance is inseparable from thought, temperament, and emotion. Listening to the authorial voice requires openness and a kind of submission to someone else's world. Crucially, in recognizing a person's agency, the capacity to not know is as important as knowing.

If either literary criticism or medical humanities position themselves as disciplines that better understand what patients say and, as such, can teach physicians to understand patients better, we are condemned to repeat the same exclusion perpetuated by institutional medicine. The noun 'submission' used by Andrews is drastic. However, isn't a submission to a mutual worldview a way of creating community? Andrews' proposal goes beyond calling for empathy and imagines a society in which the patient is the centre and where the rigid distinction between healthy and sick people is neutralized.

The tradition of modern poetry detaches itself from the tranquillity of linear narratives to make room for texts analogous to palliative practices. The care for people's last days occurs when we recognize the failure of scientific medicine's golden dream of conquering death. In these cases, the patient becomes more important than medical knowledge. I want to take Andrews' proposition that 'to not know is as important as knowing' further. Poetry written by the sick, especially in terminal cases, shows us that one has to bear the impossibility of apprehending disease: the language and eyes that analyse, understand, and cure are defeated. To embrace this failure to control reality, modern poetry emerges from a profound principle of self-criticism: 'modernity is a sort of creative self-destruction. Since Romanticism the poetic imagination has been building monuments on ground undermined by criticism. And it goes on doing so, fully aware that it is undermined' (Paz 1975: 3). Modern poetry is a textual corpus conscious of the repetitive and insurmountable failure of language to succeed in verbalizing utopian desires. However, poets continue to attempt to depict new utopias.

Texts written by patients or direct witnesses have an undeniable aura of truth. Illness is an unclaimed area for fiction writers, unlike dystopian futures in science fiction, women's psychology in texts written by men, Machiavellian plots in detective stories, or historical novels. The most illuminating texts on disease have been written by patients or ex-patients, such as Susan Sontag, Audre Lorde, and Anne Boyer. Likewise, caregivers and bereaved offer powerful testimonies, as we can find in Paul Monette or Victoria Guerrero's poetic work. Leaving behind the author, as suggested by Barthes, does not correspond to an ethical approach to books written by sick people. Likewise, authorship exceeds the classificatory function proposed by Foucault. When a text is written *through* the body, we must close the book for a minute and consider the author.

How does the autobiographical tendency of texts of illness fit in with the depersonalizing and self-destructive impetus of modern poetics? The sick body in a deep crisis requires a radically disruptive language in order to approach its reality through death. The linguistic alienation that poetry generates is a starting point for achieving one of the goals Bleakley and Neilson (2021: 115) set for lyrical medicine: 'the release of words from imprisonment in cliché and pedestrian, normative prose'. In this respect, the abstruse language of poetry is perhaps the best medium for embracing chaotic experiences of illness.

To exemplify a modern poetics of disease, I will analyse *Diary of Death*, written by Enrique Lihn (in 2018) six weeks before his death from cancer (all translations from the Spanish are my own). The first lines explore a well-known theme of poetry, the insufficiency of language, and apply it tragically to the experience of terminal illness:

> Pain has nothing to do with pain
> Despair has nothing to do with despair
> The words we use to designate these things are vitiated
> There are no names in the mute zone
> . . .
> All our ways of designating things are corrupted
> And this is just another way of vitiating them.
>
> (Lihn 2018: 325)

The fragment shows the cycle of creation and self-destruction of a modern poem. The text begins with the statement that the current words are useless. This awakening of consciousness would seem to be an announcement of a new triumphant language, but the poet quickly declares that his poem is also a failure. Thus, the text is not an illuminating statement about his condition but another way of vitiating and alienating his own experience. Nonetheless, a profound truth about the self is revealed: the body has given up on its intention to communicate. Without this despairing lesson about language, the poetry of disease would be just another soothing narrative.

Terminal illness is an extreme state in which the person would like to have some certainty about death: '[w]hat else can be said about death/that is from it, not about it/It is a deaf, mute, and blind thing' (Lihn 2018: 372). Lihn contrasts prepositions in a similar manner to what Frank does about the body. This fragment calls to speak *from* death because the body cannot be separated from death after a terminal diagnosis. In one of the most illuminating phrases of the collection, Lihn (*ibid.*: 326) wishes for '[a] language like a body operated on in with all its organs'. Hence, the ideal language for illness and death must bear the scars of previous wounds and failures.

Failure is illustrated dramatically through the author's dehumanization: '[m]y words obviously cannot cross the barrier of that unknown language/before which I am like a baboon called by aliens to interpret/human language' (*ibid.*). In the face of death, the author–patient is an animal that cannot speak the language he wants to. Lihn's poetics lacks reassuring images. Even when *Diary of Death* can imagine a language to talk from death, defeat is recognized: 'the first pale echoes/of an unprecedented description of what is not would be heard' (*ibid.*: 339). These lines are one more testimony of how language – even in a hypothetical case – can only be a pale echo so flawed that it is not even an echo of what *is* but of what *is not*. At this point, the linguistic utopias of medicine and human communication collapse: there is no language possible for terminal illness.

When we silence biomedical promises of curing, accepting failure allows healing. Frank (2014: 1399) explains that 'healing is what remains after what can be specified is done but neither suffering nor care are finished'. It is only when the pernicious metaphor of health care as was promoted by scientific medicine is exhausted that the possibility of a radical collaboration between the dying person and the listener emerges. At this point, the author's presence becomes indispensable. The commitment of the medical humanities should not be to understand the metaphors of pain but to read in such a way that we approach the other's unshareable suffering, even if that openness requires us to relinquish, painfully, our own reassuring narrative worldview of progress and improvement. As a result, Lihn's book offers little information about his specific diagnosis or his wishes before dying. Instead, the poems deliver ambiguous, contradictory, and unconnected scenes; the semantic complexity makes communication difficult. However, if suffering and pain bring the person to a pre-language state (Scarry 1985: 4), then non-communication may be the closest language to those pre-linguistic experiences.

Biomedical language and methodology are also abstruse, contrary to widespread belief. Lisa Diedrich (2007: 150) analysed the testimony of Dr. Atul Gawande in *Complications: A Surgeon's Notes on an Imperfect Science* and concluded that 'He contends that fallibility, mystery, and uncertainty are characteristics of modern, Western medicine in general, not just in the particular case of emergent and deadly infectious diseases'. This critique is not aimed at closing hospitals or stopping biomedical research. Diedrich imagines a new medical worldview based on the limitations and errors of medicine. Moreover, she proposes that a new modern medicine has the possibility of standing on a fresh principle that she calls an ethics of failure and defines as follows: 'an ethics that emerges out of, or along with, an experience of failure, be it of the body, of (conventional and alternative) medicine, or of language' (Diedrich 148). It is from this ethics of failure that the poetry of disease gains a valuable space in health care.

The poetry of disease is a feasible medium for a medicine that embraces an ethic of failure while maintaining the author as a fundamental element. Barthes (1977: 149) sees authorship as a constraint: 'To give a text an Author is to impose a limit on that text, to furnish it with a final signified, to close the writing'. Nonetheless, a sick author guides us towards an experience that is radically opposed to Western narratives of progress.

First, authorship becomes an unexplored door rather than a limitation. If medicine under capitalism places the responsibility for health care on the shoulders of individuals, our submission to others' suffering, disorientation, and perplexing metaphors liberates us from the narrative anxiety that considers disease a pause or wreck in an otherwise positive timeline. Considering the author strengthens the necessity of including racial, gender, and economic disparities when reading texts of illness.

Second, the tradition of modern poetry allows to preserve the authorship but in an extreme version. Modern poetics can shape the defeat of biomedical mythology because the acknowledgment of failure resides within modern poetry. This language of defeat allows author–patients to embrace and portray pain and existential crisis without embedding them in a larger linear story. The authorship, now, does not offer stability to the reader. When we do not impose our narrative anxiety, a poetics that does not communicate emerges as an ethical way to approach disease.

References

Andrews A. Lean Forward and Listen. Poetry as a Mode of Understanding in Medicine. *Perspectives in Biology and Medicine*. 2015; 58: 9–24.

Aryan A. 2020. *The Post-War Novel and the Death of the Author*. Tübingen: Palgrave Macmillan.

Barthes R. 1977. The Death of the Author. In: *Image, Music, Text*. London: Fontana, 142–48.

Bleakley A, Neilson S. 2021. *Poetry in the Clinic. Towards a Lyrical Medicine*. Abingdon: Routledge.

Culler J. 2015. *Theory of the Lyric*. Cambridge/London: Harvard University Press.

Derrida J. 2002 (originally pub. 1970). Structure, Sign, and Play in the Discourse of the Human Sciences. In: *Writing and Difference*. London: Routledge, 351–70.

Diedrich L. 2007. *Treatments. Language, Politics, and the Culture of Illness*. Minneapolis, MN: University of Minnesota Press.

Eagleton T. 2008. *How to Read a Poem*. Oxford: Blackwell Publishing.

Foucault M. 1998. What is An Author? In: JD Faubion (ed.) *Aesthetics, Methods, and Epistemology.* New York, NY: The New York Press, 205–22.

Foucault M. 2003. *The Birth of the Clinic. An Archaeology of Medical Perception.* London: Routledge.

Frank A. 1997. *The Wounded Storyteller. Body, Illness, and Ethics.* Chicago, IL: The Chicago University Press.

Frank A. 2014. Healing. In: B Jennings (ed.) *Bioethics.* Farmington Hills: MacMillan, 1399–406.

Friedrich H. 1979. *The Structure of Modern Poetry from the Mid-Nineteenth to the Mid-Twentieth Century.* Evanston: Northwestern University Press.

Heath C. 2006. Body Work. The Collaborative Production of the Clinical Object. In: J Heritage, DW Maynard (eds.) *Communication in Medical Care. Interaction between Primary Care Physicians and Patients.* Cambridge: Cambridge University Press, 185–213.

Leveen L. Metastatic Metaphors. Poetry, Cancer Imagery, and the Imagined Self. *Perspectives in Biology and Medicine.* 2019; 62: 737–57.

Lihn E. 2018. *Poesía reunida.* Santiago: Ediciones Universidad Diego Portales.

Marston J. Metaphorical Language and Terminal Illness. Reflections Upon Images of Death. *Literature and Medicine.* 1986; 5: 109–21.

McEntyre M. A Short Long Story: Mapping the Course of Pain. *Genre.* 2011; 44: 277–91.

Paz O. 1975. *The Children of Mire. Modern Poetry from Romanticism to the Avant-Garde.* Cambridge, MA: Harvard University Press.

Reisz S. 1986. *Teoría literaria. Una propuesta.* Lima: Pontificia Universidad Católica del Perú.

Romero Suarez DA. Latin American Cancer Poetry: Medicine, Political Violence and Collective Memory. *Modern Language Notes.* 2021; 136: 292–312.

Scarry E. 1985. *The Body in Pain. The Making and Unmaking of the World.* New York, NY: Oxford University Press.

12

NOURISHED BY EXPERIENCES

Meaning without metaphysics in
the poetry of Dannie Abse

W Richard Bowen

Introduction: a question of depth

Dannie Abse was one of the most prominent and prolific literary figures with strong associations with Wales during the second half of the twentieth century and the early part of the twenty-first century. His extensive literary work – especially poetry, and also plays, novels and memoirs – was widely read, and his poetry readings were very popular. He played significant roles in the literary lives of both Wales and London. Two features of his life led to the subject matter of his poetry having distinctive characteristics. Firstly, his upbringing in a Jewish family led to his being well versed in the traditions and literature of his heritage; yet, as a secular Jew, he was also aware of the paradoxes of faith in an era of the ascendancy of science. Secondly, his medical education and his extensive experiences as a practising medical doctor gave him an acute sensitivity to the fragile, bodily nature of our lives, and also a heightened awareness of the limitations of scientific approaches, particularly in the alleviation of suffering. His outlook was strongly influenced by the tragedies experienced by Jewish people in twentieth-century Europe.[1]

In view of the scope and quality of Abse's writing, it is curious that his work has received relatively little serious consideration. The writer Vernon Scannell has referred to Abse as a writer who, 'while being given respectful notices in the literary press, has never been awarded the deeply considered evaluation warranted by the seriousness and consistently high quality of his poetry'.[2] Abse's most systematic commentator, the poet and academic Tony Curtis, has described him as 'a writer who has not received the critical attention which he deserves'.[3] Others, while giving broadly positive evaluations of Abse's work, have suggested that his writing lacks philosophical and intellectual depth. For instance, the poet William Oxley has written that 'he needs a stronger philosophical conviction – a more positive element or cosmic commitment – to turn his poetry into really great poetry',[4] and poet and academic Tony Conran repeatedly criticises Abse's 'middlebrow' approach, seeing it as indicating 'something that can be framed and enjoyed in isolation, like a holiday snap. It tends to imply that people and worlds are knowable', while at the same time recognising that '[t]he paradox is that Dannie Abse does not believe in such knowledge'.[5]

DOI: 10.4324/9781003341796-17

At least some of this criticism seems to arise from a confusion of clarity of expression with lack of depth, a phenomenon that Abse has himself noted in a discussion of poets such as Edward Thomas, Robert Frost and William Carlos Williams:

> There are those poets who present difficulty, and in doing so provide a living for critics. There are other poets . . . who are much more lucid and, therefore, don't get the attention they deserve . . . the more difficult a poet is, the quicker he'll get attention.[6]

He also wrote of how 'those poets/who write enigmatic nonsense become famously/the darlings of the professors they most despise'.[7] The lack of serious critical attention appears to have been a personal concern of his, as he wrote of himself in the penultimate poem of his last collection:

> Wide awake or half asleep you liked to be
> deceptive, yet never babblative enough
> to employ the bald serious scholars'.[8]

Abse's writing certainly never exhibits the confusion that the term 'babblative' suggests. Indeed, he identifies clarity of writing and stylistic accessibility as being a characteristic of the work of accomplished doctor-writers. This he attributes to their training in 'decoding mysterious signs and symptoms' and their concomitant impatience with those who 'muddy their own waters so as to appear more deep', as Nietzsche expressed it.[9] Yet, the clarity and accessibility in his own poetry can also be deliberately deceptive, as he explains in the Introductory Note to his first volume of collected poems:

> For some time now my ambition has been to write poems which appear translucent but are in fact deceptions. I would have a reader enter them, be deceived he could see through them like sea-water, and be puzzled when he can not quite touch bottom.[10]

This intriguing description of a reading experience shows that Abse certainly aimed at intellectual depth. Moreover, he regarded commitment to both accessibility and depth – or, as he put it, a 'duty to communicate person to person' and being 'unashamed of soul' – as also being characteristic features of Anglo-Welsh poetry, with which he identified.[11] Abse's commitment to depth is also apparent in his expression of dissatisfaction with a tendency to banality and superficiality in some of the 1950s work of the 'Movement' writers, such as Philip Larkin and Kingsley Amis, whose work was in part a reaction to the richly evocative poetry of W. B. Yeats and Dylan Thomas:

> The new choir that moves in is neat and sane
> and dare not whistle in the dark again.
> Proudly English, they sing with sharp, flat voices
> but no-one dances, nobody rejoices'.[12]

In contrast, as the examples in the present article will illustrate, Abse's own poetry shows openness to a rich diversity of human experience, including its religious, professional, scientific and interpersonal aspects. Abse has written that as his poetry matured he sought a 'conversational' tone,

> rooted in common reality . . . I looked outward to start from the visible and I was startled by the visible . . . Abstract ideas as a partial source for poems ceased to interest me; instead my

poems were nourished by experiences, imagined and factual, my own and others', ordinary and extraordinary.[13]

This conversational tone characterises Abse's personal poetic voice, and it becomes increasingly apparent from his work of the late 1950s and onwards. What follows in the present article is an exploration and analysis proposing an understanding of how Abse did indeed achieve profundity, without the need for an explicit, abstract metaphysical framework, by considering two major aspects of his mature work: his engagement with his Jewish heritage, particularly through its literature, and his sensitive portrayal of medical experiences and the insights that arose from them. These are topics with which he continually engaged, with a deliberate awareness of an element of repetition: 'perhaps without repetition there would be no character, no style'.[14] Where appropriate, I consider Abse's approach in the context of the writings of leading modern philosophers, particularly Emmanuel Levinas and Ludwig Wittgenstein, and the literary analyst Susan Handelman, providing comparisons that demonstrate the depth of his thinking.

Faith in literature

Though both of Dannie Abse's parents were Jewish, his mother was practising but his father was not.[15] As a child he took part in the life of the local synagogue, including Hebrew classes, the latter apparently without great success.[16] Indeed, though he valued having been taught biblical stories and listening to sermons referring to current affairs, both in English, his overall view of the synagogue was not positive: 'I did not like the synagogue. I could not understand the Hebrew address to the one God which the elders there uttered so devoutly. Their chanting seemed so ineffably sad and, like God, inexplicable'.[17] By the age of fifteen he had ceased to attend synagogue or to say Hebrew prayers, becoming interested rather 'in the green ordinary world where God only existed because He was absent'; except that, for the young Abse, the ordinariness of the world itself was extraordinary and he already had a resolve 'to start with the visible and to be startled by the visible'.[18]

Despite this early renunciation of Jewish practices, Abse's relationship to religion was one of the most pervasive and complex influences in his search for meaning. At one level, he maintained a clear and frequently expressed alienation from organised religion, evident in his vehement dislike of conventional religious practitioners, whom he described as 'God's robots', and in his reaction to religious buildings: 'Inside soaring places of worship – Jewish, Moslem or Christian – I feel not just secular but utterly estranged like one without history or memory'.[19] However, alongside such rejection there are many other, often subtle, levels of interaction with religion in his writing. At a fundamental level, Abse's vocational commitment to writing is itself quintessentially Jewish. The prominent French writer Edmond Jabès has described Jews as the 'race born of the book', 'for Judaism and writing are but the same waiting, the same hope, the same depletion'.[20] Moreover, Joseph Cohen has seen Abse's writing as being consistent with central aspects of Judaism, suggesting a relationship to a key concern of Jewish mystics, 'to fathom the mystery of Creation by determining the mysterious relationship of language to it'.[21] There are certainly in Abse's writing parallels with rabbinic thought patterns, with the 'relentless skepticism of the Rabbis – manifested in the constant search for alternative explanations' and with the uncovering of meaning in the physical world 'without the abstracting, idealizing movement of Western thought'.[22] The Jewish literary analyst Susan Handelman has further observed that historically for the rabbis 'the primary reality was linguistic; true being was a God who *speaks* and creates *texts*, and *imitatio deus* was not silent suffering, but speaking and interpreting'.[23] Abse showed his engagement with this linguistic reality of Judaism by his multifaceted interaction with its texts. He engaged seriously, if sceptically, with Scripture and even advised his granddaughter to do likewise. His advice to her was that such writing provides access to a valuable kind of experience and that it is not necessary to be devout to learn from the narratives of the Hebrew Bible. He wrote: 'They do not stale or fade/and may fortify and mollify', but added that it is best to forgive the 'triumphalism and the pride' and to avoid the 'curses and the ritual stuff'.[24]

It is particularly the moral complexity of biblical texts that fascinated Abse as he showed, for example, in his extended and complex poetical retelling of the story of David and Bathsheba, which combines elements of the laconic original with a commentary that has been described as sometimes being in the modes of the Music Hall, *Carry On* films and modern tabloid newspapers.[25] The original story tells of how an innocent, everyday activity, such as King David taking an evening stroll, can have grave consequences, including an adulterous relationship and the murder of Bathsheba's husband. Abse's interpretation also imagines the complicity and moral slide of Bathsheba:

> Of course she hankered for the Palace.
>   Royal charisma switched her on.
> Her husband snored at the Eastern Front,
>   so first a kiss, then scruples gone.[26]

This exhibits the humour that is characteristic of Abse's mature writing, yet variations on a refrain, 'their teeth like milk were white,/and their mouths like wine were red', repeatedly draw attention to the moral complexity of the actions, indeed to their deadly consequences through allusion to Coleridge's 'The Rime of the Ancient Mariner'.[27] There is a sense of darkness even at the most light-hearted moments, such as the imagined breakfast following their first encounter: 'the apple-flesh as usual/after the bite turned brown'.[28] This is an ominous phrase which, typically for Abse, includes further biblical reference, to the Eden narrative. Thus, beneath the humour are serious considerations of the original text, an example of depth in Abse's thought – in this case ethical reflection – that the outward lightness of his writing at first disguises.

Abse also had a fascination with Jewish tales outside the Bible. Indeed, in keeping with a living tradition, he created some himself, such as several stories about Itzig, a kind of religious fool: 'My neighbour, Itzig,/has gone queer with religion'.[29] Itzig's dog also appears in poems, and can apparently be an important link in his prayerful relationship with God: 'when I say please God this/and thank God that,/then God always makes, believe me,/the dog's tail wag'.[30] For Itzig, God can answer in mysterious ways. Abse seems in such poems not so much to be making fun of religion as to be seeing the humour in religion. Indeed, Jewish tales often combine truth, tradition and humour, with the latter being an unexpected component of an approach to truth for those more familiar with the dry approaches of Western academic philosophy. Such a synthesis occurs in a poem of Abse's in which a woman asks a rabbi where the God who once appeared to her as a child has been since:

> Rabbi Shatz turns, he squints,
> he stands on one leg
> hoping for the inspiration of a Hillel.
> The Holy One, he answers, blessed be He,
> has been waiting, waiting patiently,
> till you see Him again.[31]

Here Rabbi Shatz imitates the ancient Jewish sage Hillel, who was asked to explain the Torah while standing on one foot. Abse has said that in this poem he was trying to catch the 'wry flavour' of certain Yiddish tales.[32] The importance of stories in Jewish thought is an aspect of a cautious attitude to generalisation, so that tales applying principles have a priority over direct statements of principles, described by Handelman as 'the priority of the concrete embodiment of a thought over its abstract representation'.[33] Abse imaginatively engaged with such traditions but was also aware of the diminishment which they have experienced, as he described in an account of a Kabbalistic rabbi, Baal Shem, who, when he had a difficult task to undertake, would 'go to a certain place in the woods, light a fire and meditate in prayer – and what he had set out to perform was done'. Generations later neither the place nor the prayers were known, nor was the fire lit – all that remained was the story of how it was done.[34] This expresses a key aspect of Abse's attitude to his Jewish heritage – that engaging with the literature provides a valuable approach to exploring meaning in our existence, but that the practices of organised religion have lost much of their spiritual significance.

Abse was also knowledgeable about Christianity, in the first instance at least because he had attended a Catholic secondary school, as 'the only Jewish boy' at St Illtyd's in Cardiff.[35] He writes that he did not feel much alienated there, but he seems at times to have been subject to 'inquisitions' by the Christian brother teachers to which he could reply, 'All I believe in, Brother, is wonder'.[36] His poem 'The Abandoned' unusually uses explicitly Christian imagery to explore a central theme of post-Holocaust Jewish thought, the apparent withdrawal or hiddenness of God. The importance of this theme to Abse is shown by his repeated revisions of this poem: it appeared in his *Poems: Golders Green* (1962), in revised form in *New and Collected Poems* (2003) and in further revised and expanded form in *Ask the Moon* (2014).[37] The original version is prefaced by two quotations from George Herbert, 'Where is my God? what hidden place/Conceals thee still?/What covert dare eclipse thy face?/Is it thy will?', and 'thy absence doth excel/All distance known'.[38] The position described in Abse's poem is not atheistic; it is not an absence even of absence. Indeed it refers to hiddenness rather than an absence: 'we have to hold our breath to hear you breathing'. Furthermore, Abse suggests a double abandonment: God has abandoned his people and his people have hence abandoned God:

> Dear God in the end you had to go.
> Dismissing you, your absence made us sane.
> We keep the bread and wine for show.[39]

Just as the tale of Baal Shem suggests that the practices of organised Judaism have lost much of their significance, so this reference to the Eucharist, the central aspect of organised Christian worship, suggests that, for Abse, the practices of Christianity have suffered a similar loss of spiritual content.

Even so, Abse's writing also expresses a persistent worry that he may be missing something about religion, that he is 'like the deaf man/who knows nothing of music or of dance//yet blurts out, observing musicians play/and dancers dance – Stupid, how stupid'.[40] His poetry sometimes expresses longings for religious experiences, 'Let me believe in angels for an hour.//Let long theatrical beams slant down/to stage- strike that hill into religion. Me too!'[41] Indeed, he occasionally seems to have had such experiences:

> There are moments when a man must sing
> of a lone Presence he cannot see.

. . .

There are moments when a man must praise
The astonishment of being alive[42]

The language here – 'sing . . . Presence . . . praise' – is evocative of key aspects of the expression of religious faith. This is characteristic of Abse's alertness to the world around him and of his open-ness to all types of experience: he does not replace religious dogma with a dogmatic secularism. However, sometimes his descriptions are more ambiguous:

Repeated desert, recurring drought,
sometimes hearing water trickle,
sometimes not, I, by doubting first,
believe: believing doubt.[43]

This poem intriguingly appears to refer both to spiritual experiences and to the writing of poetry. More frequently, any expression of experiences of ultimate reality in his poetry is deeply uncertain, as in the dialogue poem 'Hunt the Thimble' based around the children's game of the same name:

Is it like that? Or hours after that even:
and darkness inside a dead man's mouth?

No, no, I have told you:
you are cold, and you cannot describe it.[44]

Here the bleak imagery of the phrase 'darkness inside a dead man's mouth' indicates an intimate knowledge of death that reflects Abse's medical background. The uncertainties about liminal experiences which such a background can induce are also apparent in a line in a late poem, 'I was close to Eternity the other night', which, though it evokes Henry Vaughan's famous 'I saw Eternity the other night', describes the side effects of a drug following a medical emergency.[45] Indeed, it is Abse's knowl-edge and experiences as a medical professional that are a second source of pervasive and complex influences on his mature poetry, and another key aspect through which his writing achieved profundity.

A suffering doctor

A doctor-poet has been described as 'a creature rare enough in nature to be worthy of special notice', though they include such fine poets as Henry Vaughan, John Keats and Robert Bridges.[46] It is exceptional for doctor-poets to write explicitly and extensively about their medical experi-ences in their poetry; indeed, Abse's assessment of Keats is that he 'turned away from his fearful experiences at Guy's . . . his poetry . . . is almost free of medical references'.[47] In modern times, the leading American doctor-poet William Carlos Williams only occasionally made direct use of his medical experiences in his poems; and the influential Czech doctor-poet Miroslav Holub wrote about medical science rather than medical practice, for his career was mainly in research.[48] Abse's extensive and explicit incorporation of medical themes in his poetry is thus very unusual: by his own reckoning, twenty-eight out of the 180 poems in his second extended collected poems 'were (are) indisputably medically coloured'.[49] The collection was itself entitled *White Coat, Purple Coat*, referring to his dual personal commitment to medicine and poetry.[50] However, like Keats, Abse found his medical training and early experiences as a doctor traumatic: 'as a medical student, I was spiritually bruised by what I had witnessed in Casualty or in Outpatients at Westminster Hospital'.[51] It was only from 1962, with an increasing conviction that 'poetry should immerse itself in common reality, not be an escape from it', that he began to write poems that 'touched strenuously' on his medical experience.[52]

The first of these poems, 'Pathology of Colours', shows how profoundly such experience could influence his outlook, for whereas rainbows often give rise to feelings of wonder and beauty, for a doctor such colours may be bleakly associated with acute medical conditions:

> So in the simple blessing of a rainbow,
> in the bevelled edge of a sunlit mirror,
> I have seen, visible, Death's artefact
> like a soldier's ribbon on a tunic tacked.[53]

Here there is no Wordsworthian leaping heart, nor is there mention of the covenant with Noah: this rainbow is associated with death and violence. Even in the late 1980s, the memories of his early medical student experiences in the dissecting room at King's College were still sufficiently intense for him to write a long poem meditating on the unpleasantness of such activity and its relationship to life and death:

> You, anonymous. Who were you, mister?
> Your thin mouth could not reply, 'Absent, sir,'
> or utter with inquisitionary rage.[54]

Abse regarded this essential component of medical studies as a violation of a once living person, and it troubled him greatly. A medical education gives students encounters with suffering and death of an intimacy and intensity rarely experienced by other young people. Abse's writing shows that the resulting 'spiritual bruising' – itself a description of unusual intensity – can have a profound and long-lasting effect.

Abse's poetry becomes especially intense when later in life he looks with his doctor's experience at the suffering of those closest to him, such as his dying father:

> he's thin as Auschwitz in that bed.
> . . .
> so like a child I question why
> night with stars, then night without end.[55]

The reference to Auschwitz in such a personal context is likely only appropriate for a writer of Jewish heritage. Yet, the final lines of the quotation, which are also the final lines of the poem, confirm that such heritage does not provide definitive answers for Abse: in this situation he feels that he has no more understanding of death than he did as a child. His experience of his mother's death was also extremely traumatic, in this case expressed in biblical terms:

> As my colleague prepares the syringe
> (the drip flees its hour glass)
> I feel the depression of Saul,[56]

As this poem continues, still with a biblical vocabulary, Abse recalls the story of David and Bathsheba, 'out of so much suffering/came forth the other child,/the wise child, the Solomon',[57] and
asks a question:

> but what will spring from this
> unredeemed, needless degradation,
> this concentration camp for one?

He can find no explanation of, or benefit from, his mother's suffering, the intensity of which is
again expressed in terms of the Holocaust.[58] When asked about death in a later interview, Abse first
replied, 'You see, I haven't any conscious attitude or *weltanschauung* now about death. I have no
view really. Death is zero plus zero', before reflecting and adding: 'Well, I have a view: I find it
repugnant'.[59] Experience of his own illness was also deeply troubling to Abse, as expressed in the
probably autobiographical 'Prayer in the Waiting Room':

> Banished from health I enter the unknown
> as the two did stumbling from Paradise.
> . . .
> Now, doctor, magic me.[60]

Here he reverts to biblical imagery to describe the powerfully troubling uncertainty of his experience: illness portends a bleak future, such as Adam and Eve faced on being banished from
the pleasures of the garden of Eden. Further, the word 'magic' alludes to the desperation often
associated with serious illness, as well as to Abse's fascination with those whose healing abilities appear to depend mostly on charisma, such as Franz Anton Mesmer, the wearer of a purple
cloak.[61] Despite medicine's many benefits, its ultimate insufficiency in the face of suffering
and death makes doctors clearly aware of the limitations of science. Abse was a doctor who
did not exalt science unduly, as he explored in a meditation on the insights achievable with a
stethoscope:

> Should I
> kneel before it, chant an apophthegm
> from a small text? Mimic priest or rabbi,
> the swaying noises of religious men?
> Never! Yet I could praise it.[62]

This contrasts with the almost religious exaltation of science expressed in the writings of contemporary scientific new-atheists such as Richard Dawkins.[63] Abse's view of science was more
balanced: he recognised and made use of its benefits in his extensive medical work, but he did not
base his world-view solely on it.

Abse was strongly affected by the extreme physical and psychic suffering experienced by
Jewish people in twentieth-century Europe. He wrote often of the Holocaust, observing that
'Auschwitz has made me more of a Jew than Moses did', and remarking: 'I often think about my
not going to Belsen'.[64] The latter quotation refers most immediately to his not being allowed to
travel to Germany to give medical treatment to survivors, as he was a Jew, but also to his own
avoidance of the fate of the victims. Abse has suggested that to continue living as happily as

possible we suppress the memory of events such as Auschwitz, with consequences of which we are unaware:

> So who can tell what psychic devastation has really taken place within us, the survivors, especially for those of us who were brought up in an optimistic tradition, heirs of the 19th century, who believed in the inevitability of human progress, and who thought that the soul of man was born pure?[65]

The latter part of this quotation refers to the teaching he received as a boy that 'man was essentially good', as expressed in this morning prayer: 'My God, the soul which thou hast given me is pure'.[66] Part of Abse's response to these issues is his play, *The Dogs of Pavlov*, dramatising the controversial experiments of Yale University psychologist Stanley Milgram, who explored the propensity of individuals to inflict suffering on others for some supposed higher cause.[67] This exploration of 'the banality of Evil' – the apparent propensity of many humans to carry out acts contrary to their conscience if instructed to do so by a figure of authority – also questioned the ethics of Milgram's own experiment, which in Abse's re-imagining was carried out by doctors.[68] He knew that doctors and scientists are also figures of authority who can claim to be serving some higher cause, scientific enquiry, which he provocatively terms 'the fatherland of Science'.[69]

The psychic damage caused by the savagery of twentieth-century life is also the subject of Abse's long poem 'Funland' and the accomplished play *Pythagoras* that developed from it, in both of which many of his key themes converge.[70] Both are set in a psychiatric hospital, so here Abse develops insights into aspects of medicine beyond his immediate personal practice. A central character of the play (and also of the poem) is a man who believes himself to be a reincarnation of the eponymous sixth-century BC Greek philosopher, whose thought combined science, mathematics and an intellectual kind of mysticism.[71] An important theme of the play is the clash between the cold scientific approach of the superintendent, Dr Aquillus, and the richer yet apparently delusional imagination of Pythagoras. Pythagoras accuses Aquillus of having no religious intuitions, of not seeing the revelation in the world around him. He expresses regret that even some of his own pupils apprehended the scientific side of his teachings but neglected the ethical and magical sides. An additional important theme of the play is the power of the medical profession: 'the doctor-patient relationship is based on the assumption that the doctor has superior knowledge to the patient'.[72] This power can be abused, as in a scene when the patients are humiliated by being displayed and questioned before medical students. However, it is not always easy to distinguish between the 'sane' and the 'insane' – a visiting journalist mistakes Pythagoras for the superintendent and the superintendent for a dangerous patient – and the doctors can also have trouble making such distinctions. Even so, at the end of the play the cold rationality of science triumphs. Pythagoras prepares to leave the hospital after receiving 'electroconvulsive therapy' to take up a humdrum job rather than his previous profession of stage magician. The last words of the superintendent are, 'Don't call him Pythagoras. His name is Tony Smith'.[73] Abse was a poet who resolved to start with the visible and to be startled by the visible, who was astonished by the 'irreducible strangeness of things'.[74] His plays, which he regarded as the work of a poet,[75] are among his most expressive accounts of the dangers of a modern world in which a reductive scientific outlook is dominant: in *Pythagoras* the denial of the autonomy, indeed the personhood, of the patients by the medical hierarchy is particularly troubling.

Meaning without metaphysics: philosophical parallels

The profundity of Abse's work can be further appreciated by considering parallels with the writings of leading modern philosophers. To begin with a key example, Abse characteristically remarked that 'Auschwitz made me more of a Jew than Moses did' and wrote of the great suffering of Jewish people in the twentieth century without finding any rationalisation. Here, it is pertinent to compare his attitude to that of Emmanuel Levinas, one of the leading Jewish philosophers of the twentieth century, who in his essay 'Useless Suffering' wrote: 'The disproportion between suffering and every theodicy was shown at Auschwitz with a glaring, obvious clarity'.[76] Levinas wrote of 'the obligation for Jews to live and to remain Jews, in order not to be made accomplices of a diabolical project'; and Abse did so through his extensive, imaginative engagement with Jewish texts.[77] For example, a poem such as 'Events Leading to the Conception of Solomon, the Wise Child', discussed earlier, could be considered to be in the spirit of *midrash*, 'a dominant mode of Jewish reading of the Bible . . . with its imperative to connect with the biblical text, its irrepressible playfulness, and its delight in multiple, polyvalent traditions of interpretation'.[78] Ancient and modern rabbis have preferred such imaginative interpretation, lying between pure commentary and creative composition, as a means of finding a text's significance for the present moment, rather than the more systematic, academic approach characteristic of Christian theologians.[79]

Abse's antagonism to the institutional aspects of organised religion is consonant with his distrust of hierarchy, but his strongly expressed dislike of non-hierarchical, practising religious believers is puzzling, particularly as he had a close relationship with his religiously practising mother. Here it is useful to consider Levinas's distinction between totalisers and infinitisers.[80] Abse may have considered 'God's robots' to be what Levinas terms totalisers, seeking control of understanding by focusing on closed orders of knowledge; indeed, the capabilities of robots are fully defined by the specific set of instructions in the computer code that controls them. In contrast, Abse was himself an infinitiser, seeking creative advance in his life by using his imagination in ways that were essentially exploratory rather than definitively explanatory. But there are also lacunae in his knowledge, such as his misunderstanding of the nature of prayer: he wrote a highly ironic poem about George Herbert's description of prayer as 'reversed thunder', and elsewhere commented, 'yet what is more arrogant than prayer? It's like looking up at the blue sky or towards the darkness behind the vast stars to exclaim narcissistically, "Here I am God"'.[81] The last phrase of this quotation resonates with the Hebrew *hineni*, an expression occurring at several key points in the Bible.

Yet, it is not an arrogant expression, as leading philosopher, and practising Jew, Hilary Putnam has explained, but is rather an offering of oneself: '"hineni!" performs the speech act of *presenting myself*, the speech act of *making myself available to another*'.[82] Abse may also have had unrealistically high expectations for the direct numinous experience in the physical world that he seems to regret lacking. In a poem echoing parts of Matthew Arnold's lament for the fading of religious belief in 'Dover Beach', he writes of looking down from cliffs 'to read the unrolling/holy scrolls of the sea. They are/blank . . .// The tide *is* out'.[83] Yet, even for the prophet Elijah the LORD appeared not in a great and mighty wind, an earthquake or fire but as 'a soft murmuring sound', 'a still, small voice' (I Kings 19. 11–12).

Each language may be considered to be 'a system of concepts as well as forms'.[84] Abse knew that the power of expression varies between languages: 'Say now in Yiddish:/"Exile. Pogrom. Wandering. Holocaust."/Say now in Hebrew:/"Blessed Art Thou O Lord"'.[85] Hebrew is a language particularly associated with religious speech, yet Abse wrote solely in the more secular English, and this may also be a factor in his decision to use his rare numinous experiences to write poems 'sitting comfortably in my study far from the thistle-eating donkey and the desert of religion'.[86]

He has also written that he believed that if one reaches 'God' it is through pleasurable experiences and creative activities: 'And writing poetry, by the way, is a kind of singing and a kind of beautiful work that names things. And the naming of things, itself, ultimately – a country, or a star, a flower or a baby – is a kind of worship'.[87] The names in this prose statement are notably evocative of Henry Vaughan's great poem of Christian faith 'Peace', again illustrating Abse's openness to the insights of religion as expressed in literature – his outlook is explicitly informed by such insights even though he rejects the practices of organised religion.[88] Nevertheless, Abse realised that poetry can also be debased, as dramatically demonstrated by the character Mr Poet in a purple plastic coat repeating solely single-word obscenities in 'Funland'.

An important philosophical parallel can also be drawn with the muted response to science in Abse's poetry. Abse was a poet with a high-level scientific education, a man who repeatedly declared his secularity and resolved to start with the visible and to be startled by the visible. He has been accurately described as 'representative of the professional in a technological world who is profoundly disturbed by and suspicious of that modern world'.[89] It is, therefore, surprising that pure science features so little in his poetry and other writings – he seeks meaning elsewhere. One of the few sustained instances is an early poem addressed to his friend, fellow doctor and poet Alex Comfort: after a description of the work of several distinguished scientists, the poem concludes:

> And the old professor must think you mad, Alex, as you rehearse
> poems in the laboratory like vows, and curse those clever scientists
> who dissect away the wings and haggard heart from the dove.[90]

These lines attribute to Comfort a profound dislike of the reductionist tendencies of science, a view which the poem indicates is also that of the poet. In a later poem that recounts the fundamental discoveries of several notable doctors, Abse describes himself as, 'their slowcoach colleague, half afraid,/incurious', and he notes that he had been so even as a boy.[91] Thus, the dearth of reference to science likely partly reflects his personal disposition, but a second factor seems to be his strong awareness of how little we know, and of the interim nature of the knowledge that we presently have:

> I should know by now that few octaves can be heard,
> that a vision dies from being too long stared at[92]

Here Abse suggests that we need to be modest about even the apparently great triumphs of modern science for there may be much beyond the reach of our senses. A further likely factor is his revulsion at the misuse of science. His acclaimed poem 'Pathology of Colours' deals not only with acute medical conditions but also with the use of nuclear weapons, 'the criminal, multi-coloured flash/ of an H-bomb', and the threat of nuclear war is apparent in several other poems.[93] Indeed, military violence is wrong, shameful and often linked to science in Abse's outlook. Furthermore, as previously discussed, his plays *The Dogs of Pavlov* and *Pythagoras* display a distrust of the application of science when associated with powerful hierarchies.

The muted response to science in Abse's poetry can be more profoundly understood by considering his work in the context of an important aspect of the writings of the philosopher Ludwig Wittgenstein. Wittgenstein was very concerned by the modern hegemony of scientific explanations, particularly as many of the most important questions about meaning and value in our lives are not scientific questions. Rather these questions require 'a form of life, a set of communally shared practices, together with the ability to hear and see the connections made by practitioners of this form of life'; that is, a culture.[94] In Wittgenstein's view, our preoccupation with science has led to a craving for generality, a generality that excludes the non-theoretical understanding available to us in music, art, creative writing, and shared life.[95]

He wrote that, 'People nowadays think that scientists exist to instruct them, poets, musicians, etc. to give them pleasure. The idea *that these have something to teach them* – that does not occur to them'.[96] He saw that such non-scientific representations had an integrity that was not amenable to general expression in scientific terms. Indeed, they might be characterised by his term 'imponderable evidence', which refers to insights arising from our full range of sensitivities.[97] Key features of imponderable evidence are: that it is seen as evidence for a particular judgement; that its value depends on the experience and knowledge of the person providing it; and that it cannot be evaluated, 'pondered', by appeal to general principles or universal law.[98]

Hence, such evidence has specific and fully personal characteristics that contrast sharply with the general and impersonal nature of science. These features, however, are analogous to the characteristics of rabbinic approaches, and they also describe Abse's use of such approaches as a model for seeking meaning in his poems and plays. On such an evaluation, Abse's writing does not lack philosophical depth or commitment; it is rather consonant with the profound insights of one of the twentieth century's most original and influential philosophers.

Abse's sensitivity to suffering was closely linked to his acute awareness as a doctor of the bodily nature of our existence and hence of the fragility of our lives and activities, even apparently refined and abstract activities: 'Poetry is written in the brain/but the brain is bathed in blood'.[99] Conventional philosophical metaphysics often neglects this aspect of our existence: a focus on our human vulnerability contrasts with the characteristic Western esteem of strength and autonomy. Such bodily fragility is perceptively explored in Abse's account of ill-fated brain surgery, where the patient apparently cries out:

'Leave my soul alone, leave my soul alone,'
. . .
                                        till the antique
gramophone wound down and the words began
to blur and slow, '. . . leave . . . my . . . soul . . . alone . . .'
to cease at last when something other died.[100]

The poem is not only an account of fragility and medical failure, it also broaches the complex issue of the relationship between mind and body. Scientific explanations of consciousness have frequently used models based on the technology and science of their time, such as clocks, telephone exchanges, computers, programmes and quantum mechanics, or in this poem a gramophone.[101] However, as science is concerned with objectively measurable properties of the world, and as consciousness consists of qualitative, subjective awareness, consciousness lies, strictly speaking, outside the realm of science, and there is also little place in science for a soul. Yet, Abse knew that it is difficult to avoid such language if we are to express the richness of life, if we are to experience well-being: ' "I've lost my soul," the sick man said/(the soul does not like a sick body)'.[102] Abse's poetry attempts no explanation of such personal suffering: his response may rather be seen in his practical contributions to the alleviation of suffering during his long medical career. This is consonant with what Levinas describes as 'the fundamental ethical problem which pain poses "for nothing": the inevitable and pre-emptory ethical problem of the medication which is my duty'.[103] Unlike Levinas, Abse had the professional skills necessary to act on this assessment, and did so.

Despite his sometimes bleak view of existence Abse has described his poems as being those of a fortunate man and he repeatedly observed that, before the tragic death of his wife in an accident, he had 'been nearly as happy as possible'.[104] Abse's writings show that he found a vital source of consolation and meaning in close personal relationships, especially that with his wife: '"He who is without a wife," the Talmud proclaims, "dwells without blessing, life, joy, help, good, and peace"'.[105] Such blessing is expressed by lines in his last collected poems:

> Love, read this though it has little meaning
> for by reading this you give me meaning.[106]

At the same time he was clear that aspects of other persons are always inaccessible, which he expressed in an early poem that seems to be about his wife: 'You raise your eyes from the level book/as if deeply listening. You are further than I call'.[107]

Such inaccessibility can decrease with time, so perhaps it is more correct to say that consolation and meaning in Abse's world were found in long-term close personal relationships. Thus, in a later poem, he meditated on how he would like to die: 'finger-tapping still our private morse, ". . . love you",/before the last flowers and flies descend'.[108] Levinas found in such intimate human encounters a 'glimpse' or 'trace' of God – his view has been succinctly summarised as 'the thought of God arises in humans in all its vividness as one relates to the other'; or, 'The human soul in search of God is referred to a different address: the neighbour'.[109] Abse sought hints of the numinous elsewhere: maybe he was not looking in the most obvious place in his visible world.

The Jewish traditions in which Abse wrote often find meaning in concrete ways without the abstract theorising that is typical of Western thought, and there are many examples of this in Abse's work. One apparently simple instance occurs in his description of an outwardly inexplicable yet meaningful act at a burial:

> I do not know why I picked up two small stones
> . . .
> and why won't I throw these stones away? Don't laugh.[110]

The taking of these stones from a gravel path also expresses Abse's originality, for the Jewish tradition is rather to place a small stone on the grave when leaving.[111] A further poignant example is Abse's description of his dying father sucking a peach, his father's favourite fruit and a gift from his wife, 'perhaps for her sake –/till bright as blood the peachstone showed'.[112] Those who see a lack of depth in Abse's writing have underestimated the significance of such uncovering of meaning without abstract conceptualisation in his work, and his concomitant rejection of the totalising strategies of Western philosophy.

One of Abse's finest representations of the significance of apparently simple things in the visible world is his late poem 'Condensation on a Windowpane' that evokes the epitaph that Keats, his fellow poet and doctor, asked to be placed on his tombstone, 'Here lies One whose Name was writ in Water':

> I want to write something simple
> that everyone can understand,
> something simple as pure water.[113]

The poem laments that to science even water is complicated, it has many structurally complex phases. Even so, Abse writes his wife's name and his own name in capitals with his finger on the glass and recalls their youthful love. Yet with time:

> Our names on the window
> begin to fade.
> Slowly, slowly.
> They weep as they vanish.

Thus, in a series of clear word images Abse captures the significance of simple things, the importance of love, the fragility of life and the tragedy of loss. As throughout his writing, he offers no totalising metaphysical perspective, but rather a sensitive and imaginative appreciation of the meaning that he was fortunate enough to find.

In Western societies we live in an age in which religion is often disparaged and in which science is revered, in which individual strength and autonomy are typically prized and in which abstract thought is cherished. In a spirit of Absean clarity, some simple yet valuable observations contrary to the spirit of our age may be distilled from the present assessment of selected key themes of his mature poetry: engagement with the literature of religious traditions continues to offer great opportunities for making sense of our lives; the practice of science has more limitations than is commonly assumed; we should always remember the fragile, bodily nature of our existence; meaning can be expressed without abstract metaphysical speculation. The profundity of Abse's thought is also apparent in other aspects of his poetry, such as his early more political work, his portrayal of the bizarre aspects of modern society, his poignant accounts of bereavement and his reflections on old age. To provide an account of such themes in his development as a poet, over more than sixty years of publication, was outside the scope of the present article, but his work offers many further opportunities for exploration of the originality and profundity of his thought.

Acknowledgements

I thank Iselin Eie Sokhi for perceptive comments during the development of this article.

Excerpts from *From Ask the Moon* by Dannie Abse published by Hutchinson. Reproduced by permission of The Random House Group Ltd. © 2014. All rights reserved.

Notes

1 Dannie Abse wrote extensive autobiographical prose, with the most accessible collection being *Goodbye, Twentieth Century* (Cardigan: Parthian, 2001). Born in Cardiff in 1923, he attended local elementary and secondary schools, the latter run by Catholic brothers. During the 1940s he studied medicine at the Welsh National School of Medicine (Cardiff), King's College (London) and Westminster Hospital (London), qualifying as a doctor in 1950. He worked as a specialist chest physician at the Central Medical Establishment Chest Clinic (London) between 1954 and 1989. From 1957 he lived with his family in Golders Green, London, and in 1972 they acquired a second house in Ogmore-on-Sea, south Wales. He spent periods as president of the Poetry Society and as president of the Welsh Academy, and received many awards and distinctions. Abse's first volume of poetry was accepted for publication whilst he was still a student and he continued to write and to publish poetry until his death in 2014.

2 Vernon Scannell, 'A Vision of the Street', in Joseph Cohen (ed.), *The Poetry of Dannie Abse* (London: Robson Books, 1983), pp. 26–38.

3 Tony Curtis, '"We Keep the Bread and Wine for Show" – Consistent Irony and Reluctant Faith in the Poetry of Dannie Abse', *Proceedings of the British Academy*, 154 (2008), 337–60.

4 W. Oxley, 'Same Coin, Different Sides – the Poetry of Dannie Abse and Leonard Clark', *Poetry Wales*, 20 (1985), 66–88.

5 Tony Conran, *Frontiers in Anglo-Welsh Poetry* (Cardiff: University of Wales Press, 1997), p. 242.

6 Dannie Abse, in D. H. Brock, 'An Interview With Dannie Abse', *Literature and Medicine*, 3 (1984), 5–18.

7 Dannie Abse, 'Perspectives', in *Ask the Moon: New and Collected Poems 1948–2014* (London: Hutchinson, 2014), p. 311.

8 Dannie Abse, 'Gone', in *Ask the Moon: New and Collected Poems 1948–2014* (London: Hutchinson, 2014), p. 342.

9 Dannie Abse, 'Authorship and Medicine', in *The Two Roads Taken* (London: Enitharmon Press, 2003), p. 12.

10 Dannie Abse, 'Introductory Note', in *Collected Poems 1948–1976* (London: Hutchinson, 1977), p. xi.

11 Dannie Abse, 'Introduction', in Dannie Abse (ed.), *Twentieth Century Anglo-Welsh Poetry* (Bridgend: Seren, 1997), pp. 13–15. The term 'Anglo-Welsh poetry' has, of course, complex connotations. Abse recognised this and his 'Introduction' is followed by a 'Prologue' consisting of twenty-two quotations providing approaches to the term by a wide variety of writers.

12 Dannie Abse, 'Enter the Movement', in *New and Collected Poems* (London: Hutchinson, 2003), p. 32.

13 Dannie Abse, 'Pegasus and the Rocking Horse', in *A Strong Dose of Myself* (London: Hutchinson, 1983), pp. 201–20.

14 Abse, 'Introductory Note', p. xi. The profundity of Abse's thought is also apparent in other aspects of his poetry, such as his early more political work, his portrayal of the bizarre aspects of modern society, his poignant accounts of bereavement and his reflections on old age. However, to provide an account of the many themes in his development as a poet, over more than sixty years of publication, is outside the scope of the present article.

15 Dannie Abse, *The Presence* (London: Vintage Books, 2008), p. 16.

16 Abse, *Goodbye, Twentieth Century*, p. 24.

17 Abse, *Goodbye, Twentieth Century*, p. 21.

18 Abse, *Goodbye, Twentieth Century*, pp. 28–29.

19 Abse, p. 88; Abse, *Goodbye, Twentieth Century*, p. 450.

20 Edmond Jabès, quoted in Jacques Derrida, *Writing and Difference* (London: Routledge, 1978), pp. 64–65.

21 Joseph Cohen, 'Introduction', in Joseph Cohen (ed.), *The Poetry of Dannie Abse* (London: Robson Books, 1983), pp. 7–14.

22 Susan A. Handelman, *The Slayers of Moses: The Emergence of Rabbinic Interpretation in Modern Literary Theory* (New York: SUNY, 1982), pp. 19, 28.

23 Handelman, *The Slayers of Moses*, p. 4.

24 Dannie Abse, 'Inscription on the Flyleaf of a Bible', in *New and Collected Poems* (London: Hutchinson, 2003), p. 377.

25 Tony Curtis, 'White Coat, Purple Coat, Overcoat: The Late Poetry of Dannie Abse', *Poetry Wales*, 34 (1998), 10–16.

26 Dannie Abse, 'Events Leading to the Conception of Solomon, the Wise Child', in *New and Collected Poems* (London: Hutchinson, 2003), p. 379. In the Hebrew Bible, the narrative begins in 2 Samuel 11.

27 '*Her* lips were red, *her* looks were free,/Her locks were yellow as gold:/Her skin was white as leprosy,/The Night-mare LIFE-IN-DEATH was she,/Who thicks man's blood with cold'. Samuel Taylor Coleridge, 'The Rime of the Ancient Mariner', in Helen Gardner (ed.), *The New Oxford Book of English Verse* (Oxford: Oxford University Press, 1972), p. 531.

28 Abse, 'Events Leading to the Conception of Solomon, the Wise Child', p. 382.

29 Dannie Abse, 'My Neighbour, Itzig', in *New and Collected Poems* (London: Hutchinson, 2003), p. 355.

30 Dannie Abse, 'Of Itzig and His Dog', in *New and Collected Poems* (London: Hutchinson, 2003), p. 201.

31 Dannie Abse, 'Tales of Shatz', in *New and Collected Poems* (London: Hutchinson, 2003), p. 176.

32 Dannie Abse, 'Conversations With Dannie Abse', in J. Cohen (ed.), *The Poetry of Dannie Abse* (London: Robson Books, 1983), pp. 151–81. Quotation on p. 179.

33 Handelman, *The Slayers of Moses*, p. 66.

34 Abse, 'Conversations With Dannie Abse', pp. 179–80. See also Dannie Abse, 'The Message', in *New and Collected Poems* (London: Hutchinson, 2003), p. 239.

35 Abse, *Goodbye, Twentieth Century*, p. 26.

36 Abse, 'All Things Bright and Beautiful', in *Ask the Moon: New and Collected Poems 1948–2014* (London: Hutchinson, 2014), p. 259.

37 Dannie Abse, 'The Abandoned', in *Poems: Golders Green* (London: Hutchinson, 1962), p. 37; Abse, 'The Message', p. 55; Abse, 'All Things Bright and Beautiful', p. 28.

38 Changes in the epigraph also indicate his continual engagement with religious thought. In *New and Collected Poems*, the first is replaced by a quotation from the Talmud, 'There is no space occupied by the Shekinah'; in *Ask the Moon*, this is replaced in turn with a quotation from Rainer Maria Rilke's poem 'Du, Nachbar Gott'.

39 Dannie Abse, 'The Abandoned', in *Ask the Moon: New and Collected Poems 1948–2014* (London: Hutchinson, 2014), p. 28.

40 Dannie Abse, 'Encounter at a Greyhound Bus Station', in *New and Collected Poems* (London: Hutchinson, 2003), p. 239.

41 Dannie Abse, 'Watching a Cloud', in *New and Collected Poems* (London: Hutchinson, 2003), p. 167.

42 Dannie Abse, 'The Grand View', in *New and Collected Poems* (London: Hutchinson, 2003), p. 66.

43 Dannie Abse, 'The Water Diviner', in *New and Collected Poems* (London: Hutchinson, 2003), p. 46.

44 Dannie Abse, 'Hunt the Thimble', in *New and Collected Poems* (London: Hutchinson, 2003), p. 84.

45 Dannie Abse, 'Side Effects', in *Ask the Moon: New and Collected Poems 1948–2014* (London: Hutchinson, 2014), p. 321; Henry Vaughan, 'The World', in Anne Cluysenaar (ed.), *Henry Vaughan: Selected Poems*, (London: SPCK, 2004), p. 113.

46 A. H. Jones, 'Literature and Medicine: Physician-Poets', *The Lancet*, 349 (1997), 275–78.

47 Dannie Abse, 'Following in the Footsteps of Dr Keats', in *The Two Roads Taken* (London: Enitharmon Press, 2003), pp. 26–45. 'Guy's' refers to Guy's Hospital in London.

48 William Carlos Williams, *Selected Poems*, ed. Charles Tomlinson (London: Penguin, 2000); Miroslav Holub, *Poems Before and After: Collected English Translations*, trans. Ian Milner et al[0]., 2nd edn (Hexham: Bloodaxe, 2006).

49 Abse, *Goodbye Twentieth Century*, p. 437.

50 Dannie Abse, *While Coat, Purple Coat: Collected Poems 1948–1988* (London: Hutchinson, 1989).

51 Dannie Abse, 'Following in the Footsteps of Dr Keats', p. 37.

52 *Ibid.*, p. 41.

53 Dannie Abse, 'Pathology of Colours', in *New and Collected Poems* (London: Hutchinson, 2003), p. 83.

54 Dannie Abse, 'Carnal Knowledge', in *New and Collected Poems* (London: Hutchinson, 2003), p. 264.

55 Dannie Abse, 'In Llandough Hospital', in *New and Collected Poems* (London: Hutchinson, 2003), p. 98.

56 Dannie Abse, 'Exit', in *New and Collected Poems* (London: Hutchinson, 2003), p. 241.

57 Solomon was the second, but first surviving, child of David and Bathsheba.

58 The use of imagery of concentration camps to describe other types of suffering has caused controversy, notably by Sylvia Plath to describe her personal, inward devastation. Abse was aware of this issue and addressed Plath's work in a sympathetic way in a lecture/essay: Dannie Abse, 'The Dread of Sylvia Plath', in *The Two Roads Taken* (London: Enitharmon Press, 2003), pp. 125–41. His own use differs to Plath's due to his close identification with his Jewish heritage and as he is describing the suffering of others.

59 Dannie Abse, 'An Interview With Dannie Abse at Princeton University', in *The Two Roads Taken* (London: Enitharmon Press, 2003), pp. 229–49.

60 Dannie Abse, 'Prayer in the Waiting Room', in *New and Collected Poems* (London: Hutchinson, 2003), p. 399. See the narrative in Genesis 3 in the Hebrew Bible.

61 Dannie Abse, 'The Charisma of Quacks', in *The Two Roads Taken* (London: Enitharmon Press, 2003), pp. 46–53. Mesmer was an eighteenth-century Viennese physician and showman.

62 Dannie Abse, 'The Stethoscope', in *New and Collected Poems* (London: Hutchinson, 2003), p. 186.

63 Richard Dawkins, *The God Delusion* (London: Bantam, 2006).

64 Abse, *Goodbye, Twentieth Century*, pp. 105, 135.

65 Dannie Abse, 'The Experiment', in *The Dogs of Pavlov* (London: Vallentine, Mitchell, 1973), pp. 13–14.

66 Abse, *Goodbye, Twentieth Century*, p. 106.

67 *The Dogs of Pavlov* was also published in revised form in Dannie Abse, *The View from Row G: Three Plays*, ed. James A. Davies (Bridgend: Seren, 1990). However, this volume does not include Abse's introductory essay, 'The Experiment'.

68 Abse, 'The Experiment', p. 55. The phrase was introduced by Hannah Arendt in her book *Eichmann in Jerusalem: A Report on the Banality of Evil* (Harmondsworth: Penguin, 1994).

69 Abse, 'The Experiment', p. 121.

70 Dannie Abse, 'Funland', in *New and Collected Poems* (London: Hutchinson, 2003), p. 144; Dannie Abse, *Pythagoras* (London: Hutchinson, 1979). The play was republished in *The View from Row G: Three Plays* in unchanged form except that the title became *Pythagoras (Smith)*.

71 Bertrand Russell, *History of Western Philosophy*, 2nd edn (London: George Allen and Unwin, 1961), pp. 49–56.

72 Abse, *Pythagoras*, p. 77.

73 Abse, *Pythagoras*, p. 80.

74 Dannie Abse, 'The Test', in *New and Collected Poems* (London: Hutchinson, 2003), p. 184.

75 Dannie Abse, 'Introduction', in *Pythagoras* (London: Hutchinson, 1979), p. 9.

76 Emmanuel Levinas, 'Useless Suffering', in Robert Bernasconi, David Wood (eds.), *The Provocation of Levinas: Rethinking the Other* (London: Routledge, 1988), pp. 156–67.

77 Levinas, 'Useless Suffering', p. 164. Levinas ascribes this expression to Emil Fackenheim.

78 David Stern, 'Midrash and Jewish Interpretation', in *The Jewish Study Bible* (Oxford: Oxford University Press, 2004), pp. 1863–75.

79 A. E. McGrath, *Christian Theology: An Introduction*, 4th edn (Oxford: Blackwell, 2007).

80 Emmanuel Levinas, *Totality and Infinity* (Pittsburgh: Duquesne University Press, 1969).

81 Dannie Abse, 'The Power of Prayer', in *New and Collected Poems* (London: Hutchinson, 2003), p. 205; Abse, *Goodbye, Twentieth Century*, p. 551.

82 Hilary Putnam, *Jewish Philosophy as a Guide to Life* (Bloomington: Indiana University Press, 2008), p. 74.

83 Dannie Abse, 'A Letter from Ogmore-by-Sea', in *New and Collected Poems* (London: Hutchinson, 2003), p. 356. Arnold's poem 'Dover Beach' refers to the 'melancholy, long, withdrawing roar' of the 'Sea of Faith'. Matthew Arnold, 'Dover Beach', in Helen Gardner (ed.), *The New Oxford Book of English Verse* (Oxford: Oxford University Press, 1972), p. 703.

84 Jonathan Culler, *Literary Theory: A Very Short Introduction* (Oxford: Oxford University Press, 1997), p. 59.

85 Dannie Abse, 'Of Two Languages', in *New and Collected Poems* (London: Hutchinson, 2003), p. 280.

86 Abse, *The Presence*, p. 17.

87 Abse, 'Replies to an Enquiry', in *The Two Roads Taken* (London: Enitharmon Press, 2003), pp. 221–28.

88 Vaughan, 'The World', p. 80. The poem includes the lines, 'My Soul, there is a Countrie/Far beyond the stars,/. . ./And one born in a Manger/. . ./There growes the flowre of peace'.

89 Tony Curtis, *Dannie Abse* (Cardiff: University of Wales Press, 1985), p. 113.

90 Dannie Abse, 'Letter to Alex Comfort', in *New and Collected Poems* (London: Hutchinson, 2003), p. 6.

91 Dannie Abse, 'X-Ray', in *New and Collected Poems* (London: Hutchinson, 2003), p. 194.

92 Dannie Abse, 'Mysteries', in *New and Collected Poems* (London: Hutchinson, 2003), p. 115.

93 Abse, 'Pathology of Colours', p. 83.

94 Ray Monk, 'Wittgenstein and the Two Cultures', *Prospect*, 43 (1999), 66–67.

95 Ludwig Wittgenstein, *The Blue and Brown Books* (Oxford: Basil Blackwell, 1972), pp. 17–18.

96 Ludwig Wittgenstein, *Culture and Value* (Oxford: Basil Blackwell, 1980), p. 36e.

97 Ludwig Wittgenstein, *Last Writings on the Philosophy of Psychology*, vol. I (Oxford: Basil Blackwell, 1982), p. 119e.

98 Ray Monk, *How to Read Wittgenstein* (London: Granta Books, 2005), pp. 102–4.

99 Dannie Abse, 'Sixth-Form Poet', in *New and Collected Poems* (London: Hutchinson, 2003), p. 345.

100 Dannie Abse, 'In the Theatre', in *New and Collected Poems* (London: Hutchinson, 2003), p. 144.

101 J. E. R. Squires, 'Mentality', in Ted Honderich (ed.), *The Oxford Companion to Philosophy*, 2nd edn (Oxford: Oxford University Press, 2005), pp. 586–87. Gramophones were still current technology when the poem appeared in 1973; consumer CD players first became available in the 1980s.

102 Dannie Abse, 'Among a Heap of Stones', in *New and Collected Poems* (London: Hutchinson, 2003), p. 399.

103 Levinas, 'Useless Suffering', p. 158.

104 Abse, 'Portrait of an Old Poet', in *Ask the Moon: New and Collected Poems 1948–2014* (London: Hutchinson, 2014), p. 279.

105 Abse, *The Presence*, p. 228.

106 Abse, 'Postscript', in *Ask the Moon: New and Collected Poems 1948–2014* (London: Hutchinson, 2014), p. 286.

107 Dannie Abse, 'The Moment', in *New and Collected Poems* (London: Hutchinson, 2003), p. 33.

108 Dannie Abse, 'Last Words', in *New and Collected Poems* (London: Hutchinson, 2003), p. 214.

109 Renée D. N. van Riessen, *Man as a Place of God: Levinas' Hermeneutics of Kenosis* (Dordrecht: Springer, 2007), pp. 150, 191.

110 Dannie Abse, 'Two Small Stones', in *New and Collected Poems* (London: Hutchinson, 2003), p. 99.

111 Ronald L. Eisenberg, *The JPS Guide to Jewish Traditions* (Philadelphia: Jewish Publication Society, 2004), p. 91.

112 Dannie Abse, 'Peachstone', in *New and Collected Poems* (London: Hutchinson, 2003), p. 123.

113 Dannie Abse, 'Condensation on a Windowpane', in *New and Collected Poems* (London: Hutchinson, 2003), p. 300.

13

DEBRIDING THE MORAL INJURY

Tolu Oloruntoba

Everything Must Go

In an inversion of the crucifixion of Christ,
my father crucified his mother.

I know it was love. When the nerves below her stroke
shriveled her arm and leg into granite spasm

he came home with medicine men that carved tallies
into her flesh behind arcane doors,

rubbing night, and somehow no tetanus, into the cuts.
It must have been love, how he tried to bludgeon

her hand into obedience. Given hundreds of years, his invention
of physiotherapy might have become medicine.

He did know how to work a captive audience, though,
starting where all surgery began: carpentry.

The bandage, the crossbar he strapped one spastic hand,
and one writhing other, to, recreated the upright

rack he asked our help stretching her out upon; to outrace
the balled fist, the frozen elbow,

the bent knee beyond repair, on daily schedule, her screams
a primal language beyond crumpled speech

DOI: 10.4324/9781003341796-18

cortices. She had pleaded for our help with her eyes,
wondering at our strange cruelty.

Below her cross, in the corridor upstairs, was the scaffold
we built to receive her, the one we tore down,

quiet and urgent, two years later. After the morgue was the fire.
We bagged it all, uprooted her bed

clothes; trinkets of war; castles of pillbottles; the spoons,
even plates   we took turns feeding her with.

The foam mattress, bandages pungent with menthol,
cushion chair. Everything went   quickly

to the pyre   by the banana trees
behind the house.

To the last one,   a wait broken, we were soot, that night.
And after the furnace,

rainstorm collecting her memory through the windows,
rifling the one sepia photo we kept,

there was a lighter patch where her bed had been,
and silence.

The hurricane lamp was an eye we gathered
around as the questions we hurled up

fell outside, worrying the roof, and *we*, buried
hurriedly inside, burned.

Medical Séances

Acolytes, we filed into a darkened temple,
luminous film of arcana below the false priest
at the lectern, casting visions overhead.
In the projection we learned to listen
for the murmurs of hearts that wanted to speak,
and the dead we did not allow to.

Pa James, he with the ligature of his hanging
still on, was our cadaver. We stripped the gnarly
windbreaker of his skin, his fleece of fat, for anatomy.
Routinely felled by formalin fumes at night,
it was worse later, in morbid anatomy, too-gleeful
residents brandishing sternal saws like breadknives.

All the dead could teach was the fear of life, and how
it can end. Benign sturgeons-general, schools in tow,
swam us past tufted-ear stingrays but we drowned still,
hydrophobic. Resuscitated after medicine, I remember
little but the Latin, an oculus being the grasp of a brain
on stalks. Pick your colour. Forgive me, father,

I am not the Esau you sought, with a stethoscope beard
to make you proud. Had I listened to spirits of dead
doctors who named everything after food — bread
–and-butter pericardiums, *café au lait* skin, *poma facies*
with nutmeg liver on a cribriform plate —
you might have liked the meal I made you.

Gulliver, Braided to the Ground

Some are felled by brain bleeds, others by the brain injuries
cannonballing through Nigerian roads. They cannot turn

in half-sleep, so we turn them two-hourly to ward ulcers,
and also to say: *awake from the grassy knoll, the ICU-green*

sheets, before you grow roots. Thus my people tell the sick:
do not leave your body on the ground. Because hell is: other

people, those that could not rise from the bed; the ones melded
to the little mouths of green; the ones caught in conspiracies

of gravitropism. Another saying: *may we be kept indoors*
whenever the road is hungry. But these roads be: replete,

but still eating. We know vagrants were the ones who ate sacrifices
travelers left for òrìṣà at crossroads: the half-gourd, the meals

of white–eggs and starch–spattered with libations of palm oil.
At other crossroads, on left turns, travelers presented cracked pans

of skull, broken in near-death beside palm trees: trees withholding
their saving oils from the hydraulic springs below. People pray

to deities; surgeons pray to the body, willing those hemispheres
they can scoop back to germinate, grow toward consciousness.

Also: to save them from smothering families. We'd heard:
of hemiplegics predictably drowned by their lunch;

by families that would check tattooists in as visitors,
who'd pick a divine number of incisions, strike with the razor blade,

follow with the medicine before the nurse could see: ashes
of incantatory passages, slurried and smeared into the wake of blood.

Malign forces, and countries: they have not been appeased;
but they must be bad at their jobs if all they do

is eat their own.

Divination

I was a misattribution at my physician's desk:
a false oath. Patients thought me an oracle

in those rooms. I had fled from a Cronus
that would puppet me. I would flee again.

I was too warm behind the masquerade,
which Yorùbás say hide the faces of gods.

Another saying: *whoever betrays the earth,*
will go with it. Legend told of traitors swallowed

into sudden-cracked earth, where Anubis
had spliced a lion, a crocodile, a hippopotamus.

Those fates may catch me yet, but I've been
slippery. And I *did* pay some of their due.

Like Ifá's priests would prescribe a sacrifice –
I gave requisitions for tests; I asked blood

of my supplicants. I fed people into the jaws of MRIs.
I cut things out of them. I stabbed things into them.

I drew people into the world; I cracked their ribcages
as they left it; I put others to sleep, faithful to the guild.

And I listened to the instrument of my divination:
a tablet, not with scrying camwood but formularies;

I repeated the doctrines of prognosis whispered
by the fates. If Macbeth's Sisters – the lawyer, the doctor,

the engineer – who prescribed their own professions,
find me, I will tell them I left, had had to, to heal myself.

In Fetu

Here's the city, dying twin, papyraceus
siphoned from navel siege ramps,
neighbors smuggling petrol
out of the country and Kalashnikovs in.

Here, I, anointed, teach preformation—
from miniature homunculi
we sprout, premade in costly condominiums,
grown like Lugard's bad seed.

I deliver mothers of their children,
sending Leopold maneuvers
to warn them of this place. It is
their partners that are hysterical, gripping

my shirt collar, their migrant uteri
roughing me up. Sympathetic pregnancy
we call it. And yes, I'm aware of the absurd
history of hysterics and obstetrics.

Perpetually *in fetu*, midwives ride
the mountain of my mother in vain.
The cut under is fluvial, a Y-confederacy,
disbanded. I bustle to bind the infirm

with mortar dust, who want me to bind
faster, who must never know my work
is not science yet. We have re-turned
to dark arts: burial-shroud children

guarding the perimeter. They bivouac
in the charnel barracks; they lob
their fast-forward wilt into domes above us.
My guild is fled. Succor me, winch me now.

Niacin Creed

I believe in doubt.
Apostasy is all I have.
I believe in beauty.
I believe (I want to believe)

it remains, or means something.
Yes, I still believe in repair.
The fog is, at heart,
a cleansing water.

I believe there's some wisdom
in the fear of hospitals
and their indentured wardens.
One of my grandmothers,

faced with surgery, asked
Dr. Jesus to do it instead.
In Ibadan, many with fractures
chose the bonesetters,

with branch splints, and ointments,
and herbs, over ortho. They believed:
that the singular promise of hospital,
for them, was amputation.

Easy to deride those who choose
gangrene. Harder to explain non-survivorship
bias to those holding on to limb,
and livelihood. Having lived this decade

without the pillars of my beliefs,
I understand the fear of skeletal loss.
I am far from the labs where I studied
the structure of vitamin B3.

If only it could save me now –
help me convert nutrition to energy,
collect the lipids of North America from me,
but I digress . . .

I believe in the one holy
and apoptotic clutch of disillusion.
I believe its ouroboros. I will plumb the depths
of disbelief. I will find some faith

Maitre'D

In the citadel of bleeding tendencies and ammoniacal breath,
the coffin boxcart came often to receive its procession.
The flapping hands waved hello, goodbye, all too quickly.
That hepatocellular ward was more hospice than hospital,
more motel than infirmary. I was little more than its concierge, then:
Hello, goodbye. I don't know what it was for, but I guess
people must try.

I was empowered by new love. I felt secretly obscene, like an angel
of death must. The abdominocenteses could have been death
sentences. I felt like the duct tape holding a national health system
together. The idealists in these scenarios need more grief counseling.
I received none.

Mercy: the body produces its own hallucinogens at those
end stages, their minds changed irreversibly before the end.
They did not see things as they were before.
I am too far gone now.

Ọ̀kàakan ni á ò jí

Another saying: *May we wake one by one*, said at bed time.
This did not apply during nights on call when strident shrieks

rent the hospital. Parents, who had been ninepin-sprawled
outside the wards, were asking for their children; casting

their bodies to the ground to break the temple of medicine.
Not waking all at once: May the fire alarm of medical

emergencies pass us by. Febrile seizures could be
the smoke signal of malaria. My uncle knew nothing

of left lateral positioning or aspiration risk, so he hoisted
my jerking brother and ran with him out of the house,

toward the clinic down our street. Here's how folk wisdom
can be deadly: the belief that once a person having seizures

locks their jaws, they can never come back. The antidote?
Spoons. They wedged the metal into the grinding mouth,

churning teeth loose. Some others placed the feet of children
on kerosene stoves to wake them up. One part was intuitive:

ice cold water from the fridge poured rapidly on the head.
To shock them back? Good for a febrile meltdown.

Otherwise iffy. But what did we know of neuroscience?
All my nightmares involve being back in Ibadan

in some form or the other. I have fond memories of my home.
I do want to say good things about it.

But if we are to be woken from somnambulance,
why not all at once?

Side effects of medical practice include:

1. Trigeminal neuralgia, rising like the biological wars
   of permafrost, the vengeance and reward of varicella;
   the twinge, the slap on the wrist from the occupying forces
   of viruses in nerve endings; carpet-bombing shingles
   on the hillside of the face; the memory of the child
   with papules, and the physician's gift of calamine.

2. Unplanned (to the pilot) exits from the ascending craft
   of a career; resignations of one's commission as golden child
   in a dysfunctional vortex of family; desertions of one's
   conscription as a child (17) into wars of advantage
   in a desolate country; refusal to want the excellence
   one strove so hard for. Consult the things you are sure
   you do not want, if you notice a persistent and adherent
   suspicion of your foolishness. Remember, also:

3. dizziness at the suffering of others.
   Not from blood geysers or degloving injuries; yes from
   descriptions of infibulation, and while changing dressings
   of those one had mummified, while living, on burn wards.
   Remember the knowledge, later on, of vasovagal responses,
   a simple name for the boom of fusillades against one's
   constitution, faithfully obeying the plentiful triggers
   of medical practice. Remember that video of Paul Alexander,
   in iron lung for 50 years, a relic of polio. Three minutes in,
   the discomfort, then the nausea. He'd been describing how,
   with his diaphragm paralyzed, he had to consciously remember
   to breathe, and would occasionally get tired. Then came the patches
   of white encroaching the visual field, the need to lie down
   till the trembling subsided. Remember the not-knowing
   how to fully exist in a world that insists on a currency of grief,
   how to manage the chromatography of an empath,
   with the rising aquifer of ink reaching your quivering knees.

Reports

I wonder what Ṣọ̀pọ̀nná, Yorùbá god
of smallpox, did when he was retired
by the needle. Perhaps he lives on
in the last cryo-tubes of himself
in Novosibirsk, and Atlanta,
gathering his return.

Grappling his rafters, Sàngó
Olúkòso cannot land in towns
thick with spired thunder catchers.
The crying egbére, with broom sheaves
and Faustian stock tips, are silent now.
There are no metaphors left.

Mami Wata: eaten by plastic,
and mercury; her filigree immiscible
with oil spills; her mangrove blanket
asunder; her cowries betraying
ambiguous constellations. What say
the striations of time-lapse stars

on an Ọ̀ọ̀ni's head?
My legion machetes are
beaten into shields and then
a suite: of butterknives,
of windchimes, planters,
golf tees, and accordion slats,

spoons, and shot glass, tweezers.
Not everything must become ash.
I remain. A parasol spine for Greco-
Roman suns can come.
In shade will be the mythos
that should have been mine,

another house where there'd been
none for me, because some things
are compostable, in a plot
beyond the forest of demons,
and the leatherfaced
heroes that kill them.

Bloodletting

The theory of in-flow and out-go
made physicians of old
bloody indeed.
Whatever went in to ail
must be brought out again—exorcising
lance and blade, leech and purge,
plumbers bleeding valves off two millennia
of sick. How else to deal with poison?

This is what Ayurvedic deans,
Sufi saints and charlatans knew
of poetry,
why we drink diluents,
potent books to wash us out,
poured through activated charcoal
pencils filtered again in paroxysmal
dialysis twice a week.

At sedentary workstation, things pool
decubitus toward my bottom
and I must descant them
before they make me mad. Crab-like,
I scrabble abracadabras on my desk
to disappear into the caffeinated pools
spurting from my wrists.
How else to deal with poison?

Later the antidote, first the purge.

Portrait of the artist with patricidal fantasy, having dug two graves

At the clinical trial of my father,
I will ask him why he did it.
But even if I vanquished my unmaker,
I would still bear his marks.
I would like to raid the master's house,
but he'd probably be irradiating me already,
from when I enter below the lintel.
He'd done a Tuskegee on me once;

I would be arriving weakened
and syphilitic, skull punched-through.
I'll be delirious for my HeLa, my infirmity
taken and made global.
I will not use the master's tools, so
I will not be using the hypobaric chambers,
or retconning J. Marion's speculum
into oropharyngeal airways.

I'll be wanting to acquaint him
with duende. Give me my frontal lobe,
and the neural maps of my back alleys,
I'll call from the door. He'll use my poems
to try to commit me. I'll dunk his head
in the stream of all the
conscious he has dammed
with empiricism. If the elixir
is other people, do we want it?

I'll want the heads of everyone
who answers yes, too.

And speaking of human sacrifice,

every society has their Moloch,
the things they like to feed their children to:
the Aztecs had Tlaloc, and Ehecátl Quetzalcóatl.
The Phoenicians gave dozens to Cronus.
The Americans have firearms, and automobiles.
There's lead water, and cholera, and malaria run
rampant, clusters of lung disease around factories.
They do it to appease a powerful being,
or industry, or inertia. In exchange for rain,
and the promise of sustenance. Yet we say
we are not cannibals. This is how healthcare
is inherently political: in the things we allow.
I am probably too angry for policy work.

The builders of North America, and Australia,
modern Mexico and Venezuela, demanded
the sacrifice of residential schools. They buried
those children for their society. This, too, is health
policy, by substitution. Sometimes the witch doctors
promised wealth, or health, or more witch power
in exchange. Nollywood gleefully produced
their versions of this. You can fortify your tap water
with fluoride, but you can never purify the calcium
from the children in your groundwater, settling
into your bones. You will carry this body of death.
You will not understand the grief of your body.

The futuristic Soylent Green will be the children
of others. From the universal border of your care system,
blockaded blackhole mouths will expel meteorites
and prehistoric retribution upon your skies.
You will call it wormwood as air quality sirens go off.
You will attempt, as is your custom, to use tiny hands
of infants to unlock forgiveness for yourselves.
It will be denied you. You will pay, at last,
with your own lives.

Kneecap

I was born without a kneeling plate in my legs,
the patellae, came later. The sesamoid demand
for obeisance came with the age of reason:

three to six years old. First I learned to stand,
then genuflect, then stand on my own.
The first to go was the tendency

to be allegiant. I am faithful only to my own promise.
I am, myself, sesame: seed in the gristle;
leavened in the warm of joints, kneaded till I rise

hardened. I become fulcrum for a pulley of connective
tissue. Rub me the wrong way for some tendinitis.
Ask me for genial flexion of my body

toward your orthodox will. I retain some capacity
for jackknife movements: the headbutt, the axehead,
the nunchaku. An abecedarian after my unlearning:

be atypical, birefringent, contralateral; dilated
and efferent. Fistulate, with gamma knives,
the hypoechoic mass; be the idiopathic jamais-vu.

I am keloidal, yes, labile from meiotic side effects.
Nosocomial oligemia has me craving the occult blood
of an accessory circulation. But paroxysmally,

this quickening: reperfusion, from salvage therapy,
unicornuate upregulation, presenting volar for the
vulnerary, the water-borne xenobiotic yielding

a reverse zoonosis, my return to the primal.

The Glory

After Galen's millennium, in which he watched the exposed pigeons
of gladiator hearts cooing their last, full of metal, came Harvey's.

When William was excavating those cities of the body,
their arterial aqueducts and sluice gates, their one-way traffic,

their Venetian waterways betrayed their maps. He thus found
the pumping stations of the body, their gargantuan feeders

and receivers. The heart, juggler in the big tent of the chest, moved
more than it could carry at any time. He intuited the deltas of capillaries

beyond the Main Street, linking fingers through islets of flesh. He mapped
the route the miners would take, the irrigants the landscapers depend on,

the red and blue bandages of barbers, the amen of plumbers
and civil engineers. Even the carpenters, bone doctors, washed their hands

in its streams, praying for the union of pieces. If the Book said
It is the glory of God to conceal a matter, and the glory of kings to search it out,

do we, standing on the shoulders of vivisectionists and grave robbers,
hallow the earth, or profane it, with our groundbreaking of its stretched body

on the rack? There are capsule probes that we send now into the internal
caves; to make a movie and send back word. There are laparoscopic claws

for the morcellation of its secrets. There are ouija turbans for the speech of brains.
There are voodoo-doll farms with the sacrificial mice studied for their index.

We have dissected the geology, and archaeology; the electricity and hydrology;
the architecture of this body. We have its recordings but no confession.

We have occupied the city but its quarters refuse to dance for us.
Its citizens sabotage our answers with more questions.

We have the maps but no true way in. I and the poets chisel
at the metaphysics of the city: its personality and desires,

seeking audience in its mystic temple, which no one has seen
but we guess the dimensions of, the cubits of an avalanche of mouths,

the unified theory become law, the thing all our ravaging and beauty
are divisible by, investigating the final why of the body.

Consider the history

Alas, I must retain my mistrust of parents
of specialties, and those who would be magi.
A person needs belief, yes, but blasphemy too.
Question the unquestionable. Grasp the pristine
hem with bloody fingers. I have no use for saints,
or their hagiographs, since they do not exist.

There will be no shortage of praise singers.
Blessed be the gadflies. My rosary has the names
of criminal physicians, ones who rose from oaths
to be murderous.

I carry the clanging non sequitur as counter
to the hyperemia of beneficence. You said
you'd be good, they said you were good,
but if *your sin will find you out*, you may
or may not be good in the end.

"Furies waste angels"

> (From Shane Neilson's poem, 'Every Age, the Erinyes', in *On Shaving Off His Face*)

Are you tender, or were you tenderized?
I asked this once. I know the answer, in your case.
Would that I could make medicine repay its debt to you,
which would involve time travel. But what's the best
one could make of what should never have happened?
To comfort others with the comfort one has received,

                                                   if any.

Aristotle said *primum vivere deinde philosophari*.
Galenus said that the best physician is also a philosopher.
Ken Poirot has said: "You have not lived until you have fled
a city in a country where you do not speak the language
in the middle of the night." That last bit is postcard wisdom,
because you could have fled that country of sudden
and persistent terror, but are the one who stayed on staff,
who stayed as staff planted in the grass, with resident
snakelets leaving mounds of sloughed scales, reaching forks

                                         for the brain.

Why serpents? Some say an avatar to look upon.
Which would be appropriate, since seeing another
is the greatest kindness one could ask.
Some are reductive and kill all snakes;
others in a curious irony, repel them with tobacco plants.
But there's a reason venom remains the costliest liquid.
Few have the skill to collect it   (and some do within themselves)
and enrich its proteins   (and some do within themselves)

                                              into medicine.

a coast is not the same as a land

(a cento from Alan Bleakley's *Lull*)

The body's drawstrings are undone.
A lung swelling with ventilated drizzle
of the bristling red engine
hardens as the heart's spark fails
permanently startled
the dough of the liver rests in rusting blood
as wood is petrified, where the soft tissue
stripped of diction and restored to flatus
and memory creeps in against time like two seahorses
a tangle of sinews for dogs to worry
The once springy muscle as flat as old beer.

heavy Head
Spoiled like wet pepper.
spending flame, emitting
With sudden force as a near-gyre
Of electrical recollection
Sinking upwards into a rainstorm

Hydrosphere

We are in a struggle to keep the sentient congress of cells together – in union, in a confederacy – in a war to the death. Why do most living things (and this includes committees and nonprofits) fight to survive? A superstition of my people says you must never call people "heavy." Only the dead are heavy, cell walls crumbling under the weight of water, interstitial tributaries forming a styx of purge and liquefied fat. In an abolition of paradise lost, we therefore reject the waters of kaos. The hospital in which I learned medicine had first saved me as a jaundiced child. When I was given to that same temple, I ran saline oceans into the bloods of others; bled lumbar geysers from prawn-folded children; anything to preserve the armistice of 60% water. Wade in the water, but in the shallows. Make the dose   of the poison. Titrate the sink, and the float.

PART 4

Neurodiversity and the colonizing of the other

14

ALDA MERINI AND THE MAKING OF LYRICAL PSYCHIATRY

Marta Arnaldi

Introduction: if poetry could have a word

In this chapter, I explore the idea that lyric poetry – understood as non-narrative accounts of experiences, understandings, emotions, and feelings often spoken in the first person – can be a primary source of psychiatric knowledge.[1] My starting point is the perspective of Alda Merini (1931–2009), an Italian woman poet and patient who was incarcerated in a mental asylum for 10 years following a diagnosis of bipolar disorder and schizophrenia (1964–74).[2] Historically, this period precedes the enactment of the Basaglia Law, the Italian Mental Health Act of 1978, which contained directives for the closing down of all psychiatric hospitals in Italy (Foot 2015). This event – which had enormous impact on a number of countries, from Brazil to Sweden and from the UK to the USA – is considered 'the most radical mental health legislation ever passed in any country' (Burns and Foot 2020: 62). Merini's poetic imagination foresaw the main political and scientific ideas substantiating this revolution. This chapter engages with some of these preoccupations and predictions, in the process illuminating poetry's critical role in the evolution of psychiatric practice and knowledge in Italy and internationally.

According to different sources, Merini was given between 46 and 57 electric shock treatments during her hospitalization and was sterilized at age 39 (Zinnari 2021: 427). Two decades after this period of confinement, Merini described her experience as a patient in two works: the collection of poems *La terra santa* [The Holy Land] (1984) and the memoir *L'altra verità. Diario di una diversa* [*The Other Truth: Diary of Another*] (2007b), whose lyrical prose is interspersed with 11 poems and seven letters addressed to a fellow patient and lover. The present study focuses on the latter work as an example of the complexities linked to the recounting of the psychotic experience.

I chose it fully aware that neither this type of narrative, nor such experience, can be pinned down to a single genre, register, or medium. This is why the composite structure and style of Merini's memoir presents itself as a privileged site where psychiatric storytelling and episteme converge. One may object that using a mixed-genre memoir to discuss poetry is counterproductive or even illogical. In this situation, however, I believe that the opposite is true: poetry and the lyrical necessitate a theoretical and conceptual expansion through which we may be able to fully grasp their potential as art forms, art works, and practices. Conceiving of poetry as a technical discourse

DOI: 10.4324/9781003341796-20

for elite literary experts or passionate hobbyists is a double outlook error that places us at the two extreme ends of the reality spectrum.

As Werner Wolf (2005: 23) points out, 'lyric', an umbrella term used for 'most versified literature (except for the epic and verse drama)', has become 'a synonym of "poetry" tout court'. In the present study, I use the terms 'poetry', 'poems', and 'lyric' interchangeably, and the adjectives 'poetic' and 'lyrical' to refer to Merini's non-narrative, non-linear, and non-chronological storytelling, one that can be defined at once as poetry, prose, fragment, memory, clinical report, psychiatric textbook, and philosophical essay.

If it is true that patients do not generally use poetry and/or literally inflected speech to communicate with one another, their families, and health providers, it is nonetheless important to critically investigate the lyrical qualities (broadly understood) of their utterances. These include metaphors, silences, omissions, rhythmic pauses, nonverbal gestures, and oneiric elements as well as the embodied, performative aspects that are typically found in poetry more than in any other genre. If we fail to attend to the inherently lyrical speech of the sufferer – that is, if we fail to tune into the psychotic and poetic 'wavelength' generated by their words (Pearson et al. 2022: 2) – we risk oversimplifying, if not misunderstanding, patients' discourse, with consequences that can be significant at diagnostic and treatment levels.

It has already been demonstrated that, in psychiatric settings, poetry writing and reading can support meaning making (Pearson et al. 2022), suggesting novel understandings of psychosis (*ibid.*) and sustaining creative modes of recovery (e.g. Pennebaker 2004; Punzi 2021). Moreover, by way of its semantic obscurity (a difficulty that invites us to deeply engage with words), poetry can help us better understand 'individuals' illness experience as a grounding for the ethics of the clinical encounter' (Kirmayer 2007: 21).

I draw upon these findings to develop the intuition that poetry can contribute to psychiatric science in a substantial fashion. Poetry, I argue, does not simply offer personal and invaluable insights into the lived experience of illness in general and of mental distress in particular; neither is it solely a creative activity that can complement pharmaceutical therapies while accelerating recovery and enhancing wellbeing. Poetry has an active role in psychiatry, and it should be considered on an equal footing with science.

When produced and considered in contexts of mental distress – as Alda Merini's diary reveals – poetry is a source of psychiatric knowledge that asks to be beneficially exploited. By the same token, psychiatry has a submerged poetic nature whose presence, forms, and functions have remained secondary in the shaping and development of a discipline that despite having a solid interdisciplinary core privileges biomedical approaches at the expense of the poetic (Bleakley and Neilson 2021). Merini's memories offer important testimony to what I see as psychiatry's lyrical underpinnings and workings.

The idea I propose here – where poetry provides a primary, non-ancillary perspective to the creation of psychiatric knowledge – does not take us on unscientific routes. In line with the principles of 'critical medical humanities', it rather highlights a methodological and programmatic correspondence that enables us to pursue an endeavour that is as scholarly rigorous as it is clinically relevant. My appeal to consider lyrical psychiatry (as I define it) an integral part of psychiatry tout court, not in opposition to, or in substitution of, it responds to critical medical humanities' invitation to abandon the belief that humanistic knowledge is secondary or supplementary to medical knowledge. In fact, as Merini's diary discloses, poetic knowing provides a compatible, comparable, and intersectional epistemology that has a similar authority to medicine's (Whitehead et al. 2016: 35–36; Bleakley and Neilson 2021). As a result, poetry – as practiced by 'lay' subjects and providers – and biomedicine – practiced by experts – jointly contribute to better understanding psychiatric suffering in a way that erodes epistemic hierarchies.[3]

I first examine three distinct and interlaced processes of epistemic 'Othering' at work in the production of psychiatric knowledge: the epistemic exclusion of the patient, the marginalization of psychiatry as a discipline, and that of poetry as practice and discourse. Second, I link this discussion to the study of Alda Merini's memoir – where the three processes are concurrently present – by considering some of the nuclei of epistemic creation emerging from the analysis, namely: diversity, obscurity, and incommunicability. Together, I intend to demonstrate 1) that there is a continuum between the seemingly irreconcilable discourses of poetry and psychiatry and 2) that in some of its forms, a lyrical psychiatry may help us to circumscribe epistemic injustice perpetrated in mental health care by showing ways of embracing degrees of unknowability. I also suggest that psychiatry and poetry are similarly disruptive sites of knowledge production rather than the strongholds of opposite epistemic forms.

The triple Othering of knowledge: on patienthood, psychiatry, and poetry

Paradoxically, the first epistemic Other in the creation of medical knowledge is the patient, whose capacity as knower of, and contributor to, the diagnosis and treatment of their disease is often undervalued, if not all together ignored or displaced. This is particularly true in psychiatric settings due to the 'persistent negative stereotypes that affect people with mental disorders', who are often believed to be 'cognitively impaired or emotionally compromised, [. . .] existentially unstable, [. . .] or psychologically dominated by their illness in a way that wraps their capacity to accurately describe and report their experiences' (Crichton et al. 2017: 65–66). This unfortunate situation leads to a 'credibility deficit' (*ibid*.: 65) that is as widespread as it is alarming. Despite having 'direct access to and knowledge of their experiences', psychiatric patients have a certain epistemic privilege (Drozdzowicz 2021: 1), yet as has been pointed out, they are susceptible to even greater epistemic exclusion than people with physical illnesses (Crichton et al. 2017: 65), provided that a distinction between bodily and mental suffering is still one that we should consider.

This form of 'epistemic injustice', to evoke Miranda Fricker's (2007) pivotal concept, harms psychiatric patients as well as their families and providers, who cannot come to terms with a practice that is elusive and often unsuccessful. At the same time, the epistemic marginalization of the patient produces unhelpful knowledge hierarchies that, in turn, generate significant epistemic losses. It has 'detrimental effects on individual psychiatric patients' in that it obscures their epistemic contributions to appropriate diagnosis and treatments (Crichton et al. 2017: 65). At an institutional level, epistemic losses of this kind limit the funding of psychiatric services while cultivating a dangerous distinction between, on the one hand, the 'hard' or objective evidence provided by the methods and results of biomedicine (e.g. randomized control trials, systematic reviews, X-rays or MRI scans) and, on the other hand, the 'soft' or subjective evidence offered by patients and their families (*ibid*.: 66; see also Engebretsen et al. 2020). As is often the case, fictional literature – from poetry to memoirs to, more recently, blog writing to tweets and Instagram posts – captures these methodological, conceptual, and disciplinary dissonances that reflect the dominance of certain epistemic, social, and/or political paradigms at work in the production of science and knowledge. The reading of Merini's work will help us glimpse this key, lyrical substance of psychiatry.

The dominance exercised by 'hard' science (that studies measurable facts and bodies) over 'soft' science (through which we attempt to examine emotions, perceptions, and the life of our minds) has led to the imperialism of numbers over stories and of quantitative approaches over qualitative ones, with destructive consequences for psychiatry as a discipline. It is a well-known, yet unspoken, reality that psychiatry is 'itself stigmatised within medicine' (Crichton et al. 2017: 68) because it is thought not to rely upon or generate medicine's objective truths. From this perspective, psychiatry is an epistemic Other in itself, thus representing the second type of epistemic Othering examined in this chapter. Crichton and colleagues (*ibid.*) observe that 'despite the lack of objective truth in psychiatry, many psychiatrists are influenced by their general medical [and biomechanical] training and import this bias into the field'. Even though they acknowledge the 'biopsychosocial model' of mental disorders (Engel 1977) and, therefore, the need for a holistic approach when diagnosing and treating mental illness, 'they often [and counter-intuitively] retain their biological orientation' (Crichton et al. 2017: 68).

This diagnostic, conceptual, and epistemic inconsistency causes moments of friction between, and across, mental health professionals and sufferers, whose voices remain covered and/or distorted by dominant, biological paradigms. The situation is aggravated by the fact that psychiatry – as a body of professionals, a discipline, and an institution – 'continues to be seriously challenged in the face of recruitment difficulties, unfilled posts, diagnostic controversies, service reconfigurations, and public criticism of psychiatric care, in addition to other difficulties' including 'criticism concerning the medicalisation of normal behaviours and states of mind', 'anti-therapeutic ward environments', and the 'denial of patients' families as partners in care' (Yakeley et al. 2014: 97).

In a ground-breaking editorial published in the *Psychiatric Bulletin* in 2014, Jessica Yakeley and colleagues announced that 'psychiatry is on fire'; for them, the sovereignty of positivism (as in hard science), accompanied by the dismissal of subjectivity and emotions in psychiatric training and practice, had compromised the credibility and sustainability of the discipline. To contain this critical and clinical damage, they promoted a double intervention, or movement, whereby the subjective (e.g. patients' knowledge) could be objectified and the objective (e.g. clinical reasoning) could be subjectified (*ibid.*: 100). They continued by saying that 'promoting awareness of the subjective and emotional aspects in psychiatric training and practice' does not mean to 'undermine the position of psychiatry within the natural sciences, nor erode the still fragile evidence base for the aetiology of mental disorders or efficacy of their treatments' (*ibid.*).

Rather, what the authors suggest is that a 'better integration of the subjective and objective paradigms' will help us address 'unhelpful splits in our epistemological thinking, increase our tolerance of uncertainty and ambiguities within [. . .] clinical work', and 'enhance creativity and innovation in psychiatric research' (*ibid.*). Such integration has the potential to increase not just clinical benefits for patients but also forms of disciplinary, societal, structural, and/or personal stigma, considering that 'people with mental illness often accept and internalise [the] negative stereotypes' attached to them (Crichton et al. 2017: 68). As Merini's experience will show us, this unified paradigm represents a valid way forward in that only a truly interdisciplinary effort can enable us to capture, and respond to, the complexities of mental disorders, their management, and their societal impact.

The integration between biomedical, research-led perspectives on the one hand and subjective, patient-produced knowledge on the other is a creative act not just because it reveals a largely unknown territory, one that asks us to try different and/or new explorative tools, but also because it continuously posits the question of reinvention. Each person is different from another, not just genetically, as personalized medicine shows us, but also culturally. Each one of us is also different in relation to her-/himself throughout the course of our lives in that our identities are in flux, ever-changing and evolving (a description of this process is offered, for example, by Julia Kristeva's theorisation of the *subject in process* in her 1979 essay 'Le temps des femmes' ['Women's Time']). As a result, prevention, diagnosis, and treatment strategies should reflect biocultural diversity in all its forms – genetic, biological, linguistic and/or cultural – especially in the case of psychiatric disorders in which the boundaries between the somatic and the psychological, the biological, and the cultural blur.

By keeping in mind the creative energy necessary to, and resulting from, the encounter between the apparently opposite realms of the biomedical and the subjective, I now introduce the third epistemic Other as part of my analysis, that is poetry. Lyric writing has long been marginalized not just in the literary domain, where novels have more popularity and generate better revenues, but also in the field of narrative medicine (Bleakley and Neilson 2021). Having emerged to 'skilfully receive the accounts persons give of themselves', narrative medicine challenges 'a reductionist, fragmented medicine that holds little regard for the singular aspects of a patient's life'; in doing so, it protests 'the social injustice of a global health care system that countenances tremendous health disparities and discriminatory policies and practices' in order to develop 'increasingly nuanced view of the workings of the narrative, relational, and reflexive processes of healthcare' (Charon et al. 2017: 1). The impact of this narrative revolution has been transformative; yet, as has been observed, 'non-narrative poetry has not simply been overshadowed, but rather eaten whole, by narrativist approaches' (Bleakley and Neilson 2021: 3), with the unwanted result that narrative medicine and reductive biomedicine have often produced identical epistemologies instead of diverse, complementary visions (*ibid.*: 43 et passim). This is even more surprising given the similarities between poetic speech and patients' words in the vernacular.

Among others, Julia Kristeva has consistently described patients' discourses as inherently poetic in that we, as patients, often use devices that are typical of poetry as a genre, such as embodied metaphor. Poetry's absence from the scene of narrative medicine is also striking if we consider another level of similarity: the 'shared characteristics' between lyrical poetry and clinical practice. In their seminal volume *Poetry in the Clinic: Towards a Lyrical Medicine*, Alan Bleakley and Shane Neilson (2021: 138) list and discuss eight categories of juxtaposition between the poetic and the clinical: 1. character, achieved through approaching subjects 'slantwise'; 2. intensity, depth, and brevity with focus on particulars; 3. Epiphany or sudden insight; 4. Use of metaphors, with focus on invention and expansion; 5. Subjectivity and confession stressing emotion, mood, and passion or embrace of affect; 6. tolerance of ambiguity embracing empathy; 7. beauty (privileging quality over quantity and form over function or the purely instrumental); 8. orientation to here-and-now space and place rather than there-and-then time.

In the second part of this chapter, I will discuss Merini's creation of psychiatric knowledge by engaging with some of these categories. I will use the triple framework of epistemic marginalization that I have just introduced as foundational ground for examining Merini's (and other poets' and patients') psychiatric knowledge. In doing so, I challenge the distinction between hard science (biological, mainstream psychiatry) and soft science (poetry) to suggest the idea that the subjective is as rigorous a method as the objective, especially given that all sciences both hard and soft retain a degree of interpretation (see Engebretsen et al. 2020), unknowability, and opacity.

As mentioned above, Merini's writing samples are not used as a case study; they are a primary source of psychiatric knowledge offered by moving, accurate accounts of what it means to need, receive, and provide care. They are also more than a call for the reconceiving of care precisely because they fundamentally contribute to the making of psychiatric knowledge. From an epistemic angle, this approach has radical consequences; it implies that the vision of the disabled and sick is a valid one and that we should seriously take it into consideration when trying to help the sufferer in their healing process.

Not a case study: Alda Merini and/as psychiatry

I examine here three main areas of contribution to the making of psychiatric knowledge by Alda Merini. In her memoir, they are presented through the triple marginalized lens of the poet–sufferer: diversity, obscurity, and incommunicability.

Before referring to processes of Othering often perpetrated against people suffering from mental illness – Othering that leads to stigma as well as to social and physical segregation in the confined space of the mental hospital – in Merini's diary, diversity is first and foremost a diversity of vision. The poet–patient's understanding of the world is in tension with that of others, be they health providers, friends, or family; their alternative perceptions function as epistemic diversity, that is a type of gnoseological dissonance or divergence with which it is important to attune. In the 'pandemonium' (Merini 1984: 15), 'infernal chaos' (*ibid.*: 14), and 'grave hell' (*ibid.*: 20) that is the asylum, diversity becomes a mode of survival, the ontological differentiation of which manifests itself through a spectrum of stories, world visions, memories, dreams, and traumas that deeply challenge our expectations about who the patient is and what their role is in illness.[4]

Merini investigates epistemic diversity by offering the alternative perspective of the poet–patient as gnoseological agent, a type of epistemic Othering that I call 'patienthood'. By challenging the often-undisputed authority of health providers, she claims at various points that mental suffering is often misdiagnosed and mistreated, possibly because of lack of attention towards the words and opinions of the patient. On the diagnostic level, she maintains that 'mental illness does not exist' (*ibid.*: 137); what do exist, according to her, are 'nervous breakdowns . . . family issues, the responsibility and effort of raising children, and the difficulty of loving' (*ibid.*). The list could potentially go on to include other aspects of what is generally considered a 'healthy' life. However, Merini is not implying that cases in which mental distress proves to be pathological do not exist; her narrative is punctuated with episodes in which psychiatric suffering is detrimental for the individual to the point of altering and/or impeding the functioning and flourishing of their life. Rather than denying the existence of mental illness, the author denounces the misunderstanding of its nature, thus offering an alternative epistemic perspective 1) on the aetiology of so-called mental diseases, which for Merini generate from affective and social disorders; 2) on the essence of so-called neurosis, which in one of the poems that crisscrosses the memoir she defines as a form of science (as in valuable understanding of facts and emotions); and 3) on the diagnostic sensitivity that is necessary to approach 1) and 2) – namely, a holistic gaze that is often lacking among her health providers: 'I wish that mental illness can be finally debunked and led back to its original foundations, that is the reality that it is an emotional disorder. I am not a psychiatrist, but I would have wanted to be one' (*ibid.*: 120).

Merini (*ibid.*: 117) continues, 'In reality, there is no folly without justification, and each gesture that normal and healthy people doom to be crazy involves a mystery of unheard suffering that men and women have not grasped' and 'Man is socially evil, an evil subject. And when he finds a turtledove, that is someone who speaks too softly, someone who cries, he throws his guilts on them, and, in this way, the mad are born' (*ibid.*: 123).

Thus, says Merini (*ibid.*: 41),

To each one of you I ask for a grace:

> To be still for an hour
> On the starry face
> Of a normal party's clock
> Then neurosis is science
> [. . .] Aren't we all mad?

She continues,

> Despite all the drugs that we took each one of us managed to remain oneself. We were promised happiness, the stabilization of our instincts. But our instincts were the instincts that anyone else had, they were only distorted by a lack of love
>
> (*ibid.*: 98)

and

> Our nurses . . . made us believe at every occasion that we were 'different' and that therefore we could not take part in their discourse or in their way of life. . . . They spent hours shut in Dr. G.'s office to come out of it with enormous files full of strange and absolutely wrong treatments to administer to the poor patients.
>
> (*ibid.* 30–31)

As this last example reveals, Merini denounces forms of epistemic and psychological violence committed against the sufferers who ended up being Othered by their providers as well as being assigned, again, 'strange and absolutely wrong treatments' (*ibid.*: 31). A discussion on the acts of violence, psychological and physical, described in the book falls out of the scope of this chapter; what matters here is to take them into consideration when examining epistemic injustice as a form of violence itself.

Merini repeatedly denounces processes of misdiagnosis resulting in inefficient and/or erroneous therapies based on biomedical approaches such as psychotropic drugs, narcoanalysis, and electroconvulsive therapy. On the topic of mistreatment, the following passages offer but some cases in point:

> Drugs deprived us of all contact with reality. My personal doctor, doctor G., argues that this was the case because of my illness. But I maintained the opposite.
>
> (*ibid.*: 118)

> Certain beasts [as in people], under the effect of the poison of the drugs, had completely lost their identity.
>
> (*ibid.*: 28)

> Under narcotic drugs my behavior was extremely negative and I screamed like an obsessed in the grip of the worst delirium.
>
> (*ibid.*: 30)

> Naturally, in our ward soft therapies were inconceivable, therefore [the patient] was forced to receive an interminable series of electroshocks, after which the poor woman came out completely mad.
>
> (*ibid.*: 51)

> In that asylum there existed the horrors of the electric shocks. From time to time we were crammed into a room and they would cast those horrible 'spells' on us. I call them spells because the only effect they had on us was that of brutalising our spirits and minds. On more

than one occasion, doctor G. grabbed me by the arm and took me away from that torture. I used to start crying and then I wet myself because of so much fear.

(ibid.: 71)

The room where the electric shocks took place was narrow and terrifying; even more terrifying that this was the antechamber where they would prepare us for this sad event. They would give us a premorphine, then some curare so that our limbs could not move anxiously and disproportionally during the electric shock. The wait was agonizing. Some cried. Some urinated on the floor. Once I took the head nurse by the throat, on behalf of all the fellow patients. The result was that I had to undergo the treatment first, and without the preliminary anesthesia, so that I could fell everything.

(ibid.: 87–88)

In reading these passages, it is important to stress that, while pointing out the limitations of biomedical approaches, Merini does not dismiss them all together; rather, she believes them to be useful at times, for some people, and under specific circumstances. What she condemns without reservations is violence committed against the sufferer.

There are instances in which Merini's lyrical psychiatry engages more closely with biomedical discourse, thus making a direct contribution to psychiatric literature; this is apparent, for instance, in the passages mentioning the inefficacy of specific drugs to treat and/or alleviate patients' suffering (e.g. Serenase, Pentothal, Leptonizal). Here, psychiatry, bolstered by pharmaceuticals, resorts to literalism or the concrete, veering away from poetics. Drugs are used as blunt extensions of similarly blunt diagnoses. In the following passage, the agent is pentothal (sodium thiopental), an ultra-short acting depressant and anaesthetic, infamously known as a 'truth serum':

Doctor G., who was more and more convinced that at the origin of my psychosis was a trauma, started to treat me with Pentothal. Pentothal is nothing but the truth serum, which, administered in light doses, can provoke euphoria and push the subject to make unheard confessions; under its effect, there is no censorship. Personally, Pentothal made me shout and move animatedly claiming that a man was scaring me [. . .] up until doctor G., seeing that I was exhausted, suspended the treatment.

(ibid.: 65)

When instead they gave me Dobren (ten injections per day), I was in a tragic state, I could not sit, I could not relax. That dreadful drug would keep me continuously awake, and I did not the so-called 'long breath', which neurologically is so important for our wellbeing.

(ibid. 99)

Use of pentothal is now discontinued. For Merini, it seemed that the drug unveiled the untruths of the psychiatric institution that was treating her, the untruths that the Basaglia Law intended to unmask. One of Merini's fellow inmates warns that treatment itself can lead to symptoms that in turn call for treatment, so that the patient is caught in a vicious cycle:

Yesterday I received a visit from a discharged patient who told me these exact words: 'At the beginning, I was hospitalised because I had a religious vision. I was immediately given a treatment based on Serenase, then they tied me up, and I was considered mad. . . . After this episode, my cognitive capacities, my personality worsened. I did not have the perception of myself any longer. What is more, after taking the drugs I used to suffer inhumanly because, as is well known, psychiatrist drugs have violent side effects, to the point that the patient in the hospital cannot but cry for help. This request is usually met by tiding the patient up to the enclosure bed'.

(ibid.: 119)

This cycle, which RD Laing (1970) called a 'knot' and Gregory Bateson (Bateson et al. 1956; Bateson 1972) a 'double bind', itself is a product of treatment meriting further treatment:

The asylum was a place of enormous pain, one in which the hospital cart was carried around to make us believe in some help that did not exist. Like an animal, I would jump out of my resting place and ran, ran towards the cart and overturn it, and after this I would certainly be punished with a high dosage of Largatil.

(Merini 1984: 73)

[The doctor] gave me three injections of Valium [. . .] I believe that in those moments I had the perception of dying. The injection was so violent that I fainted and slept for three days. When I woke up I was tied up to the bed.

(ibid.: 103)

In an interesting and arguably controversial section of the diary, Merini maintains that whenever drugs were suspended (for example during pregnancy), she would not suffer from psychosis. This statement resonates with other patients' testimonies recorded in the book: 'When I was pregnant all symptoms disappeared and I could be back to be normal. All treatments were suspended and, without having a period, I stopped being hysterical'. *(ibid.*: 16)

Overall, what this section on epistemic diversity with reference to processes of misdiagnosis and mistreatment shows is that the psychiatric patient can be harmed in terms of their capacity as knower, especially on the grounds of their experience of detachment from reality and/or what is supposed to be considered an inability to exercise their will, which I see as a further element of epistemic discrimination. As Merini notes, 'Doctor G. maintained that for a long time I had lost contact with reality. But I have always doubted about it. Who can decide what reality is?' *(ibid.*: 121). She asks, 'What kind of truth could emerge from a such an atrocious and unhealthy place?' *(ibid.*: 142), while she poses the existential question of 'Why a lunatic cannot be in charge of their will? *(ibid.*: 16).

Such ethical reflections allow me to introduce the second epistemic principle: obscurity. This is a notion that partly explains psychiatry's and poetry's segregated positions within the disciplinary realms of biomedicine and the humanities, respectively. Despite significant advances, both the nature and insurgence of mental illness remain largely mysterious as of today, and treatments prove particularly difficult, especially where pharmaceutical companies retained vested interests. For all its attempts to be as scientific a discipline as possible, with statistical models and reduction to brain mechanisms and biochemical reactions sustaining its course, psychiatry requires a high 'tolerance of ambiguity', an aspect that is central to both the medical and the poetic imaginations (Bleakley and Neilson 2021: 159). At times, ambiguity of interpretation can generate areas of incomprehensibility and ignorance in which meaning is obscured. Merini's writing helps us to recognize 'epistemic darkness' as a necessary element of lyrical psychiatry and of psychiatry tout court:

> We came out of that hell already bewildered. This was a further proof that our folly remained an inexplicable fact and that it would have never provided a rational truth.
>
> (Merini 1984: 37)

> I had a thirst for truth and I could not comprehend how I could have ended up in that inferno. Naturally inclined to rationalism, striving to find out the 'motive of all things', I was frightened by the obscenity of the ignorance that people had in that place.
>
> (*ibid.*: 38)

> I asked my doctor the reason for my monstrosity. But my doctor has never been capable of giving me an exhaustive description.
>
> (*ibid.*: 43)

> What was incomprehensible to me was how I ended up in that place.
>
> (*ibid.*: 65)

These words echo Eduard Glissant's concept of opacity; in his *Poetics of Relation*, the French Caribbean poet and translator insists that we must 'clamor for the right to opacity for everyone', that is 'the right not to be understood' (1997: 194). Epistemic unknowability, both on the part of the patient and the provider, should at times be protected for the medically just project to succeed. This is what enables Merini (1984: 138) to say that marginalization, be it physical and/or epistemic, can be a 'social right': 'Psychiatrists should stop harassing us [. . .] just on the basis of the fact that, on an ordinary day, we lost our memories. This might have been due to the game of love, to the fatality of life or to a mechanism of self-defence. Marginalisation can be a social right'.

The opacity affecting psychiatric understanding goes hand in hand with a difficulty of speech. Using words, formulating sentences, and making meaning when dealing with mental distress can be arduous and painful. Yet psychiatrists 'depend on their patients for clinical information and are obligated to regard them as trustworthy' (Kious et al. 2023: 1). Merini registers this semantic gap by photographing moments of incommunicability, which is the third principle presented here, and once again one that applies to poetry and psychiatry alike. Patients' discourse is often nonverbal; they struggle and/or are forbidden to speak; they remain silent, whisper, or scream; they misunderstand, yelp like animals, or cry:

> For the whole day they left us with nothing to do, without cigarettes or food other than lunch and dinner; even talking was forbidden. [. . .] Screaming yes, that was allowed.
>
> (Merini 1984: 19–20)

> In the asylum they made us used to silence. In the morning they would make us stand in line on the benches, our hands in our laps, and with the command 'do not say a word'.
>
> (*ibid.*: 96)

> I got up after two days [. . .] and I began to cry, holding on to the bars of my window.
>
> (*ibid.*: 66–67)

I am still perplexed today, after twenty years I still cannot understand how a human being can misrepresent certain things.

(ibid.: 67)

I curled up by my bed and started to yelp just like a dog. In mental illness the primitive part of our being [. . .] comes to the surface

(ibid.: 68)

By way of a poetic imagination, Merini gives a difficult and important message, one that, by advocating for a lyrical psychiatry, is not always and not necessarily antagonistic to psychiatric science. This brief overview has touched upon the poet–patient's contribution to the understanding of psychiatric suffering, the formulation of diagnosis and treatment, and the necessity to accept opacity as an epistemic principle. The section has also shown that Merini's memoir does not serve here as a case study, that is as a piece of literature reporting a patient's experience of psychiatric incarceration and illness; instead, it is a primary psychiatric source that help us construct psychiatric knowledge.

Conclusions: if words could be science

The creation of clinical knowledge has been produced from the triply-Othered condition of the psychiatric poet–patient. My analysis of the production of the incarcerated patient contributes both to the contemporary debate around epistemic injustice in psychiatric settings and to the field of critical medical humanities. Both psychiatric research and literary scholarship on Alda Merini can benefit from this discussion inviting disciplines to move away from their usual foci and methods of investigation.

In this chapter, novel questions were asked, and alternative perspectives formed. Due to the richness, complexity, and gravity of the topics considered, my analysis offers but an initial insight into the forms and meanings of lyrical psychiatry; deeper discussion and attention to details are needed. I expect, and hope, that future research on Alda Merini's 'case' (through the critical medical humanities) will expand these preliminary thoughts. This will further articulate the dynamic equilibrium at work between epistemic obscurity and relativism, historical evolution (e.g. the Basaglia Law in the Italian context) and individual changes, social activism, disillusionment, and joy when we try to investigate, deeply and fully, psychiatry's and poetry's strife for meaning. I will leave the last word with Merini: 'With this volume I, Alda Merini, make my own experiences available to other people, so that psychoanalysis may have fruitful outcomes and psychiatry may undergo a humanistic emancipation' *(ibid.*: 145).

Notes

1 I thank John Ødemark, Eivind Engebretsen, and Mona Baker for allowing me to present this idea in its preliminary forms on two occasions: at the 'Translational and Narrative Epistemologies' symposium, University of Paris, 22 November 2022 and at the 'Knowledge Translation and Incommunicability' workshop, University of Oslo, 25 May 2023. This research is kindly supported by the 'Bodies in Translation Project: Science, Knowledge and Sustainability in Cultural Translation', The Research Council of Norway, University of Oslo.
2 I gathered this piece of information from Alessia Zinnari's helpful article (2021). According to Merini's daughters, during the period 1972–79, Merini's mental health alternated between states of

distress and wellbeing, an oscillation that resulted in times of sporadic internment up until 1979, when Merini was finally discharged. See the poet's biography on her official website: <www.aldamerini. it/?page_id=8#1513806848988-e8fa5e55-760b>.

3 I thank Alan Bleakley and Shane Neilson for their helpful and sensitive questioning of this idea, which invited me to look for a more sustainable and rigorous understanding of the relationship between poetry and psychiatry.

4 The English translations of Merini's Italian original are mine. I used the 2007 BUR edition of the *Diario* throughout. The page numbers of the Italian text are provided in parentheses. According to Alessia Zinnari, the *Diario* has never been translated into English (2021: 428). After an online search, I discovered that there exists at least one English-language translation authored by Serena Ferrando and published by L'Incisione, Milan, in 2007. However, since I could not retrieve a copy of this volume, I decided to translate the writing samples myself.

References

Bateson G. 1972. *Steps to an Ecology of Mind: Collected Essays in Anthropology, Psychiatry, Evolution, and Epistemology.* San Francisco, CA: Chandler Publishing Co.

Bateson G, Jackson D, Haley J, Weakland J. Towards a Theory of Schizophrenia. *Behavioral Science.* 1956; 1: 251–64.

Bleakley A, Neilson S. 2021. *Poetry in the Clinic: Towards a Lyrical Medicine.* Abingdon: Routledge.

Burns T, Foot J. 2020. *Basaglia's International Legacy: From Asylum to Community.* Oxford: Oxford University Press.

Crichton P, Carel H, Kidd IJ. Epistemic Injustice in Psychiatry. *British Journal of Psychology Bulletin.* 2017; 41: 65–70.

Drozdzowicz A. Epistemic Injustice in Psychiatric Practice: Epistemic Duties and the Phenomenological Approach. *Journal of Medical Ethics.* 2021; 47: E69.

Engebretsen E, Henrichsen GF, Ødemark J. Towards a Translational Medical Humanities: Introducing the Cultural Crossings of Care. *Medical Humanities.* 2020; 46: E2.

Engel GL. The Need for a New Medical Model: A Challenge for Biomedicine. *Science (American Association for the Advancement of Science).* 1977; 196: 129–36.

Foot J. 2015. *The Man Who Closed the Asylums: Franco Basaglia and the Revolution in Mental Health Care.* Brooklyn, NY: Verso.

Fricker M. 2007. *Epistemic Injustice: Power and the Ethics of Knowing.* Oxford: Oxford University Press.

Glissant E. 1997. *Poetics of Relation.* Ann Arbor, MI: The University of Michigan Press.

Kious BM, Leweis BR, Kim SYH. Epistemic Injustice and the Psychiatrist. *Psychological Medicine.* 2023; 53: 1–5.

Kirmayer L. Celan's Poetics of Alterity: Lyric and the Understanding of Illness Experience in Medical Ethics. *Monash Bioethics Review.* 2007; 25: 21–23.

Laing RD. 1970. *Knots.* Harmondsworth: Penguin Books.

Merini A. 1984. *La terra santa.* Milan: Scheiwiller.

Merini A. 2007a. *L'altra verità. Diario di una diversa.* Milan: BUR.

Merini A. 2007b. *The Other Truth: Diary of Another.* Milan: L'Incisione.

Pearson M, Rennick-Egglestone S, Winship G. The Poetic Wavelength: A Narrative Interview Study Exploring the Potential of Poetry to Support Meaning Making and Recovery Following Psychosis. *Psychosis.* September 2022. Available at: https://doi.org/10.1080/17522439.2022.2116475. Last accessed: 27/7/2023.

Pennebaker J. 2004. *Writing to Heal: A Guided Journal for Recovery From Trauma and Emotional Upheaval.* Oakland, CA: New Harbinger Publications.

Punzi E. Creative Writing at a Swedish Inpatient Clinic: Perspectives From the Authors Who Guided the Patients. An Interview Study. *Journal of Poetry Therapy.* November 2021; 1–12.

Whitehead A, Woods A, Atkinson S. (eds.) 2016. *The Edinburgh Companion to the Critical Medical Humanities*. Edinburgh: Edinburgh University Press.

Wolf W. 2005. The Lyric: Problems of Definition and a Proposal for Reconceptualisation. In: E Müller-Zettelmann, M Rubik (eds.) *Theory into Poetry: New Approaches to the Lyric*. Boston: Brill, 21–56.

Yakeley J, Hale R, Johnston J, et al. Psychiatry, Subjectivity and Emotion: Deepening the Medical Model. *Psychiatric Bulletin*. 2014; 38: 97–101.

Zinnari A. Alda Merini's Memoir: Psychiatric Hospitalization, Institutional Violence and The Politicization of Illness in 20th Century Italy. *Journal of Trauma & Dissociation*. 2021; 22: 426–38.

15

DEAR GP

Psychiatry in the spotlight

Elisabeth Kumar

Dear GP began its life in Twitter threads, in which the hashtag #deargp began to bring together users of services who, bemused, aghast, or furious about the care they had received, turned the medical gaze outwards and posted referral letters of their own for their psychiatric specialists and mental health nurses. In tweet-length fragments and longer prose poems, these pieces depict psychiatrists who are 'moderately well-kempt' but 'somewhat preoccupied with insignificant details' or mostly 'oriented to time and place' but 'unresponsive to pain, dizziness, risk or emotional despair'. Ultimately this movement resulted in two published collections, the online zines *Dear GP* (Dear GP Collective 2019) and *Dear GP issue 2* (Dear GP Collective 2021).

If poetry is, as Ben Jonson defined it, 'the craft of making', these pieces make and remake worlds. Many in the c/s/x (consumers/survivors/ex-patients) movement have found psychiatry itself to wield a dark poetry, shaping an identity that is hard to escape. Or, much more accurately, many identities – and not, as we will see, only for those who receive services but also for those who deliver them. The enacting of distress (understood variously as mental illness, divergence, madness, and an array of other conceptions that map only partially onto each other) gives form to suffering and difference. The reception of care opens worlds of contingency and obligation. The provision of treatment activates a call to care.

Dear GP,
I met with CMHT member, Mr Y Bother, today, a diminutive man in his late 50s. Having described his job as a 'bit of a care-coordinator that-sort-of-thing' (query: delusions of grandeur?) I had seen him a few times before and was interested to see he was attired, still, in his favourite C&A outfit of pale beige trousers, short sleeve brown check shirt with white socks and brown slip on shoes . . .

Throughout our brief appointment he sighed and fidgeted continuously (query: tapeworm? Asthma?) . . .

I am confident that the diagnosis I originally conferred upon this CMHT member of BPD (BORED of PATIENTS DISORDER) is, indeed, the correct one.

(Dear GP Collective 2019: 10–11)

Throughout these poems, the language of psychiatry and therapy is co-opted and recycled, and this itself is something of an irreverent act, a breaking down of a wall that until recently stood

DOI: 10.4324/9781003341796-21

sacrosanct between a medical specialty and its subjects. Psychiatry's language, for many reasons, is no longer its alone; democracy, perhaps, is at the gates:

> On arrival she was carrying a book entitled DBT The Gold Standard Treatment for Because Psychiatrists Discriminate, a bowl and small wooden mallet. She was dressed in what appeared to be a cheer leader outfit and greeted me with what seemed to be a forced half smile, addressing me as DEAR MAN.
>
> (*ibid.*, 13)

This is a theme that runs through both collections – both as a sense of parody directed towards aspects of clinical care and as a sly directive to uncomfortable clinicians who may find these pills hard to swallow. The poems point out the psychiatrist who 'arrived for the appointment slightly late, which may be indicative of problems with her executive functioning, or may demonstrate a reluctance to engage with the service' (*ibid.*, 16) and one for whom 'Gentle disagreement and the presentation of new evidence cause visible discomfort, and the suggestion that two experiences could be interlinked was met with scorn and disbelief' (*ibid.*, 18). They report that 'Dr Y has a mobility impairment, and I have decided that this irrelevant detail is a useful piece of information to communicate, despite it having no bearing on the reason for assessment' (*ibid.*, 30) and have an eye out for strengths: 'Her manner was empathetic without being vomit-inducing, forced or false' (*ibid.*, 50).

Both volumes of Dear GP address practitioners directly, acknowledging that these pieces have sharp things to say and may be difficult to read – 'Perhaps eat a raisin mindfully' (*ibid.*, 3) – but ultimately positioning the poetry at a slant; these words, in their bent and sharpened forms, belong to those who have first received them:

> Please use your distress tolerance skills to manage any uncomfortable feelings that arise from reading these letters. Remember these are only thoughts you are having and nothing to do with systemic problems that need challenging. Focus on your breath and mindfully accept the feelings that arise. Remember, you MUST take responsibility and only be the right amount of distressed in order for us to help you. We've heard making a cup of tea, having a bath and other naive coping strategies are guaranteed to help.
>
> Unfortunately, we can't offer you any support or reassurance as it may encourage dependency.
>
> (Dear GP Collective 2021: 3)

These pieces, while original works, take the found forms used for clinical documentation within psychiatric services. They construct referral letters from the language used throughout mental health care, from face-to-face conversations between clinicians and patients (the 'consumers' of care, as the saying often goes, as if psychiatric services are leisurely purchased and eagerly gobbled rather than accessed out of necessity, with difficulty, or unwillingly) to the running entries that document each instance of care. These, breezily known as 'notes', track each professional's interactions and interpretations. Perhaps professionals think of them as sort of grocery lists: to-do, to tick off, to have been ticked off with, never to be repeated. But the metaphors extend. They can become 'notes' as in criticism, stage directions, instructions to do a bit better, and they're also 'clinical', which means you need to take them lying down. Or maybe they're the same 'notes' as in perfume – attempts to summarize the whiff emitted in the brief passing, to record whatever may hang in the air.

But let's step back for a moment and consider the notes. Throughout modern Western medical history, doctors and nurses of the mind have recorded their impressions of their patients' mental states (the word 'state' already carrying overtones of position and rank). They may document the person's own words and actions; see, for example, this record from Bedlam hospital in 1910, which conveys the patient's condition a few days into his admission:

> This morning he tried to do an addition sum but failed to do it in the right way – He states that in Ireland he can buy young pigs for nothing. Also, if you go to the right places you can get any number of young elephants for nothing, because they simply run into your arms.
>
> (Waddington 2015: 2)

They may also provide evaluative judgments of the person's temperament and conduct: 'Eats and sleeps well . . . cheerful and willing to help' (Jones et al. 2012: 158), as a Maudsley patient was described in the 1920s. A New Zealand doctor–poet recalls nursing in her youth at the Seacliff Mental Hospital, where new patients 'were invariably described as "pleasant and cooperative" or "sullen and resentful"'; she goes on to add that 'Most of the nurses would also fit the latter category' (Varcoe 2020).

A consultation letter or referral 'is an official doctor-to-doctor communication', says a journal article from 1982, going on to point out that the psychiatrist's letter

> is meant to be read, for clinical and educational purposes, by many people and is available, for currently unavoidable reasons, to many others, who may read it for insurance or review purposes, out of idle curiosity, or even out of maliciousness.
>
> (Garrick and Stotland 1982: 849, 851)

The genre's suitability for malicious usage is not news: another study taxonomizes professionals' offensive written comments as 'patronizing', 'stigmatizing', 'flippant', and 'lay terms used pejoratively', noting that the categories are united by 'an over-readiness to use clichés' (Crichton et al. 1992: 675).

Traditionally, however sensitively it is phrased, the psychiatric record necessarily 'tells a radically simplified and thoroughly mediated story of an absent person's experiences' (Glew 2022: 3–4). It is a complex act of translation, tailoring a narrative that will, if all goes well, make sense of the person's needs for funding and services; it may grant or deny help, highlight, or downplay distress and cement or question explanations, smoothing the way for the person to be understood or at least categorized usefully: 'If madness has been perceived historically as uncontrollable and excessive, paperwork is its opposite – deliberate, methodical, systematic' (*ibid.*, 5).

More recently, of course, it has become possible (and in some areas mandatory) for patients to have access to their documentation, and so psychiatry has turned its attention to the language clinicians use. Opening the record to those who have hitherto been merely its object is indeed poetic; an itchy fear seems to rise in some clinicians, frequently expressed beneath a calamine layer of ethical concern. 'Health data in each area of medicine is sensitive', explains one practitioner, considering the possibility of sharing the record with patients,

> but in psychiatry, these are special data, which sometimes contain a whole life story of the patient and involve a family history . . . and of course, such information is very explosive data, if this kind of information fell in the wrong hands, the outcomes can be incurable.
>
> (Chivilgina et al. 2022: 6)

The 'transition toward the patient "seeing the practitioner, seeing them" comes with the benefit of transparency and openness' (Smith et al. 2021: 2) but opens, perhaps, a cavernous Pandora's box of vulnerability and risk: 'What concerns me is the patient sitting alone reading it and misconstruing my language' (Chimowitz et al. 2020: 163). Whether this risk is primarily upon the practitioner or the patient is arguable, complicated, and unclear.

What is wanted from the patient is not poiesis, not a new creation, but a repetition of the psychiatric interpretation – adoption, agreement, concordance, an epistemic compliance. At the most, a riff. This has come to be known straightforwardly as 'insight', defined in a recent textbook of psychiatry as 'the patient's understanding of how they are feeling, presenting, and functioning as well as what the potential causes of their psychiatric presentation may be' (Sadock et al. 2017: 50), though, of course, it is not; an understanding at variance with the commonly held will hardly qualify. Mad scholar Cath Roper likens the concept of 'lacking insight' to being cast as a child: 'Many will sympathize' with the person deemed to lack insight into their condition, 'but the sympathy locates itself around the incapacity to grasp "obvious" truth, which all adults know but the child does not yet know' (Hamilton and Roper 2006: 420).

One philosopher of medicine argues that 'psychiatry, as a body of knowledge and as a set of institutional practices, lacks the conceptual resources to handle' a person who rejects the psychiatric explanation 'and accommodate the person's view (notwithstanding individual clinician's experience and wisdom in doing so)' (Rashed 2020: 601). This is not to say that a rejection of psychiatry underlies every instance of protest, in Dear GP or more generally – far from it – but to point out the stifling effects of a system that really prefers the patient's performance of illness and recovery to stay on-book.

'When we talk about what's going on for us in the dominant language of mental illness and symptoms', an artist and activist explains, 'it's likely we'll be described by professionals as having insight into our experience. Whereas when we speak outside of these terms we'll be described as lacking insight' (Loren 2022). In his classic study *Patient as Text*, Petter Aaslestad (2009: 8) noted that 'an insane person's behaviour and their perspective on life is often understood to be an integral part of their illness'; nowhere is this truer than in the psychiatric record, where even the minute, otherwise trivial details of the patient's dress, hygiene, eye movements, and time management take on a sense of gravitas and import. On the other hand, as Aaslestad observed in clinical notes from immediately before and during the Decade of the Brain, the 'medical-scientific jargon' has taken root in culture – psychiatry has, in many ways, provided explanatory constellations that scaffold our very experience. We may, he argues, suffer in novel and medical ways, bringing terminology and technical schemas to our practitioners: the 'doctor is, in other words, responsible for a greater part of the patient's story than a traditional sender-receiver model should imply' (Aaslestad 2009: 30). Mad scholar Beth Filson (2016: 22) explains that there is a problem when the language available to people who are ready to tell their story is 'far too needy, too thin and wasted' to be of use:

> In the context of the medical model, the story we learn to say is that we are *ill*. We begin to see ourselves as *ill*. We tell stories of illness, and the psychiatric system and, by extension, society accepts illness as the story of our distress. Being able to tell your own story – not the illness story – sets a new social context – one in which mad people are seen in a new light.
>
> (*ibid.*)

But it is time for a poem. Both volumes of *Dear GP* are attributed to the 'Dear GP Collective', with the authors of some individual pieces identified by Twitter handle or first name. Some, for example this user, are now inactive and difficult to identify, while others are anonymous. In this chapter I have chosen, in the spirit of this collective authorship, to err on the side of preserving anonymity. Twitter user @goodnewsfrombad introduces the *Dear GP* project by describing a letter her psychiatrist sent to her doctor, filled with details she found beside the point:

> Eventually the phrase 'she has no hair' made me laugh. Not only is it irrelevant, I didn't know why my GP would need this pointing out! In my frustration at not being able to do anything about it, and need for some relief, I shared the absurd statement on Twitter and swore I too could write a ridiculous clinic letter for that session (including assumptions, inaccuracies and missing information).
>
> (Dear GP Collective 2019: 4)

Several of these details, taken up by various writers across the Twitter platform, recur throughout the two collections: 'Dr H is reasonably well kempt. She has plenty of hair, no freckles and her teeth are normal size for her face' (*ibid.*, 7). Over and over we hear authoritative analyses of clothing choices, facial features, and eye contact; we are invited to consider practitioners' level of attention ('seemed to be preoccupied with a clock mounted on the wall behind me' [*ibid.*, 28]), emotion regulation ('affect was congruent with his mood which he described as "very well, thank you"' [*ibid.*, 29]), and social skills ('struggling to contain her laughter when discussing the topic of sexual activity' [*ibid.*, 24]).

Among the most heartbreaking pieces within the collections are those which gather verbatim quotes from actual psychiatric letters and notes. These range from the inexplicably tangential (the patient 'spotted in a pet shop' [Dear GP Collective 2019: 26]) to the ridiculous ('dressed in a non-depressive way' [Dear GP Collective 2021: 24]) to the frankly cynical: 'This lady has some background knowledge of psychiatry which she may use to her advantage' (*ibid.*, 25). These lines are presented in isolated fragments, gathered on a couple of pages within each collection. Some are photographed or scanned from paper letters, preserving the sense of institutional copy-paste carelessness experienced by many and reinforcing the collections' ethic of punk protest:

Dear GP,

Thank you for referring me to this delightful consultant psychiatrist. Our appointment was over the phone due to the Covid-19 pandemic but I will assume he is a balding middle-aged man. Apologies if he does in fact have a full head of hair, or indeed, a hair piece.

Dr G seemed orientated to time and place, phoning at the time he said he would. This is a rare trait and not one I've experienced in my clinical history, so did take me somewhat off guard. In our previous consultation he phoned five minutes late and both acknowledged AND apologised for this, which is highly unusual. GP to check that Dr G is not in fact a mythical being . . .

My only concern is that Dr G was so good at his job that it has been difficult to satirise in this letter to you.

I will not be seeing Dr G again owing to the fact that his position is temporary, as it's required to be under Sod's Law. I would be grateful if you could continue monitoring Dr G throughout his career to check for any signs of burnout or progression to Regular Psychiatrist Syndrome. Early symptoms include arrogance, condescension, poor time-keeping and a fast-growing sense of entitlement. This can then develop in the later stages into the wearing of a waistcoat or bow tie.

Yours sincerely,

Nell (Dear GP Collective 2021: 23)

These pieces stand, if awkwardly, in a long tradition of writing by patients; it's true that the lived stories of profound mental suffering, and perhaps especially stories of receiving treatment, have often been, to borrow Jane Hillyer's (1931) title, 'reluctantly told'. Phenomena that are somewhat ineptly captured in the word 'stigma', from outright discrimination to a vague lack of social nourishment, are at play in the absence we find for the mad within the literature of the world.

'Silence is not only a noun. It is also a verb. To silence, to censor: not just individuals but whole groups over time have been left largely unacknowledged, unseen, unheard' (Gittins 1998: 47). Psychiatric patients are far from the only group to be dismissed in this way – women, children, ethnic and sexual minorities, those in poverty or displaced from their homes or outside of the norm in an endless array of other senses, in fact those whose predicaments are often listed as vulnerability factors for mental illnesses of all kinds, have long been left without a voice where it matters: 'the struggle to be heard is ongoing, as is the power to silence' (*ibid.*).

Nevertheless, the voices of writers outside the stream of sanity, if I may borrow a highly troublesome term, have broken through. Margaret Cavendish was referring mainly to her gender when she admonished her readers to remember not to dismiss her writing on its account: for 'all is not Poore, that hath not Golden Cloaths on, nor mad, which is out of Fashion' (1653: 121). Without question, though, her madness was part of both the glamour and the resistance that surrounded her in her lifetime.

Emily Dickinson expressed what has become a somewhat tired trope when she wrote that 'Much Madness is divinest Sense' (n.d.). Elsewhere, poets whose unusual mental conditions have shaped their work, from Christopher Smart and Mary Lamb to Anne Sexton and Sylvia Plath, from Ivor Gurney to Theodore Roethke – poets of war, confessional writers, those feeling the anguish of love and those haunted by fears, and more recent poets, like Pamela Spiro Wagner, Janet Frame, Neil Hilborn, Jeanann Verlee, Elizabeth Morton, and Wes Lee – have spoken with energy and authority about things no diagnosis can quite touch.

To cite just one example of a psychiatrized view of patient poetry, it has been argued that what one psychiatrist calls 'morbid poetry', or poetry written by people experiencing psychosis when at their most unwell, 'may offer a glimpse into the ebb and flow of chronic psychosis' and illustrate disorder or dysfunction, presumably for the benefit of clinicians. 'As individuals progress in treatment', he goes on, 'their words may move from disorganization and chaos to self-reflection and healing. When this shift happens, a new form of expression, called insight poetry, emerges' (Bakare 2009: 223). In this conception, poetry is useful to professionals as a way of encouraging people into treatment and as a method of therapeutic surveillance – a window into illness and a funnel into further care, but the poems in Dear GP reveal quite a different purpose.

They speak up not as a way of requesting further intervention (though some, certainly, do want medical help with ongoing struggles) but in protest. They are poems of 'coping', not in the current definition of putting up with more and more, withstanding whatever comes, but in the earlier sense – to strike, to cut, to come to blows. This is poetry of self-defence, of action. In his breathtaking book *Language for Those Who Have Nothing*, Peter Good (2001: 206) explores the interplay of voices within the psychiatric encounter: 'often, the energies of the clinical interaction are taken up in responding to a set of choices and the burden is placed firmly on the patient to refuse an offer'. Amid the language of laughter, mocking, and irreverence, he argues, power shifts; marginalized voices find each other in fellowship, and meaning of all kinds is finally celebrated.

What of practitioners themselves? Within the psychiatric record, Aaslestad (2009: 22) again argues, the 'patient's background, problems and behaviour are rarely presented in such a way as to be incomprehensible for the outsider. This does not acquit the texts', or, by implication, their medical authors, 'of their potential to manipulate. There are of course numerous seemingly neutral, "innocent" text passages designed to activate certain pre-programmed reactions in the reader'. To join in the production of this genre must raise questions for the clinician – for this writing, however mundane it may seem, *is* poetic, is creative. But creative of what? The psychiatric process at the same time observes and organizes suffering: 'Doctors find a category first – what class of trouble? – and begin to narrow down partly via complaints of the patient, symptoms – the word from Greek, "that which befalls, a departure"' (Boruch 2015).

Miriam Larsen-Barr is a New Zealand clinical psychologist and researcher with lived experience of mental distress whose publishes her poetry under the name Miriam Barr. Her poetry beautifully holds the tension between these varied roles. She has written at length about the experience of trauma in *Bullet Hole Riddle*, a collection that explores selfhood and suffering, shared predicament, shared pain: she writes, 'Bartering our existence/we exchange small pieces of ourselves/ until the lines blur' (2014: 62) as wounds well up and subside. For Barr, the truth is in connection, in the far-from-empty places between:

> you can find me
> in the patterns we make
> my lines spread out to join you
> here then, between us
> we are not numbers and anatomy
> we are summations
> (*ibid.*, 59)

In this piece, 'Statistics for the Social Sciences', she faces her complicated roles as a clinician and lay human – a multifaceted existence in which she moves through the world as potentially helper and hurter, whatever that might mean:

> I had this idea I could join the system
> and change it from the inside
>
> but you can't join the system
> and not join the system

Barr suggests, through a series of metaphors about (not) 'rocking the boat' that we should rock the boat but not tip it, playing the game, where we

> do not redesign the boat
>   definitely don't point out
>   the ocean isn't deep here at all
>   and hey we could walk
>   if we don't mind getting our knees wet

But, we musn't get our knees wet and if we do, then 'keep it to yourself'. This is not just the patient voice, the one accustomed to suffering, the one that knows it must wait; it is also the voice of one who has had to pick a side, or at least to give up the naïve idea of occupying a place in the psychiatric system while remaining completely free of the linguistic violence it is, in part, built on. Barr laments the silence she, too, experiences, where

> I am full of bias in a boat
> of balanced, nodding quiet
> swallowing my reactions back like stones . . .
> (Barr 2018, edits poet's own)

Drawing on statistical metaphors, Barr says that we can be insignificant, outliers with no power, or we get 'trimmed off':

> so we become swallows instead

> A cloud of silent swallows
> billowing out across the sky
> and our feet, our knees
> are perfectly dry.

Is it enough? It would be hard to argue that *Dear GP* doesn't partially exist to demand better, to pound at the door to the table of those who make decisions on patients' behalf. There are lessons to be learned – painful ones, perhaps, but not really difficult – and the editors acknowledge that this message is already reaching practitioners: 'we have heard from professionals that the first issue . . . has made them reconsider the overused tropes and phrases used in clinical writing' (Dear GP Collective 2021: 3).

But, as I hope we have seen, there is far more purpose to this poetry. As Stephen K. Levine (1992: 15) says, 'Expression is itself transformation'; there is a kind of social change that already inheres in the cries of protest, in the laughter of exasperation, and in the raucous insubordination of those who speak out openly. The awkward abuses that have become the mundane architecture of psychiatric record-keeping stick out, gain presence, when those who stumble against them don't hide.

Painful as it may be for those of us working in the psychiatric field to turn our gaze around, to pay attention to the language we deploy in the course of our profession, this may be unavoidably vital to the vocation we had better have: to care about patients' stories, their treatment and predicament – to care about the worlds that we create for those who suffer. In the ancient sense of the word, to care, to grieve, bewail, lament. To begin the poiesis of new and safer and more vulnerable worlds. And perhaps, as we allow ourselves this care, the elephants in the room – not for nothing – will simply run into our arms.

References

Aaslestad P. 2009. *The Patient as Text: The Role of the Narrator in Psychiatric Notes, 1890–1990*. London: Radcliffe Publishing.

Bakare MO. Morbid and Insight Poetry: A Glimpse at Schizophrenia Through the Window of Poetry. *Journal of Creativity in Mental Health*. 2009; 4 (3): 217–24. https://doi.org/10.1080/15401380903192671.

Barr M. 2014. *Bullet Hole Riddle*. Wellington: Steele Roberts Aotearoa.

Barr M. 2018. Statistics for the Social Sciences. *Mad in America*. Available at: www.madinamerica.com/2018/08/statistics-social-sciences-miriam-barr/. Last accessed: 10/8/2018.

Boruch M. Diagnosis, Poetry, and the Burden of Mystery. *New England Review*. 2015; 36: 23–36. https://doi.org/10.1353/ner.2015.0063.

Cavendish M. 1653. *Poems, and Fancies Written by the Right Honourable, the Lady Margaret Newcastle*. London: Printed by T.R. for J. Martin, and J. Allestrye. http://name.umdl.umich.edu/A53061.0001.001

Chimowitz H, O'Neill S, Leveille S, Welch K, Walker J. Sharing Psychotherapy Notes with Patients: Therapists' Attitudes and Experiences. *Social Work*. 2020; 65: 159–68. https://doi.org/10.1093/sw/swaa010.

Chivilgina O, Elger BS, Benichou MM, Jotterand F. What's the Best Way to Document Information Concerning Psychiatric Patients? I Just Don't Know – A Qualitative Study About Recording Psychiatric Patients' Notes in the Era of Electronic Health Records. *PLoS One*. 2022; 17: 1–18. https://doi.org/10.1371/journal.pone.0264255.

Crichton P, Douzenis A, Leggatt C, Hughes T, Lewis S. Are Psychiatric Case-Notes Offensive? *Psychiatric Bulletin*. 1992; 16 (11): 675–77. https://doi.org/10.1192/pb.16.11.675.

Dear GP Collective. 2019. *Dear GP*. Available at: https://deargp.home.blog/download-the-dear-gp-zine/.

Dear GP Collective. 2021. *Dear GP Issue* 2. Available at: https://deargphome.files.wordpress.com/2021/04/dear-gp-issue-2-2.pdf.

Dickinson E. n.d. Much Madness is Divinest Sense – (620). *Poetry Foundation*. Available at: www.poetry foundation.org/poems/51612/much-madness-is-divinest-sense-620. Last accessed: 1/12/2022.

Filson B. 2016. The Haunting Can End: Trauma-Informed Approaches in Healing From Abuse and Adversity. In: J Russo, A Sweeney (eds.) *Searching for a Rose Garden: Challenging Psychiatry, Fostering Mad Studies*. Monmouth: PCCS Books Ltd, 20–24.

Garrick TR, Stotland NL. How to Write a Psychiatric Consultation. *American Journal of Psychiatry*. 1982; 139: 849–55. https://doi.org/10.1176/ajp.139.7.849.

Gittins D. 1998. Silences: The Case of a Psychiatric Hospital. In: M Chamberlain, P Thompson (eds.) *Narrative and Genre*. London: Taylor & Francis, 46–62.

Glew L. Documenting Insanity: Paperwork and Patient Narratives in Psychiatric History. *History of the Human Sciences*. 2022; 35: 3–31. https://doi.org/10.1177/09526951211068975.

Good P. 2001. *Language for Those Who Have Nothing: Mikhail Bakhtin and the Landscape of Psychiatry*. New York, NY: Kluwer Academic/Plenum Publishers.

Hamilton B, Roper C. Troubling 'Insight': Power and Possibilities in Mental Health Care. *Journal of Psychiatric and Mental Health Nursing*. 2006; 13 (4): 416–22. https://doi.org/10.1111/j.1365-2850.2006.00997.x.

Hillyer J. 1931. *Reluctantly Told*. New York, NY: The Macmillan Company.

Jones E, Rahman S, Everitt B. Psychiatric Case Notes: Symptoms of Mental Illness and Their Attribution at the Maudsley Hospital, 1924–35. *History of Psychiatry*. 2012; 23 (90 pt 2): 156–68. https://doi.org/10.1177/0957154X10394306.

Levine SK. 1992. *Poiesis: The Language of Psychology and the Speech of the Soul*. London: Jessica Kingsley Publishers.

Loren E. 2022. *Meet Me Where I am: Listening to Insights into the Mental Health System. An Audio Book of Listening Experiments Co-Created With Alex, Anon, Chloe Beale, Florence, Hattie, Helen, Ninette, Sam and Shan. Illustrations by Merlin Evans. Commissioned as Part of Bethlem Gallery's Mental Health and Justice Project*. London: Bethlem Gallery. Available at: bethlemgallery.com/whats-on/meet-me-where-i-am/.

Rashed MA. The Identity of Psychiatry and the Challenge of Mad Activism: Rethinking the Clinical Encounter. *The Journal of Medicine and Philosophy: A Forum for Bioethics and Philosophy of Medicine*. 2020; 45 (6): 598–622. https://doi.org/10.1093/jmp/jhaa009.

Sadock B, Sadock VA, Ruiz P. 2017. Psychiatric Interview, History, and Mental Status Examination. In: B Sadock, P Ruiz, VA Sadock (eds.) *Kaplan & Sadock's Concise Textbook of Clinical Psychiatry* (5th ed.). Philadelphia, PA: Lippincott Williams and Wilkins, 39–52.

Smith CM, Stavig A, McCann P, Moskovich AA, Merwin RM. Let's Talk About Your Note": Using Open Notes as an Acceptance and Commitment Therapy Based Intervention in Mental Health Care. *Frontiers in Psychiatry*. 2021; 12: 704415. https://doi.org/10.3389/fpsyt.2021.704415.

Varcoe R. 2020. To Medicine Via Paradise. *Corpus* (blog). Available at: https://corpus.nz/to-medicine-via-paradise/.

Waddington K. 2015. Reading Psychiatric Case Notes: Tertiary Syphilis and Bethlem Royal Hospital. In: J Lewis (ed.) *SAGE Research Methods Datasets Part 1*. London: SAGE Publications, Ltd. https://doi.org/10.4135/9781473938090.

16

THE PRAIRIES ALWAYS SEE YOU

A poetics of psychosis

Erin Soros

The isolation room is compact – I can almost reach the walls if I stretch out my arms. A corrugated metal grid covers the entire back wall; the front wall is glass. I focus on the side walls, their stretch of beige, how the glossy paint exaggerates the unevenness of the surface. The flatness is uninterrupted by poster or painting. The beige feels close, ominous – the evidence of something gone, a mirror with no reflection, a face with no features. I can find no other clues as to how I have arrived here or why I'm being detained. I am wearing beige cotton pyjamas, hospital pyjamas. The medical staff had forced me to take off my top and my pants, my bra and underwear, and then they took all my clothing away. Now I match the walls. I could disappear. I'd been allowed one phone call and I wasted it on a mental health advocate who told me, firmly, quickly, that I can refuse to talk, as if my only chance at liberty could be found in one more form of erasure. On the other side of the glass doors, I can see no one, but I do hear the nurses declare the data of other patients, and some of the noise ricochets with my own story, shards of details that are not mine but fit – the names of places, the names of symptoms. My thoughts hit against the beige walls and slide down them.

And then I find a bond, in the stark isolation that is a psychiatric segregation unit, and this one intuitive choice is what I want to explore in this piece of writing that will remain as small as the room. I look at the wall and remember a reassuring sentence from a conversation the day before on the phone with a friend. I did not use the word *psychosis* when I spoke to this friend but instead said that my mind was *awry*. He repeated this word, and it seemed right, how I could share its meaning with him, this vocabulary of my choosing, my perspective off-kilter, cockeyed, shards of my mind turning within a kaleidoscope. I was surprised that he was speaking with me at all. I have grown used to another's discomfort when my words betray the errors of my mind. I have grown accustomed to stiff faces, expedient statements, and swift departures. But he stayed on the phone and found something to trust in my skittering dialogue, how I'd crack open one comment and veer in a new direction, still somehow reaching him, or he'd interrupt to reach me.

How am I doing? It was his question, voiced as if his halted attempts had a technique that could be appraised and as if I was the one in the position to judge.

This is helpful, I said. I meant both the connection and the words, how they were still working somehow even as I moved them too fast. I relished the respectful way the question positioned me when the madwoman is so often assumed to possess no insight. I could feel the value in my perspective, my own ability to assess what kinds of speech eased my fluster. But where to go from

        DOI: 10.4324/9781003341796-22

here? I knew he was from the prairies, and so I told him that the prairies made me feel vulnerable, singular, how I could sense the force of my verticality in the flatness.

He responded slowly, but with ease, and he said he was telling me what had been told to him, his gift already a gift – *the prairies always see you.*

I could imagine standing in the beige wheat fields and finding solace in them, held by a gaze of the ground.

He was nowhere near me as I stood facing the beige walls and then sat on the foam mattress on the metal bed, but I recalled his vivid assertion. *The prairies always see you.* I had always been a child of the woods – mountain greens, sombre firs, generous branches sieving light, rain a relentless syncopation, the smell of pine opening my chest, wide trunks offering a place to hide. Nothing within the segregation room oriented my mind to my geography, but I could borrow someone else's. I could feel seen – by the walls, by this friend, by language itself.

Psychiatrists have never asked me about such a shift, when within the confusion of my mental corridors some fulcrum enables me to find my way. I talk to psychiatrists in my beige pyjamas, once I am out of segregation but still within the locked ward, and then I talk to them when I am wearing the ordinary grace of clothing in the months that follow forced hospitalization. We review doses of medication and their various benefits and side effects, each time the dogged discussion of the pills as if only drugs can provide treatment for a troubled mind. Our meetings rarely consider the psychotic experience that led to medical capture, and I have never been asked to recount what kinds of therapeutic discoveries I might have made while deep within a threshold state.

We speak of "triggers" – those stressors that lead to psychotic symptoms. But what of the potential triggers that lead in the other direction? What might be their pattern, their form?

I want to pause at the wall, in that instant when I could have experienced psychic dissolution, separated from anyone who could have guided me back into some sense of shared reality, when I am left bereft of any clue as to what that reality might be, and instead I recalled one sentence that offered a kind of accompaniment. I want to stay with my friend's offering, its specific structure and use, how I borrowed it and why. In that room of segregation, in that state of isolated terror, I was able to recall that my friend had shared with me what had been shared with him, that I was being introduced into a relay of seeing. I returned to some kind of human connection even or possibly because I could comprehend its absence. I was not surrendering to psychotic belief but rather negotiating its cusp. I did not look at the wall and suddenly feel myself within an expanse of wheat. I did not hear my friend's voice. The experience involved no hallucination, visual or auditory, and I did not escape into a delusionary conviction that the wall magically peered at me like an animate thing. I knew that I was alone, and that the wall was beige, flat, unresponsive, yet that I could muster some sense of witnessing from my environment, just as my friend had been taught to do from his. The thinking involved returning to memory, and therefore to loss, to what was not in the room. I was reckoning with the objective blankness of a wall at the same time as I relished what my mind could make of it. When no human could see my body, when no loved one could witness my state, I found myself oriented by what the wall could represent, by what it could let me imagine. I was soothed not by psychotic plenitude but rather by the creative propulsion of an 'as if'.

In one of his more well-known theories, the psychoanalyst Jacques Lacan (2006: 75) suggests we become psychically organized as a self when we capture our reflection in a mirror. The mother holds the infant in front of its reflection, and at some point it jubilantly recognizes its own shape. Yet this recognition is a misrecognition: the infant cannot yet control its limbs and does not yet experience its own body as a distinct unity even as it is enticed by this gestalt, just out of reach. Lacan asserts that this developmental stage is not just a temporal event but a paradigm of human psychic structure – we continue to need our mirrors, to search for our reflections whether in glass or in photographs or in the faces of other people – and yet we never quite match what we behold. We are bound then to a paranoiac knowledge, and Lacan uses this specific term 'paranoiac', suggesting that delusion is not foreign to healthy human subjectivity but an inherent part of it.

In the depths of my psychotic states, I have picked up blue foil of a candy wrapper and pocketed it as a secret sign; I have watched the swoop of a bird and known immediately that the shape in the sky communicated with me in a way no one else could understand. The world became a mirror, an intimate revelation. For some people who experience psychosis, the direction is reversed – internal voices seem to come from outside, inner speech a frightening elsewhere, a foreign chorus. Some people can experience their own bodies as alien, a foot not continuous with a leg but disjunctive, attached only as a ruse.

I have turned to Lacan not to assert that these extreme states are banal and expected human experiences but rather to consider how they correspond at least in structure with the mirroring that we all encounter, every day, as we confirm who we are by finding ourselves where we are not. Can we risk offering our own knowledge of mirroring, as a form of guidance, when we speak to someone in a psychotic state? Can this guidance engage with psychotic thinking without merging with it? My friend drew on his subjective experience with the prairies. He communicated how another's words articulated a private yet shared feeling. Our conversation therefore involved multiple mirrors – the one between myself and my friend, between my friend and the other speaker, and between this speaker and my friend and the landscape. I was not being situated in an unmediated relationship with a surface but invited to join the mediation. And so, when I needed it most, I was able to find the prairies reflected in a wall.

Without this solace, I might have panicked in that segregation unit, where no one was a steadying presence, where I was denied another human face. Had it not been for the verbal connection to a prairie memory, I might have scanned the room and located not a single object that could remind me of who I was and then looked down at the muted colour of my pyjamas and found myself absent. I am a woman with a stubborn aesthetic: I consistently wear shades of blues – aqua and turquoise and seafoam – the colours of the ocean or the sky, as if such largeness could be my mirror, the place where I find my body. Who was I suddenly in these beige garments that recalled prison garb? Who was I locked away?

Without anyone to calm me, I might have begun to fall deeper into disarray like I have done before when the hospital doors shut. Without the psychic leverage of a helpful phrase, my delirium might have worsened and would have been found disconcerting, threatening, captured by the disciplinary interpretive crescendo that is carceral care. My mind and body would have been met with force. In other psychiatric admissions, the nurses have signalled for the security guards, and these men, who are trained to work in shopping malls, have tied me to that metal bed, binding my ankles and wrists in four-point restraints.

And here I was, years later, desperate again in locked seclusion. I stood in the space created by beige walls, alone, trying to understand my position, and the four hooks waited on either side of the mattress, blue rectangles empty, ready – for the straps, and then my ankles and wrists, the prone diagonals of my limbs. It could all have happened once more.

But on this occasion, I nodded at the walls. I see you. You see me.

I am grateful to have heard of the prairies, basket of my ignorance. My friend had not named the crops. He had not specified the colours. I could not find this place on a map. Did he mean grasslands? Or corrugated fields of wheat? Or those patchwork squares of canola yellow I have flown over or driven past, distance or speed turning detail into blur? His landscape could ripple green, swaying almost white in sunlight, dark blue to black in the shade, pockets of deep glistening brown when the rain finally pelted the earth. His landscape would hold smells and sounds I did not know, and stories, his own experiences or perhaps those of his friend, a childhood and adolescence of games and triumphs and taunts, and meanings that are beyond stories, familial and spiritual roots that the land braces and does not betray, and if I sensed that intricate texture in his voice, all I could see in my mind's eye was that beige, alive and stretching into the distance towards a horizon no one could touch. I turned to the wall and glimpsed that kind of freedom.

Yet I was in an isolation unit – I could know that too, as I thought of elsewhere. I recognized this reduction of my circumstances. Nothing in that stark square indicated I was in Vancouver, British Columbia, far from the prairies, but I had begun to piece together my place. My thoughts eddied and sedimented: outside, it would be raining, and the trees would be blocking the sky. Inside, the wall was only plaster and paint. Here I stood, here I sat, and the walls reminded me of a flat stretch of land – that was it; that was enough, beige invoking beige, entrapment gesturing towards a possible expanse that reflected my living body, here, in the moment. I would be alright.

I experienced a gestalt while grasping the torque of metaphor. During other psychotic episodes, I have not been able to achieve this dual awareness in which I felt seen while I conceptualized the structure of the seeing; instead, the object and the fantasy would become intrinsically bound. In the decade previous to this particular admission to the Vancouver segregation unit, I was living in the UK, renting a damp medieval flat – dumbwaiter in the bathroom, chandelier in the bedroom – and I once stayed up all night walking around my flat giving interviews to the CBC, but my actually being seen and heard was just hallucination's game. I stood alone, articulating my knowledge to the abiding darkness of my apartment, the only illumination the red light above the stove.

To me this light represented an entire radio studio and the surrounding hush of attention. All I possessed were hours of black and crimson and my own voice, arms gesturing into a void. Yet in my psychotic imaginings, the show was on the air. The host awaited my answers. The audience listened. I paced back and forth past the coffee table, elaborating my points, nodding occasionally towards the red light, its eye steady and radiant and loyal.

Whereas I grasped that the beige wall was not in fact a vehicle of observation, my red light had merged with my psychic fantasy. My performance was not evidence of creative play but surrender to delusion. The shape of this specific delusion is not uncommon in psychosis, not surprising my frantic narratives of surveillance through technological means: the camera in the ceiling, the chip in the brain. When I have heard patients describe their own beliefs, I sense their yearning to be significant but also something more fundamental, primal, a longing to be visually held and so to sense the edge of the self as it is created through the eyes of another, even if those eyes are powered by inanimate electric charge.

My internal muse had propelled me out of my apartment, in search of something only madness promised, and so I walked from my living room to the public library where the police soon captured my body with theirs, batons bopping at their hips. The police questioned me at the station in the aggressive and belligerent manner you interrogate a suspected criminal, and the three of them grew increasingly impatient with my incongruent claims. They threw me to the ground, handcuffed me, jamming metal into a body that would succumb to force in a way that my unfurling sentences would not. They dropped me off at the psychiatric hospital.

In the medieval town where I lived, psychiatric patients are not first admitted to a separate emergency isolation unit but instead dumped straight into a collective space, rambunctious clamour of voices inside the double locked doors, and so my delusions soon found company. When I was released from the handcuffs, I skidded my socked feet to the TV room of the crowded ward, the sofa's plaid lumps as desolate as the leftovers from a garage sale, one corner of the floor piled with the flash of *The Daily Mail*, royalty's composed faces the inversion of our dishevelled, forgotten state. The patients gazed at the boom-flicker of the television. *You are in the way of the TV!* That glowing box gave us the daily measure of our value. The volume blasted the room full of shame as *Jerry Springer* told of infidelity and incest, adult children waiting to come on stage to declare their truths. Patients were not allowed to lie down on the sofa, but the drugs made us slouch, legs and arms limp, just our heads upright as the light from the screen pulsed over slack mouths.

'I am in a movie', one patient confided as she swivelled her hips to sit closer to mine. 'It has Tom Cruise in it'.

Another patient proclaimed to me that I was Frasier, from the sitcom, not genuinely a patient but someone undercover in celebutante solidarity, and then she announced to the others that she had discovered who I was, the news of my role quickening the room to excitement the way one fixed bulb in a dark and broken stream of Christmas lights can suddenly turn them all aglow. If I existed as a character within the television series, perhaps we would all be seen by the camera. We would all be human. Outside the psych ward, the world continued without us.

I grasped--- that I was not Frasier but sensed my sudden responsibility to be this figure for these strangers who were now my community in this place of banging radiators and duct-taped windows. The room became a cacophony of star turns.

In his later work, Lacan (1991: 124) adds a second mirror to his discussion of the mirror stage, this developmental experience that continues to structure our days. The two mirrors, one concave and one flat, interplay together – the emphasis here on this relationship between reflective surfaces and how the eye is tricked by it. In the diagram to illustrate his thinking, a bouquet of flowers hangs upside down, beneath a table, and its image is inverted by the mirrors' interplay so that the bouquet appears upright, placed securely in a vase. The flowers are not in the vase, but because of the coordinating mirrors, the eye in the diagram sees them as so. The upright, contained bouquet is a fiction. The optical vectors, their connections, are the source of a mirage.

One can translate this diagram to an embodied circumstance by considering that an infant in front of a reflection is not just in relation to its own image but in relation to the adult who is holding the child and who is witnessing the child's dyadic revelation. The infant interacts with the adult who confirms the child's imagistic discoveries. No infant holds itself to the mirror – it relies on the adult's engagement, that looking back and forth, finding significance in the glass, and then search-ing for the child to do the same. Our relationships with our reflections are structured through the other's desire, a multiply mediated process of human correspondence.

When I was in the UK psych ward, one patient showed me photographs of a pop star on her phone and told me he loved her, reciting the song lyrics that declared this secret love. The screen of the phone showed his face together with the stark fluorescent light of the psych ward ceiling, both existing for a moment on the same plane. I accepted the force of this patient's fiction, unsure how to find solid ground beyond it. She tapped the phone along to the music, and my brain felt clumsy, numb, and thick, my doubts caught in her chimera of being loved. Neither of us could articulate that we were the ones to want another's gaze, that the fantasy illustrated not adoration but its absence. I had plucked dandelions from the tired and tiny lawn we were allowed to occupy, the fading grass bound by concrete walls and littered with cigarette butts, and I had placed each dandelion in plastic cups and handed these offerings to patients, and from their exclamations, I deduced that I was no longer Frasier to them but perhaps a beloved sister or a fairy godmother or a maiden in a pageant or just a fellow ward in our interminable capture, the dandelions bending at their stems, finally wilting until the blooms sank back into the water.

If the Lacanian flowers are not in the vase but appear so, through the relay of mirrors, then how do we distinguish between healthy, enabling delusion – the necessary organizing fantasy that helps us develop the sense of our own psychic and corporeal container and the complex interiority held by it – and the delusion involved in the tricks that our minds were playing in that psych ward, the tricks we perfected day and night as we shared our exuberant kindness? How exactly do you help someone develop the capacity, from within madness, to negotiate a delusion's contours? How does one define the moment when such finding occurs?

I don't believe any doctor can establish a fixed boundary between psychosis and what might be called stable human subjectivity, just as no solid border demarcates our delusions from our fantasies, our refusal of lack and our working with and through it, but I know I felt a visceral difference between the moments I tried to give and receive assurances in that run-down psych ward and the moments I would feel myself mediated years later by stillness, the imagistic statement gifted to me by my prairie friend. Does this difference have to do with my being able to sense the effect of the mirrors, their placement? Or my parsing of my own creative potential to transform what was blank? Or did both my friend and I grasp the psychological equivalent of the invisible diagonals that stretched between reflections – how my friend's statement was a citation, not uniquely his, and therefore never uniquely mine?

When the psychiatric patients and I spoke together, we were doing our best to affirm and to soothe each other, yet we became caught in the echoing chamber of want. We did not then know how to address how this want had caught us, how to articulate that we were the ones left wanting. We often could not see each other, especially not when each presence was fodder to continue delusion. Elated, we used each other, bodies propped quickly within a game of our undoing, the whole room a psychic pool table, whack of ball against ball.

In contrast to our discordant chorus, there is the meticulous arrangement of mirror to mirror, flower to vase, eye to mirror to the floating effect, each reflected petal as sure somehow as the real ones; these components are all precise, all intricately relational, not here the elated and flailing confusions of an infant but the organizing mind of an adult, situated within a social, symbolized world, formed as a self by being split from it, capable of simultaneously seeing an illusion created by reflection and identifying that it is one. Any careless adjustment and the image won't keep. When you look at Lacan's diagram, you can grasp how much depends on placement. You realize how still you'd have to stay.

My relationship with Lacan's diagram has for years been intimate, the kind forged when you are young and first determining what will be your chosen map of the world. Perhaps I have never had a solid sense of what is within me and what is without: I have long been intrigued by theories that give me a language for all that is insecure. I came to read Lacan independent of any lesson or guide; as I turned pages without confidence that I was grasping the meaning of the expansive yet cryptic text, my curiosity was piqued not just by the psychology but by the affective quiver induced by reading his prose. I had not yet experienced psychosis, but perhaps these were preparatory hours in how to negotiate its confusions: after a day with these dense paragraphs, language seemed to have loosened its referential grip.

I began to read aloud the work, feeling the resonance of its textures, encountering the language as one would a riddle or a statement in a dream. I would follow one assertion and then find the meaning inverted; I would dwell with an analogy or metaphor, enjoying the poetic layers of a text that didn't move in a straight line. When I have taught Lacan, I've tried to explicate his theories while I also gesture towards what resists explication. I have borrowed a concave mirror from the physics department and lugged it across campus to set it up in the classroom, quite sure I would be unable to reproduce the promised effect but pleased that I could at least make the students see the materiality of the mirrors, their shapes, and their arrangement in relation to each other and to the flowers that I had taped upside down. We could focus on the physicality of the thing, the art of the thing, spending time not just with the analysis but with the base component parts.

In that medieval apartment with the red light above the stove, I once tried to build my own version of these parts, composing objects in relation to each other on the floor. I did not have a concave mirror, but I had a pale green teacup. I did not have a flat mirror, but I knew that a piece of cardboard packaging would do. I had a red elastic band. I had acorns I'd collected in a bowl. Orange peels – these too could be tools. I placed each item carefully so that their angles could bounce off each other. I balanced books on their spine, hard covers open like double doors. As I descended into the spiralling mental vertigo that even during that long night I recognized as psychosis although I had no skill to stop its course, I diagrammed vectors of light or language or longing, gathering items on a flat surface so that these objects could communicate what words could not.

Whenever I make these displays, I believe my eyes are not the only ones to see the arrangement. I invent a watching presence, a beloved and loving presence, someone to understand what the objects mean.

Every one of my psychotic states has involved some aspect of this invention of a watching presence. But when I stood at the beige wall, instead of entering further into this fantasy until it collapsed into delusion, I was able to establish my bearings in a room where I knew I was alone.

The power of that decisive moment is most evident when compared with a more complete arc of other episodes, those years when I entered a plot when I had little awareness that I was the one writing it. After my time in the UK, I was living in Toronto, and my symptoms began to reappear, delirium soon as thick as the summer heat, my mind cluttered and clattering. I walked to my doctor's office, making sure first to lock my apartment that held not just all my possessions but the diagrams I'd made with them, the tin can and the candlestick, the cushion, and the running shoe.

Inside the waiting room, I once again felt the presence of cameras. Were they in the ceiling? My belief did not solidify into anything so technically specific – not here the beaming red light of my kitchen. I could not see any devices, only sense their power as I succumbed to a visceral knowledge of being watched, a hunch not unwelcomed. The eyes, I could tell, were benevolent: my friends stood on the other side of the camera, my beloved among them. I scanned the seats and the table and the information board that had looked authentic when I had arrived, although I now could tell that all the objects of this waiting room had been arranged specifically for me. I needed to identify and decipher the code.

The hardcover book with the giant print, the cover torn off – did it not tell of romance that had been ripped from my days? And *Little Red Riding Hood* – was that story not a warning of what could happen or a message about what had already happened to a child who had made the mistake of trusting someone garbed in a robe of care? Was some benevolent, unseen consciousness attending through these planted pages to my liminal state? The glossy magazines invoked those of the psych ward, and these were my beloved's way of telling me he knew of that extended entrapment, those days I had quickly folded and tucked away so I could return to school. A pregnant woman entered the room, and then another – bellies bulbous and taut, arms wrapped protectively around what I would never hold. I began to laugh because they were actors, weren't they? I grew surer: these performers were hired by my friends and my beloved to create this simulacrum of my life, my grief. It was too late for me to have children of my own, but I could have two pregnant women sitting so near, one beside me and one across, wishes caught in a funhouse mirror, my own slim body less substantial but connected, interdependent, rounded in theirs. The vibrancy of a day increased, and these women's bodies reflected my pain back to me, and the cameras would hold their shapes. Here, the lesson. My beloved would see my life, shattered, whole.

When I left the doctor's office, the Toronto street glinted, noisy and crowded, buses and street-cars emitting exhaust like the street's own sooty breath, and I passed homeless people who muttered to themselves the way I was muttering to myself. I could feel the hovering presence of my beloved as I walked past storefronts that he had orchestrated, somehow – a turquoise book, a turquoise dress – each display like a wink. I needed to find the wedding where he would be waiting, as a groom waits, as a groom watches, his eyes finding the bride. I knew ours wouldn't be a traditional wedding because I had to meet a friend at Shoppers Drug Mart, and she would show me the way, rag-tag through the summer city streets, heat reflecting off metal and glass, and coins in a paper cup, and empty bags lying crumpled as hope, and around a corner there'd be a book launch or a party or a protest or some other robust gathering that would become a wedding. When I walked through the drug store, all the products gave me clues about how to find this event. But I did not need these beauty products any more than I needed a white dress. My beloved had chosen me, as I am. Through the overhead speakers, Sarah McLachlan told me I'm in the arms of an angel, and my beloved had picked out this song, for this moment, and I read *sane* in *sanitary* and I begin to laugh because he would understand the joke.

Spend all that time waiting for a second chance, for a break that will make it okay.

He was there, somewhere – eyes in the ceiling or in these packages or maybe gazing through the window bright with sun. My laughter was not alone.

Place these two scenes next to each other: first, a woman spins in a Shoppers Drug Mart, toothpaste and shampoo and lipstick and her ebullient words to a beloved no one else can see. And then the sadder scene, the quieter scene, some years later: a woman stands still in a psychiatric segregation unit, staring at a beige wall, saying not a word. In both scenes, she is a solitaire. In both, she displays recognizable attributes of madness.

We have all walked past someone speaking with great determination to an intimate who is not there. And when a patient stands still, facing a wall, in a locked space, in beige pyjamas, there is little doubt to the nursing and psychiatric staff that her mind should not be trusted. But inside that troubled psyche where madness sometimes harbours its logics, these scenes in fact evidence two diverging mental states. On that heated afternoon chasing a wedding in Toronto – like my night performing to the red light in my UK flat – I possessed no distance from the fantasy's lure. I sincerely believed my groom was waiting for me, at some ad hoc and unconventional wedding that the stereo speakers in a drug store could announce.

What distinguishes my experience in segregation from this delirium in the store is that at the wall, I knew I was creating a sustaining interpretation of it. I could recall the recent past with my friend on the phone, just as I could imagine a future in which I might one day tell this friend about the soothing effect of his speech. He did not become an imaginary eye behind a camera. He was no spectral groom hovering in a drug store aisle. His sentence enabled me to see an image, and to see the seeing. The encounter with that beige wall felt neither sane nor insane but something in between, an intermediate realm I name poetry. I could feel observed without believing that the wall possessed eyes.

It would perhaps be no accident that my friend is a poet, although our conversation brimmed full of accidents, beginning with the chance of my phoning him that vulnerable day and then the haphazard journey our dialogue would take before we turned to the synchronistic talk of the prairies, his statement like a line that closes a poem, that jolt of rightness and surprise. There was no way to predict when I first called him what I would hear; he had no comprehension of the specifically romantic fantasy of my previous delusions, that invisible but oddly reliable beloved who mysteriously returns over and over again to wait and to watch, and my friend would not know that

I'd soon be caught in a lonely and frightening circumstance where I would encounter a surface that glinted flat and beige and blank.

My helpful friend possessed no medical expertise in diagnosis, nor had he undergone training in crisis intervention. He hadn't offered the prairies' mysterious ocular powers as a psychological treatment. He had simply done his best to follow my bouncing speech without yoking it too tightly to reason. He had spoken back in words that did and didn't make sense. And his chance statement acted as a pivotal catalyst, invoking past longings while enabling me to accept a solitude unaltered by the comfort of fixed delusion.

The prairies always see you. I have focused here on the prairies and their strange powers of seeing, but the *always* of my friend's statement also provided its reassurance, the security of a constant truth. As did the *you*, a pronoun not bound to my friend or to his friend or to me but open, as wide as the land. The statement could be directed to another and then another still, the way song lyrics or the lines of a poem resonate to each listener or reader, catching us in our moments, words, and syntax unchanged, beacon unchanging and yet becoming our own.

This statement would leverage an initial shift away from psychotic delusion, whereas our echoing dialogue together in the psych ward did not seem to realize this ameliorative purpose. An element of neutrality informs my friend's statement, the unmarked space and the sturdiness of *always* and the impersonal *you*. I could not co-opt it as uniquely mine, and in fact what sustained me was perhaps the very relationality of the teaching, the friend remaining distinct from my fray but aligning himself with me just as he had once been structured through speech by his own friend. He too possessed solitude that needed steadying. The prairies reached out with absence – no one breathing near – and yet in that uninterrupted enormity, one could be witnessed and feel it. With the ballast of this configuration, my own agency became crystalline, my mind pivoting with and through a prairie encounter as I tolerated my separation from it. Alone, I did not fall into a cascade of need within a phantasmagoria of mirrors but saw what was wanting, experienced it, so elemental, now, here, at the wall. I knew how I could answer.

When I invoke the possibility of a guide, I mean the innate worth of even this kind of tentative, serendipitous, creative exchange, my new orientation made possible by an instant of connection on the phone. I suggest taking that chance. I hope for such discoveries to occur, in dialogue, for those of us whose minds veer. What if we were to greet psychotic speech with the gathering poetry of sensuous things? Could you hear a word and turn it in the light? Could you risk the accidental ways that associations sometimes meet? Could you speak of what has held you, what has been offered you, the coordinates that have made you feel seen? We are none of us so securely ourselves that we do not need the glance of the world.

Those patients who announced to me their movies and their pop stars, their microchips and hidden cameras – the observed and therefore valuable scenes of their lives – all deserved guides who could listen and speak in unexpected way, who could think on fantasy's edge. By this I mean an intuitive process, collaborative, one that may pause to speak of the process itself. I mean responding to madness with an intimate mirror and naming it as such, not just introducing a prop but sharing some element of how you understand it. Purple gowns, and apple trees, a grandfather's silver lighter, a red stick-shift truck, a blunt haircut in a gleaming salon – in psych wards I have been privileged to hear a litany of items, each privately symbolic, each in some way a looking glass, and I know now that it's possible to work with the specificity of the object while also offering my own perspective, thereby providing another angle, a structuring angle, the one that turns the looking glass into a flower in an optical illusion, the sustaining illusion you come to recognize as itself. I know too I can name my own objects – the colour turquoise or the sea's lapping of the shore or how sunshine falls through cedar boughs – and I can say on an afternoon like today I look through the window at the hop of a robin and I feel my breath syncopate with this hop. We can speak with madness without entering its grip. We might not be able to teach the gift of lyrical and spontaneous response – that accidental play of words that enables a psychotic person both to feel seen and to see the seeing, to witness the very poetry of a struggling mind – but we could begin to try.

How am I doing?

References

Lacan J. 1991. *Seminar I: Freud's Papers on Technique 1953–54*. New York, NY: Norton.
Lacan J. 2006. *Écrits: The First Complete Edition in English*. New York, NY: Norton.

17

THE CAPACIOUSNESS OF UNCERTAINTY

From standing over to becoming alongside

Jiameng Xu

Hans-Georg Gadamer (2004: 298) writes, 'For what leads to understanding must be something that has already asserted itself in its own separate validity. Understanding begins . . . when something addresses us' (for an extended commentary on this see Laurrauri Pertierra 2022). In this chapter, I build on Gadamer's observation by engaging with the lived experience of psychiatry patients through a combination of my own observation as ethnographic researcher and critical reflection as clinician. I move between registers of creative writing and ethnographic accounts.

I begin with poetry. As Bleakley and Neilson (2021) write in *Poetry in the Clinic*, poetry has an advantage over conventional prose by not directly signifying to a larger truth. There is intentional masking, not for obfuscation but to signify varieties of meaning capturing the complexities of human experience. But my focus in this essay (and in terms of my own praxis) is different. I relate poetics to action in my life and work. While representing poetic experience through ethnographic thick description, and then by means of lines of poetry, I highlight the repetition of small units that constitute an action as a kind of 'being-held'. I purposefully experiment with form to give this essay a concrete sense of the clinical encounter's shifting forms and uncertainties, as poetic work *enacted*.

The anthropologist Cheryl Mattingly (2010) has written about the significance of recognizing the lived worlds of patients, placing at the centre what tends to become marginalized by biomedical regimes. Part of these lived worlds includes making a connection, and going on a journey, with patients. The journey can be extensive or fleeting and episodic, momentary. For me, medicine concerns such fleeting things that go on to constitute larger practices, as described in ethnographic thick descriptions by Arlene Katz (1996, 2023) of conversations between physicians and patients; Cheryl Mattingly (2010, 2014) of clinical encounters between the families of children with disabilities and their health care teams; and Melissa Park (2008, 2010) of the imaginative practices of children on the autism spectrum in a sensory integration clinic.

What is significant can be apparently minor – details, silences. Here, I build upon Katz's social poetics (2023), Mattingly's attention to *peculiar particularities* (2019), and Park's theorization of *embodied* significance to conceive of the poetic form as an opportunity to capture how 'regimes of significance' (Katz 1996) are at play in the clinical sphere: not only the powerful, received practices of biomedicine but also the small actions that lie outside of dominant ways of doing

 DOI: 10.4324/9781003341796-23

which Mattingly (Mattingly and Lawlor 2001; Mattingly 2010) has termed 'underground practices' to reflect how the small, fleeting, and *subversively* healing actions often go unnoticed – and perhaps need to remain hidden – to survive. In this move, I revise the doctor–patient relationship. I move away temporarily from rational diagnostics into embodiment and affect. What is it to *feel* the worldview of a 'patient' beyond technical empathy, a patient who in turn is responding to my presence? How will I enter and dwell in another's world? How will I engage the experience of the Other, especially where that person's experience is already judged clinically to be 'abnormal'?

Methodology: ethnographic and hermeneutic approaches

The philosopher of hermeneutics who introduces this chapter, Hans-Georg Gadamer, wrote in *Truth and Method* (Gadamer 2004) of understanding as nothing less momentous than an event that is brought about by interpretation. This requires a working out of potential meanings as reckoning with the foreknowledge and prejudgments that one inherently brings to the task of understanding. Gadamer lays out a theory of interpretation in which human beings are capable of *being addressed*, for that which we are seeking to understand always has something purposeful to say to us. Gadamer delineated his theory of hermeneutic understanding using examples of interpreting the meaning of a work of art or of a religious text considered in the present. Authors have a claim to truth, even if the meanings are not readily apparent to the reader, acting as interpreter and interlocutor. Or, in the clinical context, the health care provider – observing, interpreting, and forming an understanding to inform action.

During my ethnographic fieldwork for doctoral study, and subsequently in medical school, I could not help but ask the question: how does allowing oneself to be addressed by the claims to truth of other persons play out? Alongside other human beings, as Mattingly (2010) writes, experience is prospective – it unfolds moment to moment and is not fully bound by prior prediction. When released from classrooms into the field alongside other persons and other communities, I learned that my initial instinct had often been not to remain open but to flee when I was being addressed by a truth I could not readily grasp. I needed to cultivate a stance of being open to uncertainty while remaining in relationship with others – a poetics of uncertainty alongside others whose worlds I had entered – to complete my task as ethnographer. This poetics of uncertainty surely describes the essence of the clinical encounter. And while in health care delivery, uncertainty itself may be regarded as unsatisfactory, undesirable, or lacking in usefulness, in hermeneutics, uncertainty is the starting point of interpretation, of any understanding that can be gained; its epistemological status is a positive one.

What I did not anticipate at the time, but now in my position as a resident doctor have recognized, is that my comportment as ethnographer – this poetic stance based on aesthetic, affective, and philosophical elements – crossed over into the clinical sphere in my being alongside patients as health care provider. Below, I offer 'thick descriptions' of two clinical encounters, both with patients in an inpatient psychiatric unit, to illustrate how the values proposed by Gadamer's theory of hermeneutic understanding can come in to play, in turn deepening the quality of medical work as a poetic praxis.

The first encounter occurred during my ethnographic fieldwork and the second during clerkship as a fourth-year medical student. In the analyses, I highlight the aesthetic, affective, and body-sensing dimensions that undergirded a stance of openness to uncertainty. From my ethnographic fieldwork, I trace how my growing capacity to listen was related to changes in how I saw 'Adam', an inpatient service user, shifting from understanding his world as one dominated by loss, in which he is a patient at risk of suicide, to one containing several possibilities, in which he is a person in search of his heart. The further I am introduced into Adam's world and share scenes with him through ethnographic engagements, the more I am returned to his world as I seek to generate meaning from the elements that have significance for him.

Holding multiple possible understandings about Adam allowed me to continue to go into his world and listen more closely to his experiences that do not have closure. It is as though I had been falling into the cracks between his words, in the spaces, the silences. We think we are falling, but we are letting ourselves be held by these spaces to see what is possible – as well as letting the other person pull both of us out from such in-between spaces. I step into these spaces also so that Adam might give me his hand. I step lower than myself – and find myself plunging within.

In defence of what is fleeting (and repeats)

Arlene Katz's (2023) article outlining a 'social poetics' allows the patient's idiosyncratic voice of relating to their own world to be heard. Of many observations that she has made, the one that stands out for me as a physician concerns the 'structure of narrowing'. She notes that what matters is what appears to be fleeting. In my own practice, I have seen that the structures of poetry are found within such spaces and gaps. Such gaps are not intrusions but an invitation, and a holding, to come into something new. They resemble Heidegger's theorization of truth as a 'clearing'.

Mattingly (2010) enunciated the moral importance of such (in)actions, occurring in tandem, and prospectively, in terms of how it is to *accompany* one another in activity, forming meanings. This, in the pursuit of a life, an alternate future, at times an alternate identity, one worth striving for. I am reminded of what Heidegger said of 'comportment' or Bourdieu of 'habitus' – as forms of indwelling spaces. This, a way of being in the world that influences what it is that we see, and of specific resources being more open to us, within touch or just out of reach but sensible.

I would see this, poetically (drawing on metaphor and enjambment) as:

Where the fleeting has an insistence, of meaning
That causes oneself to be held in the moment
There is a dramatic component to significant things
Which I sense in my body
What can I hear if I allow the gaps to open
So I can step through them to the other side of understanding?
Might there be an epistemic porousness
If I listen into the spaces between things
And allow what is fleeting to happen
As the poetic and ethnographic imaginations
Flow into the clinical sphere – I might go
On journeys alongside the Other, together

The poetry interrupts, inserts. Rudely perhaps. There is a capaciousness of uncertainty in poetry, and flux, a fluctuating quality. This is built into the very structure of poetry yet is sought to be minimized in health care delivery. I think of Gadamer's (2018) reflections in *The Enigma of Health* on the technologizing of health care and what is missing there. In opening a space, a clearing, we turn what was presumed to be certain into knowledge that once more is at risk and thus has the potential to change, to be revised, in light of new needs. I found this form of attention in both ethnography and poetry, but it is squeezed out in clinical medicine.

Yet there is a wariness towards coming alongside, towards entering uncertainty. How can I let myself be held by uncertainty rather than overwhelmed by it? What can draw me to stay and let myself become addressed by what uncertainty is trying to say rather than turning away from it? When there is not a cure, and when the answer is not known, there remains care: 'presence' is something that we can offer. A shifting of perspective, perhaps, a movement to 'go alongside' the Other. The 'call' to attend to the fleeting is the repetition of something small and simple. In poetry, repetition gives a force, and it is not redundancy but the *insistence* of something that has not yet been adequately heard, has not yet been fully seen and met upon its own terms. And, as Park writes, our bodies know how to attend to significance, how to be alongside others. Perhaps the receding horizon of meaning is not a sign that understanding necessarily eludes us or remains out of reach but rather is an invitation to journey further alongside the Other and one's own interpretations which are nascent and developing.

There is a capaciousness in uncertainty

What of the poem
Of the voice, of the image
Of the compression
A place where gaps, silences, can live.

The compression of the poem – and the dramatism of the clinical moment as captured by Cheryl Mattingly's fieldwork in clinical spaces

Where the missing piece, the missing note
That which is not there, can come into being.

When what is expected does not arise
A porousness of Being
An hermeneutics of uncertainty

These three bold headings promise much. This is how some patients experience their worlds – as the tipping out of bold headings. Exclamations! But what is the subsequent text? Of health care as conferring an *experience* of healing, so that *the encounter itself is medicine*, has the potency of transformation – as much as it had been, in the spaces of rituals – to offer a sense that something could be otherwise than it is presently?

I am in search of something with the capaciousness for uncertainty, as poetry has. And in poetry, the importance of spaces in between, of silence, the pause. Where lines are left hanging and are picked up – salvaged – by another. Lisa Stevenson (2014: 13), in her ethnography of a complex – of a phenomenon and experience and topic as complex as suicide in the Canadian Arctic – says, 'We do not always want the truth in the form of facts or information; often we want it in the form of an image. What we want, perhaps, is the opacity of an image that can match the density of our feelings. We want something to hold us'. What does it mean to allow oneself to be held by uncertainty, rather than overwhelmed by it? In the following sections, I play with the structure of the ethnographic thick description to highlight momentary interactions during which elements can become rearranged, creating a gap in which the voice of the Other emerges. The first encounter, 'The Song of the Broken Piano', was originally described in a dissertation of persons living with mental illness and their family members (Xu 2019).

The song of the broken piano

An upright piano, lidless and battered, sits against one wall of the day room of the ward. Its white wooden keys bear words written in fine black ink: 'Not OK'. 'Not OK'. 'OK'. Leaning across this labelled terrain, I press a 'Not OK' key, listening for any sound. Where I expect a note to emerge, there is only quiet; the sound I wait for does not arrive. There is only the expected tone ringing in my imagination. 'The piano is broken', says a man, walking past. 'So much in here is broken'.

One morning Adam, a patient diagnosed with schizophrenia whom the staff fear will take his own life, is sitting at the piano. He begins to play a song from memory in the key of D minor. The notes circle one another; his song has a haunting quality. It does not seem to matter that the piano has several missing keys. I do not anticipate the song's end until he stops playing. 'Would you like to play a song?' he asks. Seeing my nod, he asks further, 'What songs do you know? Maybe you can play the song you know without the notes? I would like to hear it before I go'.

I bend my head and begin to play the only song that I know by heart. When the notes that I expect do not ring, my fingers falter on the next ones. My hand struggles to continue, carried forward by intention or muscle memory, to span the gap of the missing notes. My playing comes to a halt. To my ears the song sounds broken, almost unrecognizable, against the melody that I remember so clearly.

Seeing my anxiety, Adam offers, 'Maybe you can play it at a different place, so you won't have to use the missing notes'.

Closing my eyes, I shift my right hand to a higher octave. There are still some broken keys at this range, but the notes now take on a familiar contour. At the song's end, Adam says, 'That sounded really nice. You played it even though notes are missing. I know that song. It's from the movie Amélie'. The embodied sensation of unexpected gaps appearing, of the playing of the next note depending on the ones before, has remained with me.

Subsequently, other patients on the unit begin referring to me as 'the player of the broken piano'. 'No one plays that piano', they say. Yet it is Adam who first played on the piano the song he had composed. He stood next to me when I froze, offering encouragement that prompted my hands to move again upon the keys, telling me that if the playing is shifted to a different register, a song is still possible. I was stuck. I was stuck. I was stuck. But then Adam invited me to come alongside him. My fingers no longer seemed to trip over the gaps between the notes of the broken piano but rather to sweep them up into another melody. Perhaps, as with the missing notes, it is with attention to the spaces in between where one might invite the voice of the other, alongside one's own voice, to come through.

[ ]

When the sound I expect does not arise.
I am anxious.
The notes: Not OK. Not OK. Not OK.
I am falling into the gap
And he says – what if you play in a different register?
What do we do, how can we learn
When what we expect does not arise?

'Not OK'. 'Not OK'. ' OK'.
I press a 'Not OK' key, listening for any sound.

Where I expect a note to emerge there is only quiet; the sound I wait for does not arrive.
There is only the expected tone ringing in my mind.
It does not seem to matter that the piano has several missing keys.
I play the only song that I know by heart.
When the notes that I expect do not ring, my fingers falter on the next ones.
My hand struggles to continue, carried forward by intention or muscle memory, to span the gap of the missing notes.

My playing comes to a halt. To my ears the song sounds broken, almost unrecognizable, against the melody that I remember so clearly.
'But maybe you can play it at a different place, so you won't have to use the missing notes', Adam offers.

Closing my eyes, I shift my right hand to a higher octave.

There are still some broken keys at this range, but the notes now take on a contour familiar to me.

'But you played it even though notes are missing', he said.
There may be value in the silences and in allowing them to hold us.

From standing over to becoming alongside

Three years after meeting Adam as ethnographer, I return to Hillside Hospital, now as medical student. Yet the comportment of an ethnographer – to observe, to not take for granted received w ways of doing – has become ingrained in me by then.

The ward has been newly renovated. There is more natural light coming through the windows. The walls are decorated with images of forests. Where two, even four, patients had once shared a room, now every room has single occupancy, providing privacy as well as space for a large armchair for one's own, or a visitor's, use. The occupational therapy room that many patients had earlier said was the heart of the ward was made bigger, with a shiny new oven, refrigerator, and microwave. The artwork made by patients year after year that had adorned the cabinets and walls of the occupational therapy room of the old ward had not followed into the new one; not yet, or perhaps it was time to start anew.

Even on the unit where I had met Adam, which had been a 'higher care' unit, the renovations had wrought a difference. The common area for patients was no longer a single long table but a series of round tables with chairs surrounding each. The nursing station was no longer a single small square room but had been elongated. There was now a set of computers by the hallway, separated by glass, where patients would walk. Sitting there, you could see what people were doing, and there was no longer a need for cameras in each patient's room. Still, privacy was limited.

I heard of Mr. Tremblay before I met him; as so often happens, patients' medical histories precede them in the act of handover between health care providers. Meant to inform by drawing one's focus towards pertinent clinical signs, this kind of clinically constructed foreknowledge can restrict understanding only to deficits, dysfunction, decompensation, rather than allowing for a view of the whole person. In the hallway, at a computer on one side of the dividing glass, I read the photocopies of his chart sent ahead from the previous hospital: he had been there four weeks before being transferred today to Hillside; he had been diagnosed with suspected catatonia, been treated with lorazepam, and apparently improved momentarily before having a decrease in his symptoms once more.

Alongside the senior psychiatric resident, I wondered what clinical picture his constellation of symptoms might make. He had had an infectious illness that could affect the nervous system but that was treated and cured, no longer active, and unlikely to be a contributory factor to what was going on in the present. Clinical questions aimed at arriving at a hypothesis came through my mind. A first episode of major depression at Mr. Tremblay's age – 60 – is rare but not unheard of. What other episodes might he have had in the past that could clarify what he was going through in the present?

The senior resident sat with me. He had made cue cards of the symptoms of catatonia: waxy flexibility, negativism, mutism, automatism. Yet one element jumped out from Mr. Tremblay's chart: in his social and personal history, he had had only one significant romantic relationship in his life. It had been with a man but ended decades ago. My senior resident turned to me: 'It must have been very hard to be a man who loved another man, during that time, harder than it is now'.

The following day, not yet 24 hours since his arrival to the psychiatric unit at Hillside Hospital, Mr. Tremblay was brought to the interview room for a diagnostic interview. We hoped it would lead us somewhere, but we felt stuck. Dr. Bouchard, the staff psychiatrist, asked this question:

'Have you felt love?'
Mr. Tremblay's expression stilled.
'Have you been in love?'
He got up and left the room.

Upon our unit, others referred to his symptoms as a diagnostic mystery. We waited and watched. During this time, I sought to converse with Mr. Tremblay, but our daily interactions were limited to him giving me a thumbs up while lying in the hospital bed, closing his eyes, then smiling slightly before turning his head away, seemingly to rest or to sleep. Sometimes he asked me when he can go home. During his initial days on the ward at Hillside, Mr. Tremblay had spent time in the common area, seated beside other patients who carried on conversations around him. These days, he was no longer seen outside of his room. Hoping for insight and more information, I called Mr. Tremblay's brother. He described Mr. Tremblay as someone who has mostly kept to himself all his life. I felt at a loss.

What to do? In other fields, I might touch the patient, I might place a hand, to signify my presence or request the beginning of a connection, but in psychiatry, we seem to use our voices first. *I was stuck. I was stuck. I was stuck.* I stood still at the doorway.

One day, from the foot of Mr. Tremblay's bed, I was imploring him to come talk with us, to come to our activity groups, he said suddenly,
'I bet you are good at doing laundry'.
Caught off guard, I replied automatically, 'Yes. I am good at doing other things too'.

Outside of Mr. Tremblay's room, behind the glass of the nursing station, I pondered his words. I could not help thinking of the time we had asked him about being in love and he had responded by getting up and walking out of the room. Were we in a kind of tit-for-tat? What drama, what narrative, were we both caught within? How were we reading one another, and misreading one another, as Mattingly explores in her ethnographic accounts?

As the week passed, Mr. Tremblay spent more and more time alone in his hospital room. I could no longer catch glimpses of him in the common area or in the hallways as I walked around the ward to meet other patients. On the last workday of the week, nearing evening and the distribution of supper, as I was gathering my own belongings from the nursing station and preparing to go home for the weekend, I caught sight of Mr. Tremblay retreating as he walked to the shared washroom. Except this time, he was no longer wearing his own clothes as he had done earlier this week. Instead, he was wearing the standard hospital issued gown, patterned blue and white, tied at the neck and, in Mr. Tremblay's case, almost fully open behind, leaving his back and legs exposed. His moved quickly from the hallway into the washroom.

The psychiatric team spent less and less time with Mr. Tremblay. We continued to go from task to task. These are our rounds: we assess someone; we hold them until their situation changes. But Mr. Tremblay had stopped engaging with us. We started speaking of doing a pharmacologic washout, of discontinuing his psychiatric medications, to see if there might be any change we might observe in his symptoms. But when facing uncertainty, I try to draw upon readily made frameworks to allow something to speak for itself – he is certainly not broken – with the piano, playable music, just hanging out. When I returned on Monday morning, I went first to the nursing station. A nurse approached me with quick strides: 'Mr. Tremblay – he has been refusing to get out of bed for anything. Not even to use the washroom. He has been soiling himself in his bed. We don't know if he's doing it on purpose, or if he is getting worse'.

That morning, the clinical team of which I was a part stood once more at the doorway to Mr. Tremblay's room.

'Mr. Tremblay', said Dr. Bouchard in a clear, loud voice. 'We need you to come with us to the interview room. We need you to get up'.

'Can't we talk here?' responded Mr. Tremblay, sitting upright in his hospital bed.

'No, we need to do it in the interview room', repeated Dr. Bouchard.

Mr. Tremblay shook his head. Silence filled the room. As Dr. Bouchard started turning to leave, I turned to leave. At that moment, I felt a pull into the room.

'Mr. Tremblay', I said, walking to his bedside. 'We really want you to go home too, but we're missing something, there's something we're not getting. We really need you to tell us what is missing'.

A moment passed before Mr. Tremblay spoke, his voice stronger and clearer than I have heard in days. 'Can you get me a pair of pants? Then I will come out with you'.

The orderly who had been standing with our group at the doorway leaped into action. 'I'm on it!' he said. I followed him into the hallway, beyond the nursing station, to a closet. The orderly pulled open its door and reached to the very top shelf to take a set of folded, green pants, cut of a thicker fabric than the standard issue hospital gown.

When we returned to Mr. Tremblay's room, he was already sitting upright on his bed, his bare legs over the side, his feet touching the floor. He was ready to go, waiting for us. I waited outside as the orderly stepped within and proceeded to help Mr. Tremblay put on the pants. Once dressed, without effort, he stood up. His shoulders straightened, and Mr. Tremblay walked into the hallway in his green pants, pink foam hospital slippers, and the blue-and-white hospital gown still worn around his neck, covering the top of his pants.

'Let's go', he said, stepping ahead of me. As we made our way to the interview room at the end of the hallway, Mr. Tremblay offered a smile and a wave to another patient passing by. I asked him if he would attend the music therapy group this afternoon. He responded by telling me that he liked 'oldie' bands, and he proceeded to name them as we walked together.

Clinical implications: when we allow uncertainty to hold us and to address us

Something insists upon itself – over, and over, and over again. To be able to listen for the question, for what is not said.

How are you?
How do you feel?
How did you sleep?

The questions we habitually ask in the same cadence:

> *What are we missing?*
> *What are we missing?*
> *What are we missing?*
> *Can you tell us what is missing?*

The way the uncertainty asks us to stay and asks us to linger. As Gadamer had written, to tarry. More: to pose to our own understandings and interpretations questions that might hold no answer. Perhaps that is listening: to tarry just a bit longer beyond our threshold of understanding when another person gives us an invitation to stay.

> *There is poetry wherever there is a detail that stands out.*
> *There is poetry whenever there is a feeling in my body that arrests me.*
> *There is poetry whenever there is a gap; whenever I feel there is something that seems missing.*

It is an invitation to wonder what is on the other side of the threshold of understanding.

These ways may be fleeting. There may not yet be a language in which to chart them in medical records, in the explicit regimes of significance within clinical medicine. How will the chart record a capacity for tolerance of uncertainty in the name of the Other?

[   ]

It is close at hand – it is within my body. Into the microworlds, where I see others' efforts – and my own – in making a world, in making significance, wherever we find ourselves. We do not presume that the Other and the physician come from the same world, but we often communicate as though we do. The Other has a capacity for world-making that needs to be recognized though it is often overlooked. Actions and meanings we did not know of. The 'I' embodied, allowing oneself to be addressed. The detail, the detail that persists, the object that persists in an orderly environment. That which seems to insist upon its own being. That which repeats. That which does not quite fit. You create an experience for another; you create an experience for yourself. And my own embodied self, responding to the embodied selves of others.

If as lines calling to one another, like music, in the temporality of a poem:

It meant something to bring a presence
Not only a meeting of horizons –
But horizons which are called forth from one another

Waiting, skipping over, being off balance
To be caught by uncertainty, to surrender to it, to step into its vulnerability.
There is a fundamental duty to recognize the world-making of the Other.
Is it the unspoken that speaks the loudest?

A widening, an opening
Allowing oneself to be held by uncertainty

Rather than overwhelmed by it.
Even in anxiety

There is a power in attending to the particularities
Capturing significance in its own right
A place where gaps and silences can live
Where the missing piece and the missing note
That which is not there
Come into being

[   ]

Bringing to consciousness one's affective, bodily-sensing, aesthetic reactions – as an enacted poetics of uncertainty – helps us to be attuned to other data, other forms of knowledge, already in experience. These knowledges outside of received ways of understanding may be obscured or overshadowed by a singular attention to technological, procedural ways of engagement in clinical encounters. Their impact has been greatest when I could no longer avail myself of the procedural, technologically derived resources that occupy the most visible position in medical training. There is a peculiar power in attending to particularities.

More meaning is available, and more is given to us, than perhaps we might ever know. A listening for what is not being said, what has not yet been included in a frame of understanding. My experience as an ethnographer, a medical student, and now a junior health care practitioner is that the urge to flee in the presence of meaning – of meaning that might at first seem mysterious, conflicting with what I think I already know, not readily fitting with the knowledge of other actors around me, particularly if they are in positions of authority – is at times immense.

Cultivating a stance, a comportment, that treats ruptures and unexpected moments in understanding as a starting point to understanding itself, as valuable data, can be an aid to remaining with these moments in which something new is coming forth and addressing us with its claim to truth – which we may be capable of understanding if we do not turn away. Though I have presented an analysis, using philosophical, anthropological, and literary resources, to elucidate affective, body-sensing, aesthetic–*poetic* and narrative–phenomenological – dimensions, it may be the work of each person, each practitioner, to find and recognize their own, and it may be that doing so is worthwhile as it becomes embodied in our very own way of being in the world.

And Mr Tremblay – what of him? I came to stand alongside, rather than over, him. We created a clearing. We bring our presence out into the open.

References

Bleakley A, Neilson S. 2021. *Poetry in the Clinic: Towards a Lyrical Medicine*. Abingdon: Routledge.

Gadamer HG. 2004. *Truth and Method* (2nd ed.). New York, NY: Continuum.

Gadamer HG. 2018. *The Enigma of Health: The Art of Healing in a Scientific Age*. Redwood City, CA: Stanford University Press.

Katz AM. Social Poetics as Processual Engagement: Making Visible What Matters in Social Suffering. *Transcultural Psychiatry*. 2023; 60: 844–51.

Katz AM, Shotter J. Hearing the Patient's 'Voice': Toward a Social Poetics in Diagnostic Interviews. *Social Science & Medicine*. 1996; 43: 919–31.

Laurrauri Pertierra I. Gadamer's Historically Effected and Effective Consciousness. Dialogue: *Canadian Philosophical Review*. 2022; 61: 261–84.

Mattingly C. 2010. *The Paradox of Hope: Journeys through a Clinical Borderland*. Oakland, CA: University of California Press.

Mattingly C. 2014. *Moral Laboratories: Family Peril and the Struggle for a Good Life*. Oakland, CA: University of California Press.

Mattingly C. Defrosting Concepts, Destabilizing Doxa: Critical Phenomenology and the Perplexing Particular. *Anthropological Theory*. 2019; 19: 415–39.

Mattingly C, Lawlor M. The Fragility of Healing. *Ethos*. 2001; 29: 30–57.

Park M. Making Scenes: Imaginative Practices of a Child With Autism in a Sensory Integration – Based Therapy Session. *Medical Anthropology Quarterly*. 2008; 22: 234–56.

Park M. Beyond Calculus: Apple-Apple-Apple-Ike and Other Embodied Pleasures for a Child Diagnosed With Autism in a Sensory Integration Based Clinic. *Disability Studies Quarterly*. 2010; 30. No pagination. Available at: https://dsq-sds.org/index.php/dsq/article/view/1066/1232. Last accessed: 3/10/2023.

Stevenson L. 2014. *Life Beside Itself: Imagining Care in the Canadian Arctic*. Berkeley, CA: University of California Press.

Xu J. 2019. *Practices of Being Near: An Ethnographic Study of Family Members and Persons with Lived Experience of Mental Illness*. Montreal: McGill University.

18

SYLVIA WYNTER AND THE POETICS OF PSYCHIATRY

Bahar Orang

Introduction

In this essay, I want to take seriously the political philosopher Sylvia Wynter's invitation to articulate a new poesis of being human and to look at how the field of Western psychiatry reproduces colonial conceptions of the human. Wynter, in conversation with Frantz Fanon, insists that the world (our ways of thinking and being) articulates itself at the levels of language, culture, and poetics. Following this ethic, I am interested in how language is deployed in psychiatric cultures to imagine, project, and materialize what Wynter calls the biocentric genre of the human, or Man-as-Human. I want to reckon with the stakes of psychiatry's totalizing commitment to the category of Man-as-Human and think through what kinds of violence such a commitment makes possible.

If on the day that I started writing this essay (25 January 2021) you had visited the homepage of the website of the University of Toronto's psychiatry department, you would have been greeted with a banner across the page titled 'ImPACT,' which refers to 'psychiatry articles that change treatment'. On this day, if you had clicked through the featured articles, you would have read interviews with the lead researchers on three projects: 'Understanding how a key mutation influences the development of schizophrenia'; 'New research uncovers a possible cause of borderline personality disorder'; and 'Preventing the reincarceration of prisoners with mental illness'. These articles, as achievements for the department, offered – offer – an opportunity, as case studies, to consider psychiatry's agenda and psychiatry's priorities.

The University of Toronto's psychiatry department is among the most highly regarded in Canada. It encompasses hundreds of doctors, students, researchers, and trainees and is associated with several hospitals, faculties, research centres, and educational programmes. What appears on the Department's home page reveals a lot about what is being taught, learned, reproduced, enacted, cemented, and imagined about how people deemed mentally ill should be, and are, treated (clinically and beyond the clinic). What appears on the Department's home page also makes clear which stories of what it means to be human we continue to tell, indeed, which stories psychiatry has historically, and into the historical present, co-written and co-enforced. Psychiatry, I contend, is a branch of medicine that is fundamentally narratively, culturally, and provisionally inscribed. At the same time, psychiatry continually insists upon, and fantasizes after, an empirical basis even as it performs especially well, and reifies with especial violence, the biocentric genre of the human

DOI: 10.4324/9781003341796-24

(Wynter 2003). Whatever admissions of the 'psycho-social' psychiatry articulates, psychiatry ultimately further lodges, and with great anxiety, that biocentric system of knowledge.

We could call them assumptions – that which each of these articles takes as incontestable truths and against which each article props up its claim towards progress – but it may be more precise to call them omissions with an (un)ethical and political agenda. And still, omissions might suggest that simple or straightforward inclusion could be the remedial move when what is problematic is the ideological and rhetorical core and the smallest units of thought and word. The problem runs through. After grappling for a long time through my medical training with these entanglements of language and ideology and science and subjectivity, struggling to make sense of the mess that continually produces grossly uneven social relations (all the '-isms'), the writings of Sylvia Wynter, and in particular the premise of the overrepresentation of Man-as-Human, both clarified and complicated the predicament and the possibility of a radically different sociality. As for all the '-isms', in an interview with Greg Thomas (2006) in *ProudFlesh*, Sylvia Wynter explains,

> I am trying to insist that 'race' is really a code-word for 'genre'. Our issue is not the issue of 'race'. Our issue is the issue of the genre of 'Man'. It is this issue of the genre of 'Man' that causes all the -isms.

Theoretical contexts

Critical psychiatry

In a conversation between Wynter and the political theorist Bedour Alagraa, with reference to COVID19, Wynter asserts that the science we have can't give us the knowledge we need (Alagraa 2021), and such an assertion might resonate for clinicians and thinkers from the field of critical psychiatry, who might similarly argue the need for different scientific approaches. Critical psychiatry is interested in meaningfully addressing intellectual, political, and ethical critiques of psychiatry. Critical psychiatrists understand that psychiatry's dominant modes of practice are deeply flawed but also generally believe in professional services for people who are 'mentally ill'. Critical psychiatry has been interested in grappling with the limitations and problems of the *Diagnostic and Statistical Manual of Mental Disorders* (DSM), naming and excavating the profound influence of pharmaceutical companies on psychiatric clinical work and knowledge production and looking honestly at psychiatry's practices of coercion.

In 2012, a group of 29 critical psychiatrists came together to write a seminal article published by *The British Journal of Psychiatry* titled 'Psychiatry Beyond the Current Paradigm', arguing that the 'technological paradigm' which dominates psychiatry 'has not served psychiatry well'. The writers put forward that there is scant 'empirical evidence' for the technological paradigm, which privileges categorization (per the DSM) and biological reductionism (implying greater and greater use of pharmaceuticals). They suggest a post-technological psychiatry that does not abandon the tools of empirical science or reject medical and psychotherapeutic techniques but that positions ethical and hermeneutic aspects of psychiatry as primary, thus emphasizing the importance of values, relationships, politics, ethics, and aesthetics (Braken 2012). The writers of *Beyond the Current Paradigm* might therefore agree, then, that the science we have can't give us the knowledge we need.

Wynter's conceptualization of Man-as-Human (how 'he' came to be and how 'he' is continually reproduced) emerges from a specifically and essentially anticolonial study. To apply a Wynterian analysis to psychiatry is to make ethical and aesthetic claims that reference something other than the 'lack of empirical evidence' that is referenced by *Beyond the Paradigm*. A Wynterian analysis, and a careful attention to poetics, can potentially encompass critical psychiatry but only where its epistemological context has changed, expanded, or become more persistently and committedly precise in its naming and study of colonialism. It is not just that the psychiatry of the present technological paradigm has poor or bad or unsatisfactory outcomes: it is that those outcomes are a reproduction and perpetuation of coloniality and colonial violence.

So when Alagraa talks of 'the knowledge we need', our challenge is towards a liberatory science: not a psychiatry that has been renovated via a critical mode but a frightening and exciting and actual break, a radically expansive and fundamental ontological, epistemological, and poetic shift towards not just a different psychiatry but a different *genre of the human* (Wynter 2003).

Genres of the human

Our current epistemological order, dominated by liberalist scientific knowledge, answers the question of who we are as humans in purely biological, secular, and economic terms. (I understand liberalism according to Malini Ranganathan's (2016) explanation in 'Thinking with Flint'. She writes that liberalism is 'centred on the promise of individual freedoms and equality for all. Some combination of market relationship, the rule of law, moral restraint, and a minimally interfering state are all said to help deliver on this promise'.) This answer, which Wynter calls 'Man' while insisting on its total *a priori*-ness and its absolute-ness, is a descriptive statement and is therefore epistemological and subject to permutation over changing political, economic, and cultural conditions. 'Man' has emerged from the Copernican break (with the secularizing realization that the earth moves) and the Darwinian rupture (with the bio-centring theories of evolution and natural selection). Wynter (2003) tells us about Man1 and Man2 (where Man2 is our contemporary genre of human):

> The first was from the Renaissance to the eighteenth century; the second from then on until today, thereby making possible both the conceptualizability of natural causality, and of nature as an autonomously functioning force in its own right governed by its own laws (i.e. cursus solitus naturae), with this, in turn making possible the cognitively emancipatory rise and gradual development of the physical sciences (in the wake of the invention of Man1), and then of the biological sciences (in the wake of the nineteenth century invention of Man2).

Katherine McKittrick (2015), a theorist of Black feminist geographies, writes to the categories of personhood that are thus produced by Man1 and Man2:

> These figures, both Man1 and Man2, are also inflected by powerful knowledge systems and origin stories that explain who/what we are. These systems and stories produce the lived and racialized categories of the rational and irrational, the selected and the dysselected, the haves and the have-nots as asymmetrical naturalized racial-sexual human groupings that are specific to time, place, and personhood yet signal the processes through which the empirical and experiential lives of all humans are increasingly subordinated to a figure that thrives on accumulation.

In other words, a Western biological science that is underpinned by essentialized theories of natural selection, natural scarcity, and total objectivity, that is performed via classification, enumeration, and hierarchization, will always and inevitably require a *dysselected* other, who in the wake of colonialism, imperialism, and transatlantic slavery in the making of the modern world, has been the 'fallen indigenous/nonwhite/black/African' (McKittrick 2015). Western biological science enacts a racial (racist) science. [Where there are those who are naturally selected, there are also those who are naturally dysselected in the biocentric order (Wynter in McKittrick 2015: 44)].

But Wynter (2003) does not dismiss the organic bodies that we are and the material world that we inhabit; she argues rather that we are more than only 'bios' and are more so 'bios-mythos'. We are a languaging, storytelling, and bio-physical species, and these are not disparate descriptions but are utterly enmeshed, deeply entangled, co-constituting, hybrid ways of being. She explains,

> What I'm putting forward as a challenge here, as a wager, is therefore that the human is, meta-Darwinianly, a hybrid being, both bios and logos (or, as I have recently come to rede-fine it, bios and mythoi). Or, as Fanon says, phylogeny, ontogeny, and sociogeny, together, define what it is to be human. With this hypothesis, should it prove to be true, our system of knowledge as we have it now, goes.

Relatedly, McKittrick (2015) elaborates one of Wynter's scientific challenges: 'to denaturalize biocentricity and its attendant fallen/dysselected castoffs while honouring the science of func-tioning living systems'. I want to take up this challenge in the moment in which I find myself, encountering three (what I see as emblematic) psychiatric articles offered up, with no concern, by the educational institution in which I have been fixed for the past several years. I will give close attention to these psycho-scientific articles, following word and language, to understand where and how they tell the story of Man-as-Human.

The goal is to agitate, undo, and destabilize towards an 'opening up' (*ibid.*). The goal is not, as I have learned from Wynter, to simply displace the subject – 'Man' – and replace him with some other bounded or autonomous figure. Instead, the hope is to reconsider all the terms altogether towards radically reimagining and rearticulating, collectively, other ways of recognizing, address-ing, and being with each other. Wynter redirects us from boundaried subjectivity towards the realization of deep relationality.

Biocentricity and the eugenist consequence

The word 'predict' appears six times in the 2020 article 'Understanding how a key mutation influ-ences the development of schizophrenia' (https://psychiatry.utoronto.ca/news/understanding-how-key-mutation-influences-development-schizophrenia). The interviewee discusses the genetic variation 22q11.2 deletion syndrome (22q11DS), which has apparently been linked to schizophre-nia. The syndrome describes 'a condition where a small piece of DNA is missing from chromo-some 22' and phenotypically manifests as 'a range of physical and mental health issues', including schizophrenia, in 'one in four' individuals, thus making it 'the strongest known single genetic risk factor for this mental illness'. Later, the interviewee discusses the consequences of his research for clinical care,[1] and he returns to greater and greater improvements in the project of 'prediction'. He calls attention to the importance of 'thinking more in terms of early intervention for schizophre-nia'. To be clear, my close interest in language here is not to make an *ad hominem* charge against the interviewee but to identify evidence of the storying process at work in the continual creation and recreation of Man-as-Human by the psychiatry institution. Science is described, is storied, is made by word. The word 'predict' refers to a possible eugenic frontier. The highly positivistic relationship between genotype and phenotype assumes favourable and unfavourable phenotypes and therefore genotypes.

Biocentric science animates categories of selection and dysselection.[2] But this is a science whose material world ultimately exceeds it; this is a science that struggles, despite systematic elimination towards the fantasy of objectivity, to account for a complexity and a mysteriousness that resists total and closed categorization. The researcher expresses the research team's scientific curiosity about 'why so much variation exists' (even though 'the genetic variant is the same') and then says, 'we found that the information hidden in the rest of the genome can be used' to address the problem of variation.

Both the reference to 'scientific curiosity' and that to things 'hidden' are informative. In the purely biocentric worldview, there is a world that precedes the stories that are told about it, a world that can be known and manipulated through the logic of discovery, where more and more genomic data will lead to truth. Wynter thinks with the Chilean biologist Humberto Maturana, who shows that 'what is seen with the eyes does not represent the world outside the living organism; rather it is the living organism that fabricates an image of the world through internal/neurological processing of information'. What follows is that 'we fail to notice that evolution, dysselection, and biocentricity are origin stories with ontological effect' (Mignolo 2015). In what Wynter therefore calls an autopoietic system, we cannot accept biogenetic research on schizophrenia without accounting for the co-constitution of this research with the epistemic frames that produce the research.

Biocentricity, criminalization, and the sociogenic principle

The 2020 University of Toronto Psychiatry article 'New research uncovers a possible cause of borderline personality disorder' (the title already signalling biocentric fictions through the rhetorics of casualties and uncoverings), starts with the following introduction:

> Borderline personality disorder (BPD) is a mental health condition that impacts the way you think and feel about yourself and others, causing problems in everyday functioning. It includes self-image issues, difficulty managing emotions and behavior, self-harming behavior, and a pattern of unstable relationships. Using brain imaging Dr. Nathan Kolla has found evidence that an elevated amount of a chemical called FAAH may be linked to BPD, raising the possibility that existing medications could help treat the disorder. (https://psychiatry.utoronto.ca/news/new-research-uncovers-possible-cause-borderline-personality-disorder)

Later, the interviewee describes his motivations:

> I have always been curious about the brain chemistry of different forensic psychiatric populations, like those with personality disorders who show high levels of aggression and impulsivity. I am motivated to learn more about the brain chemistry in order to pave the way for new drug treatments that could effectively treat these conditions. Forensic psychiatric populations are very understudied and could highly benefit from more brain research. (*ibid.*)

The refusal/repression/resistance to our bios-mythos hybridity starts to feel immense, and a racial science, set up by a liberal mono-humanistic biocentric Western science, emerges with fewer disguises. The article does not, and indeed cannot (in a science that increasingly professes attention to race but whose language continues to covertly persuade us of post-racialism), explicitly say 'race' where it refers to 'brain research' and 'forensic populations.' But the Man vs Human struggle is an ethnoclass struggle, where the world is ordered according to a racial hierarchy that is inscribed in all the major institutions that organize our lives (prisons, hospitals, universities, laboratories).

We also begin to note where science shakes hands with carcerality (forensics and beyond): the study of brains to understand criminalized people and of science as a sociohistorical (and racial) project to psychiatrize and biologize violence, transgression, and criminality. Wynter explains, 'race and racism are logical outcomes of the biocentric conception of the human'. She continues, 'within this dangerous biological conception of the human there is life unworthy of life', and speaking directly to carcerality, she makes clear: 'This is also what is really happening to Blacks in the prison-industrial complex' (Wynter, in King 2009).

Kolla's reflections articulate and exactly manifest the fictive causal relationship between biology ('brain chemistry') and criminality ('forensic populations'). This maps on directly, though not (and opportunely not) plainly named, to race. Wynter reminds us again that 'race is really a code word for "genre". Our issue is not the issue of "race". Our issue is the issue of the genre of "Man"' (Wynter, in Thomas 2006). Wynter's project is an abolitionist project, calling for abolishing and reimagining our terms for the human: no other strategies (of, for example, equity/diversity/inclusion) will suffice.

The assumptive logic behind the researcher's biocentric descriptive codes of 'aggressive', 'impulsive', 'forensic', 'psychiatric', 'borderline' people is that the biological precedes the symbolic and that we are biological beings who create culture, discourse, language, and subjects. According to this belief, what makes people aggressive/impulsive/forensic/psychiatric/borderline is not at all related to the onto-phenomenological work of language. To recognize how a carceral culture is naturalized by 'New research on Borderline People', Fanon's concept of sociogeny and Wynter's sociogenic principle are crucially important. In 'Homo Narrans and the Science of the Word: Toward a Caribbean Radical Imagination', Bedour Alagraa (2018) writes,

> Wynter explains that there is a third, unresolved event, akin to the Copernican and Darwinian ruptures, that is the realm of possibility for a way out of our overdetermined descriptive code of the human (Man1 and Man2). This third, unresolved event is the Fanonian, which she locates in his description of a sociogenic principle. Fanon writes, 'It will be seen that the black man's alienation is not an individual question. Beside phylogeny and ontogeny stands sociogeny'.

Alagraa (*ibid.*: 168) goes on to explain how the sociogenic principle opens 'a disciplinary breach because matters of culture bear a great deal on the bios'.

Wynter (2003) writes elsewhere that we are 'bioevolutionarily prepared by means of language to inscript and autoinstitute ourselves in this or that modality of human, always in adaptive response to the ecological as well as to the geopolitical circumstances in which we find ourselves'. We are *homo narrans*, storytelling creatures. Fanon, as Alagraa (*ibid.*) points out, similarly insists on 'bringing invention into existence' because as sociogeny disrupts biological determinism, it returns 'human life into our own hands'. With this epistemic rupture, the possibility of a radically different humanity opens up as well as the realization that whatever terms we have thus far used to describe the human are sociocultural inventions.

To return to the interview about research on 'causes of borderline personality', the Fanonion thesis that beside ontogeny and phylogeny stands sociogeny radically reframes the research findings. Our carceral environment enlists biological science to reproduce carcerality at the level of psychiatric research and discourse; this reproduction therefore occurs sociogenically, where our so-called sciences are symbolically racially encoded. We simply cannot otherwise understand this research: objectivity must be abandoned. But science is still possible – though it must be a new science, a liberatory science, a science that emerges from the Third Event that only then can offer us the knowledge we need.

The writer Aimé Césaire would call such a science the 'science of the word'. In his essay 'Poetry and Knowledge', he describes a 'half-starved' science that 'enumerates, measures, classifies, kills'; that 'dominates through reflection, observation, and experimentation'; that 'knows how to utilize the world'; that 'classifies and explains, but the essence of things eludes it'; that 'depersonalizes, deindividualizes'; that is: 'gnawed from within. Gnawed by hunger, the hunger of feeling, the hunger of life' and that is produced through 'the methodical exercise of thought or the scruples of experimentation'. But alongside the 'great silence' of scientific knowledge is poetic knowledge, which, as Césaire and colleagues (Césaire et al. 1990: 19) describe, encompasses love, strangeness, intimacy, trembling, wonderment, attraction, terror, the sacred phenomenon of love, solemn encounters, emotion, imagination, precision, all cosmic force, desire, dreaming, sensuality, mind, body, all lived experience, and all possibility, where 'Everything has a right to live. Everything is summoned. Everything awaits'. For Wynter, the science of the word recognizes us as hybridly human and bios-mythos; for Fanon, the science of the word knows the sociogeny of the world. A science of the word, which would articulate poetics and science together without binary disciplining, disrupts biocentricity and all its attendant violence. Everything has a right to live. Science of the word is not anti-biological but anti-colonial.

Importantly, science of the word is not an institutionalised, and increasingly profitable, interdisciplinarity. Science of the word is not the aimless repetition that race is 'socially constructed'.[3,4,5] Science of the word is not the concluding remark in 'understanding a key mutation', which makes passing, non-meaningful, performative reference to epigenetics and 'environmental factors', so as to cover one's bases rather than to address honestly how the realization of sociogeny call into question everything else that has been said. Science of the word is not qualitative research or quantitative research's lesser funded but often no less biocentric sibling. Science of the word is not biological science at the fore but is now accompanied by social science, psychological science, historical science, literary science, anthropological science, epidemiological science, and so on, and all still return to, rely upon, and ultimately reinforce the genre of Man-as-Human.

Biocentric rehabilitations

The 2021 University of Toronto *Psychiatry* article 'Preventing the reincarceration of prisoners with mental illness', despite naming ostensibly non-positivistic, or non-empirical, research aims, is still beholden to, and does not in any way undo, biocentricity. The interviewee explains,

> This research arose from work with the Forensic Early Intervention Service (FEIS) in two jails. . . . FEIS provides assessment and intervention for inmates who have mental illness and who are on remand. We observed that many of the people seen by the service return to jail again after release, some very frequently, and we wanted to investigate how often this happens, and what social, clinical and demographic factors are associated with reincarceration.
> (https://psychiatry.utoronto.ca/news/preventing-reincarceration-
> prisoners-mental-illness)

Appeals are made, then, to the purportedly non-biological – the social, clinical, and demographic. The major 'take-home' message from the research is that

> very large numbers of people with mental illness [especially people with schizophrenia and bipolar disorder] are incarcerated every year, and many fall into a pattern of frequent rein-carceration. Investment in specific transition and community services and careful evaluation of their efficacy is required to . . . reduce reoffending.

He says that there are plans to develop community supports for 'greater continuity between mental health services in jail and in the community' and 'focused interventions before release'. This research at no point questions the related assumptions that 1) mental illness is a stable biological category and 2) that incarceration is a necessary and effective institution of Man (Foucault 1977).

In the name of care (disfigured frequently in carceral spaces and renamed as 'rehabilitation') and with social-determinants-of-health discourse as an alibi that supports nuance, the interviewee calls for more continuity between psychiatric treatment and incarceration. This call is in effect a 'reformist reform' that further entrenches the foundational, naturalized logics of mental illness and incarceration (Man-as-Human is never mentally ill and is never incarcerated). At this point, we can begin to observe how all three articles operate collaboratively to consolidate Man-as-Human. In one case, schizophrenia is stabilized as a genetically produced category of mental illness; in the next case, criminalized people are essentialized through neurochemistry; and finally, the biologically determined 'inmate' requires greater psychiatric intervention, which is never towards the delinking of biocentricity, madness, and criminalization but towards evermore biological overdeterminism.

'Preventing reincarceration' describes the crisis of a deviant population that needs to be disciplined, by both incarceration and psychiatrization. The deviant population is excluded or dysselected from the genre of Man-as-Human but can be studied and then potentially rehabilitated back into Man's circle. If the research suggests, as the interviewee states, that people deemed mentally ill are imprisoned in larger numbers, and that homelessness and drug use play a role in affecting rates of imprisonment, and that each of these dimensions produces life unworthy of life, then perhaps instead of bolstering a bio-psychiatric-complex, we might radically reconsider the interrelated stories and poetics we tell ourselves about illness and imprisonment.

In the recent interview with Alagraa (2021) referred to earlier, Wynter speaks specifically to COVID-19. I extend that here to understand the problems of (and generated by) psychiatric institutions, and here, I see parallels of medical violence. Wynter tells us that 'language is entirely the point'. For the afflictions of schizophrenia, borderline personality disorder, aggression, impulsivity, forensic involvement, incarceration, and reincarceration, the cure is to 'narrate the problem in a different way'. She goes on, 'The only cure will be a transformation of the whole society, and an entirely new knowledge order altogether'. And such a transformation must be made in the terrain of language and poetic knowledge.

As I note in this chapter's introduction, psychiatry has come to hold within itself the anxiety of the biocentric genre of the human, where it lusts after biological research to legitimize itself in our biocentric world orders of knowledge. Thereby it produces incredible violence, and still cannot escape the fact that biocentricity is a story we tell ourselves about what it means to be human. To turn to the science of the word would not merely revise but could revolutionize psychiatry, and therein, I believe, lies psychiatry's possible contribution to the broader fields of medical knowledge. Wynter again, in conversation with McKittrick (2015), says,

> So I have to be realistic and say how can I expect people whose discipline is their identity to accept this hybrid model? When what they/we are being faced with is the total removal of their discipline as an autonomous field of inquiry? But then think of the dazzling creativity of the alternative challenge that would be opened up!

It is this alternative challenge that faces us now in psychiatry, as we reckon with that possibility of the psychiatric field of inquiry as exceeding the myth of autonomous knowledge production.

Conclusions

I am curious about the unreflexive use of the word 'impact' associated with The University of Toronto's psychiatry department's article series. The department recognizes the research papers I have discussed in this paper as articles that 'change treatment'. What has impact, then, is that which changes treatment. But impact on whom? Impact for whom? What is the meaning of a treatment changed? Other than impact as having an effect or influence, impact also means the action of one object coming forcibly into contact with another. This definition for 'impact' distils certain associations that cannot be so easily dismissed. We might consider many possible forcible contacts that are made by the research articles: between patient and psychiatrist, between brain chemistry and personality, between chromosomal differences and mental illness, and so on. These are contacts forced not accidentally but for particular reasons and agendas.

In this essay, I have argued that the research articles shared by the department create impact not as any kind of change in psychiatry's course of knowledge production and not as any kind of ideological disruption but as reinforcement, entrenchment, concretization of the biocentric genre of human, Man-as-Human. What they produce is perhaps more so impaction, a medical word referring to the state of being 'pressed firmly together'. What I have also explored in this essay is Wynter's Fanonian proposal of the hybridly human storytelling species, Césaire's science of the word, and Alagraa's explanations regarding the knowledge we need and the Third (yet unresolved) Event as poetic praxis. It is the anticolonial study and impulse of these positions that is the condition of possibility for a liberatory science that could radically transform psychiatry into something exceeding the critical or the interdisciplinary (where both have been considered related interventions for psychiatry), something that could indeed be the dazzling alternative that Wynter challenges us to consider.

Acknowledgement

Many thanks to my mentors Nanky Rai, Suze Berkhout, and Mel Mikhail for your feedback, thoughts, and conversations on this essay.

Notes

1 Christina Sharpe's writing on care in the wake (that care needs to stay *in* the wake) has been fundamental to how I have come to understand much of health care, and especially psychiatric care, as state-imposed violence in the name of care. Sharpe's (2016: 10) question – 'How can we think (and rethink and rethink) care laterally, in the register of the intramural, in a different relation than that of the violence of the state?' –

makes urgent and distinct demands to all the state's clinicians. That state-sanctioned and state-imposed violence and force are cast as caring acts calls for the rigorous, unending, and deeply attentive work of disentangling care from the state's murderous misappropriation of it.

2 Mad studies and disability studies theorists have likewise made clear the historical role of psychiatry and psychiatrists in eugenic movements, the concurrent historical developments of eugenics and the 'science' of race, and moreover how eugenics continues to manifest in psychiatry's increasingly genetic determinism (Chapman et al. 2014; Burstow 2019).

3 Although the published research article makes no disclosures indicating funding from any particular drug company, the institution of psychiatry is undeniably enmeshed with the pharmaceutical industry in a manner that grossly exceeds any simple or straightforward 'conflict of interest'.

4 Alagraa writes in particular about the generative possibilities in this regard of the radical Caribbean imagination.

5 As Katherine McKittrick (2019) tells us, 'Description is not liberation'.

References

Alagraa B. Homo Narrans and the Science of the Word: Toward a Caribbean Radical Imagination. *Critical Ethnic Studies*. 2018; 4: 164.

Alagraa B. 2021. What Will Be the Cure?: A Conversation With Sylvia Wynter. *Offshoot*, January 7. Available at: https://offshootjournal.org/what-will-be-the-cure-a-conversation-with-sylvia-wynter/. Last accessed: 30/8/2022.

Braken P. Psychiatry Beyond the Current Paradigm. *The British Journal of Psychiatry*. 2012; 201: 430–34.

Burstow B. 2019. Deconstructing the Institution: Psychiatric Eugenics Then and Now-You Betcha It's Still Happening. *Mad in America*, July 31. Available at: www.madinamerica.com/2019/07/psychiatric-eugenics-then-and-now/. Last accessed: 30/8/2022.

Césaire A, Eshleman C, Smith A. 1990. *Lyric and Dramatic Poetry, 1946–82*. Charlottesville, VA: University of Virginia Pressw.

Chapman, C., Carey, A.C., Ben-Moshe, L. (2014). *Reconsidering Confinement: Interlocking Locations and Logics of Incarceration*. In: Ben-Moshe, L., Chapman, C., Carey, A.C. (eds) Disability Incarcerated. Palgrave Macmillan, New York.

Fanon F. 2021. *The Wretched of the Earth*. New York, NY: Grove Press.

Foucault M. 1977. *Discipline and Punish*. New York, NY: Pantheon Books.

King JE. 2009. *Black Education: A Transformative Research and Action Agenda for the New Century*. New York, NY: Routledge.

McKittrick K. 2015. *Sylvia Wynter: On Being Human as Praxis*. Durham, NC: Duke University Press.

McKittrick K. 2019. Description is Not Liberation. *Twitter*, January 26. Available at: https://twitter.com/demonicground/status/1089248858876661760?lang=en. Last accessed: 30/8/2022.

Mignolo WD. 2015. Sylvia Wynter: What Does it Mean to be Human? *SCRIBD*. Available at: www.scribd.com/document/556638753/Mignolo-Sylvia-Wynter-What-Does-it-Mean-to-be-Human# Last accessed: 30/3/2023.

Millenials Are Killing Capitalism. 2021. *The Third Event: Bedour Alagraa on Sylvia Wynter and Black Radical Thought*. January 22. Available at: https://millennialsarekillingcapitalism.libsyn.com/the-third-event-bedoura-alagraa-on-sylvia-wynter-and-black-radical-thought. Last accessed: 10/6/2023.

Ranganathan M. Thinking With Flint: Racial Liberalism and the Roots of an American Water Tragedy. *Capitalism Nature Socialism*. 2016; 27: 17–33.

Sharpe CE. 2016. *In the Wake: On Blackness and Being*. Durham, NC: Duke University Press.

Thomas G. PROUD FLESH Inter/Views: Sylvia Wynter. *PROUDFLESH: A New Afrikan Journal of Culture, Politics & Consciousness*. 2006; (4). Available at: https://archive.org/details/proud-flesh-sylvia-wynter/mode/2up. Last accessed: 30/3/2023.

Wikimedia Foundation. 2020. Non-Reformist Reform. *Wikipedia*, June 4. Available at: https://en.wikipedia.org/wiki/Non-reformist_Reform. Last accessed: 30/8/2022.

Wynter S. Unsettling the Coloniality of Being/Power/Truth/Freedom: Towards the Human, After Man, Its Overrepresentation – an Argument. *CR: The New Centennial Review*. 2003; 3: 257–337.

19

PSYCHIATRY'S TURF AND POETRY'S FIELD

Alan Bleakley

A sit-down Chinese meal

Back in the early 1970s, I went to an evening talk at the Philadelphia Association in London given by the South African psychiatrist David Cooper, then resident in the UK. Ronald Laing, the infamous and radical Scottish psychiatrist, was also booked to speak but failed to show. Cooper gave a passionate talk referencing his dislike of the term 'anti-psychiatry', although he had been credited with coining that term in 1967 and wrote a 1971 polemic entitled *Psychiatry and Anti-Psychiatry* (Cooper 2001) (today, the term 'critical psychiatry' is preferred). He talked about new approaches to psychiatry that extolled what we would now call 'neurodiversity', a term introduced by the sociologist Judy Singer (2017) in the 1990s, who claimed her autism as a benefit and a platform from which to speak out about issues of inequity.

Cooper called for a break after about an hour, asking if a member of the audience would nip out to a Chinese restaurant just around the corner to bring him a take-away and a beer. Somebody in the audience volunteered. The food came in an aluminium container with a lid. The session re-started. Cooper swigged the beer, then took the lid off the Chinese meal, put the container on the floor, dropped his trousers and underpants and promptly sat in the food. There was a collective gasp from the audience. This seemed like such a strange gesture. Cooper then cleaned himself up and subsequently gathered our responses. Was this a moment of 'madness', an impulse, a zen paradox, a living koan, a piece of theatre or performance, Dada, exhibitionism, an act of infantile regression, a schoolboy prank, a joke? Was it a pun on the 'sit-in', the popular student protests of the times? Was there 'teaching' in it? Well, yes, we discussed all these possibilities. The strange thing was that the act itself was innocuous, even tame, harmed nobody, could have been a piece of tomfoolery. And yet in context it was taken as the action of a rule-breaker, a norm-bender, somehow serious, even shocking or an offence to taste. Was this because it was a largely British audience, stereotypically reserved? Cooper stayed 'mum' throughout, more interested in our responses than in explaining his behaviour – typical of an analyst.

Cooper then asked us to question the legitimacy of his action as we reflected on our motives and values basis for doing so. Would we call it an act of 'madness?' Well, he said, his whole talk was indeed about the legitimacy of labels such as 'madness' and 'insanity' and how he, Ronnie Laing, and the Scottish psychiatrist Aaron Esterson had worked so hard to persuade the psychiatric

DOI: 10.4324/9781003341796-25

establishment that conventional models of madness were mad in their own right – or at least inauthentic in an existential sense (see Sass 1994). In what sense are varieties of madness any more invalid than everyday life in which we fit into prescribed roles and habitual routines that serve to make us neurotic: desensitized, anxious, and depressed?

People particularly liked the idea that Cooper sitting in his Chinese meal was a Zen paradox, a koan, a parable, or an embodied metaphor (this was, after all, the early 1970s). But most saw it as a piece of theatre to stimulate discussion. Cooper insisted, 'it is all these things and none of them', again advertising paradox. The fact that we had come up with over half a dozen possible explanations for the behaviour was the key issue. Would 'straight' psychiatry – armed with an edition of the *Diagnostic and Statistical Manual of Mental Disorders* (DSM) from this period – do the same for patients in addressing their presenting symptoms?

Sometime previously, I had been to a talk by Laing where he did his familiar party piece of soberly reading – in 'flat affect' – extracts from the latest edition of DSM for their anti-metaphorical qualities as flat text that, paradoxically, could be said to suffer from both hysteria (overblown accounts) and paranoia (seeing things that may not be there). It was like listening to a stand-up comic – exactly the point Laing wanted to make. He would show how the texts were expressly anti-poetic and then would read from his own poetic work *Knots* (1973) that described paradoxical, cul-de-sac descriptions of contradictions, or double-binds.

The notion of 'double-bind' was introduced by the English polymath Gregory Bateson (2000) in the 1950s to describe linguistic paradoxes that frustrated feedback loops. In cybernetic terms, a double-bind stunted a feedback mechanism, turned the loop on itself. Such double-binds, typically seen in families' dysfunctional conversations in Laing's model, would place vulnerable people in impossible situations where choice was removed and the only response was to freeze and potentially go 'mad'. For example, Laing (1973) writes,

> *Once upon a time, when Jack was little,*
> *he wanted to be with his mummy all the time*
> *and was frightened she would go away*
> later, when he was a little bigger,
> he wanted to be away from his mummy
> and was frightened that
> she wanted him to be with her all the time

When Jack grows up to fall in love with Jill, he wants to possess her, but then, a little older he finds he doesn't want to be with Jill all the time, but is afraid that Jill may become frightened of his new choice, so now they are in a double bind, where:

> Jack frightens Jill (that) he will leave her
> because he is frightened she will leave him.

Knots would perhaps be seen by many as 'poetry lite' – more a hotchpotch of cautionary tales and aphorisms stripped of serious poetic form. But the UK was ready for such verse in the wake of the *International Poetry Incarnation* of June 1965 at the Royal Albert Hall that celebrated the flourishing of Beat and post-Beat poetry. The event was filmed by Peter Whitehead and released as 'Wholly Communion'. Poets included Christopher Logue, Adrian Mitchell, Michael Horovitz, Allen Ginsberg, Gregory Corso, Alex Trocchi, Lawrence Ferlinghetti, and others, including the celebrated Russian Poet Yevgeny Yevtushenko.

A medical student at the time, and later to become an internationally lauded psychiatrist and expert on depression, Stuart Montgomery was also a poet and connoisseur of the avant-garde in poetry, particularly American and British poets. In 1965, the same year as the Wholly Communion event, Montgomery set up Fulcrum Press, which was to become the premier UK press for cutting-edge experimental poets such as Ed Dorn, Roy Fisher, Allen Ginsberg, Ian Hamilton Finlay, Gary Snyder, Tom Pickard, Lorine Niedecker, Jerome Rothenberg, and Robert Duncan, as well as established poets such as Ezra Pound, David Jones, and Basil Bunting; indeed, Montgomery single-handedly revitalized the career of the oft-forgotten Bunting as one of the most accomplished, if idiosyncratic, voices of UK poetry. The books sported covers designed by celebrated artists such as Patrick Caulfield. Montgomery's own poetry, such as *Sirens*, *Circe*, and *Calypso*, was influenced by Greek myth for content and the clipped style of the Koan, popular among Beat poets, for form. Who but an aspiring doctor could write of Circe's sorcery,

> First she will kiss your feet and caress
> your tired limbs as you enter her house
> seat you and feed a mixture of dangerous
> musk past your teeth like a delirious
> ghost in your throat she will rise to seize
> and anaesthetise your heart
> (Montgomery 2005: 35)

Montgomery was clearly influenced by the so-called UK 'anti-psychiatrists' – Laing, Cooper, and Esterson – although he qualified as a psychiatrist in the subsequent generation. An article from the underground or alternative paper *International Times* (*IT*) from February 1968 advertises the launch of the 'AntiUniversity of London', based in Shoreditch and described as 'a shortlived and intense experiment into self-organised education and communal living' (antihistory.org). Amongst the advertised faculty were David Cooper and Ronnie Laing, the Scottish novelist and poet Alex Trocchi (who wrote openly about his heroin addiction), and the American poet Ed Dorn, then resident at Essex University.

Also advertised were courses on poetry by Stuart Montgomery. Montgomery had completed his medical degree in 1966 and by this time was fully occupied by Fulcrum Press until its dissolution in 1976 after Ian Hamilton Finlay brought a lawsuit against the press for claiming to have published 'original' work by Finlay that had in fact been published before; Montgomery was unable to pay the legal fees, and Fulcrum Press folded, with all stock books pulped. Montgomery returned to medicine in 1976, as noted ultimately specializing in psychiatry. He would write over 500 academic papers and several books and become a major figure in the field. He was absorbed into psychiatry's mainstream, upholding the value of pharmaceutical therapies for depression, apparently shedding his early radicalism.

The original 'anti-psychiatrists', belligerently challenging the value of medications to treat psychoses, drew inspiration from the psychiatrist Thomas Szasz in North America and the French West Indian psychiatrist Franz Fanon, who was active in the liberation of Algeria from French colonial rule. Félix Guattari, a French psychiatrist – and close colleague of the philosopher Gilles Deleuze – was also an influence. Guattari set up a community for so-called schizophrenics that rejected conventional pharmaceutical and surveillance treatments to allow forms of madness to play out in a safe setting of retreat and care.

Where Laing and colleagues focused on the existential aspects of mental health and illness – the lived experience and its linguistic conundrums, such as the double-binds illustrated by Laing's poem discussed earlier – Thomas Szasz argued that no mental states (as opposed to physical states) could be called an 'illness' where this is an error of logic. Szasz saw a conspiracy between Big Pharma and the psychiatric establishment, where more symptom diagnoses equalled research development and ultimately bigger profits. Fanon focused on how persistent political oppression can induce mental illness as an unliveable condition of friction. Such critiques have themselves subsequently come under criticism not just from traditional psychiatry but also from patients who suffer from mental illnesses. Advances in medication therapies and understanding of neuroscience have taken the edge off the radicalism of the anti/critical-psychiatry movement, although there are recent fervent adherents such as the late Bonnie Burstow (2017).

The movement has now morphed into a wider political awareness movement known as 'mad studies' (Russo and Sweeney 2016), where symptoms are recognized and treatments are valued but the focus is on losing the stigma associated with so-called mental illness while valuing neurodiversity: differing mental and emotional framings of the world that draw inspiration from the radical or avant-garde arts (Sass 1994). This also parallels the critical disability movement's political stance. Mad studies draw heavily on philosophical positions of radical relativism grounded in Nietzsche's moral model of the transvaluation of all values and Gilles Deleuze and Félix Guattari's (2013) idea of boundary-free 'nomadism' (rather than its antithesis 'territorialism' that fetishizes boundary-making). Nomadism implies lack of controlled borders and fluid movement, leading to entanglements of ideas and practices. But mad studies, as noted, are also grounded in avant-garde literature such as the work of James Joyce, Samuel Beckett, Georges Bataille, Gertrude Stein, Maurice Blanchot, Thomas Pynchon, and Kathy Acker amongst many others. This work – sometimes labelled 'unreadable' and 'perverse' within conventional literary circles (Sass 1994) – explicitly sets out to undermine the standard rules of narrative and replace these with an expressive lyrical poetics (Bleakley and Neilson 2021).

The anti-psychiatry movement of the 1960s and 1970s was part of a wider, youth-inspired social upheaval that embraced radical ideas in education such as 'de-schooling' (Ivan Illich 1973) shaping alternatives to what Paul Goodman (1964) called 'compulsory miseducation'. The father of this movement was the philosopher John Dewey, who promoted 'self-direction' in children's education. Dewey's ideas influenced the classicist and educationalist Abraham Flexner (1910, 1925, 1940), the architect of modern medical education. Flexner ran a progressive school before he was invited to review and subsequently radically overhaul how medical schools operated in both North America and Europe.

Curriculum as poetic field

During the 1960s and 1970s, higher education was also in some turmoil as student 'sit-ins' became a popular form of protest against curricula and teaching and learning methods perceived as conservative and stale. Curriculum needed to be re-conceived. In the mid-1970s, scholars in the field of curriculum studies began to 'reconceptualize' what curriculum might be, critically addressing pedagogy (teaching and learning) as limited (Pinar 2000; Doll 2017). Curriculum was configured primarily as a complex process producing an identity, rather than a linear, fixed set of preconceived content. Since the 1940s, curriculum theory had been dominated by the ideas of Ralph Tyler, prescribing a functional model based on linear outcomes for learning met by such organized content as a syllabus. The means of learning was teaching, and the end of learning was a specified outcome. Assessment of learning was based on whether specified outcomes had been reached at a stated level of knowledge or proficiency. This engineering-led, closed-system model did not allow for spontaneity or difference and certainly not for positive innovation. Nor did it acknowledge the idiosyncratic or the autobiographical. It did, however, provide uniformity and was praised for its focus on consistency as fairness: again, every learner would undergo the same process and assessment, guided by objectives. This, claimed its proponents, provided equity.

The model, however, is potentially sterile, leaving no room for improvisation and innovation. It stresses conformity rather than difference and *différance* (Jacques Derrida's notion of infinite deferral of closure, that can be read as ongoing tolerance of uncertainty – a key strategy for physicians' clinical work). More, it reduces curriculum to syllabus or stated content. In its focus upon what shall be taught, it neglects differences in learning approaches and rejects spontaneity, serendipity, chance encounter, and the unexpected. William Pinar (2000, 2012) and others, in a wholesale rejection of Tyler's model and the values informing it, deeply re-visioned curriculum, starting with the root meaning of the word. 'Curriculum' literally describes the course of the Roman chariot race, but more, emphasizes the *running* of the race. Curriculum was conceived not as a noun, a thing, but as the infinitive verb – *currere* – again, a process. The curriculum was seen as the *experience* of learning of any one person within a course of study, emphasizing the process of learning rather than the content of teaching. More, *currere* expressly rejected the idea that it could prescribe a formal education in terms of teaching and learning theory and practice (pedagogy). Rather, it set out to theorize the experience of an education beyond pedagogy, drawing on existentialism, phenomenology, feminisms, post-Marxism, deconstructive and reconstructive postmodernisms, poststructuralism, queer theory, mad studies, and disability studies.

Curriculum is, suggested Pinar, a 'complicated conversation'. In essence, the present is made more complex by reactivating the past and contemplating the future. This leads to an analytic point where things are mulled over. A synthetic turn then emerges where active changes are made in developments and innovations. I prefer 'complex conversation' on the basis that linear, closed systems can be either simple or complicated (inviting straightforward feedback-correction loops) but never complex. However, nonlinear, open, dynamic systems at the edge of chaos are necessarily complex. Curriculum is an open, dynamic system that works at maximum complexity this side of chaos. It is also self-regulating. By reducing education to curriculum and curriculum to syllabus, we turn a complex system into a linear system, stunting its potential.

Returning to Laing, Cooper, and Esterson, there is a direct parallel with how 'mental illness' has been conceived within traditional psychiatry and within critical movements such as mad studies. Painting with a broad brush to highlight the epistemic differences between reductive, instrumental biomedical science and a more complex multi-values-driven approach, with ever-multiplying diagnostic categories at hand, traditional psychiatry parallels Tylerian curriculum planning as functional and objective. Of course, there will be many psychiatrists who are sensitive to the pitfalls of reductionist science, who carefully contextualize their work in relation to their patients' needs, but the epistemological constraint of the pure science will frustrate their efforts where it fails to account for the idiosyncratic and for context. Such science is content-driven (classifications of symptoms) rather than process-driven (idiosyncratic expressions of symptoms). Where, in psychiatry, this reductive approach aligns symptom classification with the need for profit of the major pharmaceutical companies and reinforces this through selective evidence of reductive brain imaging studies, psychiatry echoes Tylerian educational models. The answer to this reductive habit is to complexify the binary of instrumental and contextual science (the latter drawing on arts, humanities, and qualitative social sciences).

As a model for this transformative shift in pedagogy, the curriculum reconceptualization movement shifts the values basis for curriculum scholarship and planning away from functional, instrumental frames to aesthetic and political frames. Questions are now asked about the quality of a curriculum, such as beauty and form, elegance and aspiration, and about power – whose interests does the curriculum promote, teachers' or learners', and how are vested interests challenged and resisted? As madness is contextually sensitive, so curriculum is wholly socially engineered. There is no objective curriculum despite Tylerian attempts to make learning function through objectives. Ever-expanding classification systems for symptoms of mental illness also are not guided by aesthetic and political values; rather, such values are used as the frameworks for critiquing such loose nosologies.

Pinar's notion of *currere* sees the curriculum as context, an environment for experiencing learning. Again, where curriculum is the total course of study and syllabus the stated content, *currere* means to run the course, that is, is lived educational experience. In other words, where curriculum is the content and process, *currere* is the meta-process of experiencing and making sense of content and process. This, centrally, involves valuing – what is experienced as interesting, worthwhile, or enriching. This goes far beyond just cramming knowledge or practicing skills. It is about identity construction and values clarification, about values linked to sensuality, beauty, and love, or what is provocative about learning.

A medical student becomes a doctor, a professional. There is a shaping process at work. *Currere* is not just about what is gained but also about what is cast off, held back, rejected, or discarded. A course of study is not just crammed; rather, one indwells or inhabits its territory, and learners remake the curriculum as they study, approaching it critically and re-inventing it for their purposes. What then is the 'doctor' and the 'professional'? Are these identities identifications with the culture of medicine and its sub-cultures of specialties, or is the identity formed in the face of the Other that is the patient and her experience and in terms of transgressions of 'professionalism'? Professionalism is now persistently confounded as an ideal by the realities of work practices compromised by structural constraints such as overwork due to lack of personnel and other resources. Is the 'doctor' now defined by the identity of expertise or by mis-identities such as incidence of exhaustion and burnout?

Primarily, *currere* is poetic work, and then medical education is a poetic 'field', the same term that was used by the poet Charles Olson and the poet–physician William Carlos Williams to describe how one delimits a poem (Williams 1951/1967). A field must be set: some sense of the shape of the poem and what will inhabit it. In his manifesto 'Projective Verse', Olson (1950) says the field for a poem is set by two things: 'the HEAD by way of the EAR, to the SYLLABLE/the HEART by way of the BREATH to the LINE'. The 'dance of the intellect' captures the smallest unit of language just gone, the rhythm in the word already pronounced. This is the past in the present, reactivated. Affect moves the syllables on in groups to form the line that follows the breath. This is anticipation, future-facing, the near-future in the present. The paradox is that the form of the field morphs into the process of making. The field is nomadic and not settled.

This is not just the 'field' for the poem but also the field for the medico-diagnostic act exemplified in the forms of consultation and in expert pattern recognition (Bleakley and Neilson 2021). Where Pinar describes curriculum as 'the future in the present', so the field is the future poem's sense of both boundary and trajectory set in the now. It is the imagined poem prior to its inception, the future brought to heel. 'Field' is a metaphor, but as a delimitation of what is possible in the poem, it is also a muddy reality, a turf. Turf is also conceived within medical and surgical specialty – a neighbourhood, a precinct, a delineated district of interest – while in medicine, 'the future in the present' is the expert apprehension of the arc of the symptom in diagnosis and treatment. Often, such an arc is not so smooth, or is information interrupted by noise, particularly in mental health diagnoses and treatments, as the case study of the poet Peter Redgrove will illustrate. Here, poetry and madness intersect in meaningful ways on both literal and metaphorical turfs.

Peter Redgrove's Turf – soil, soiling, and the soiled

The late Peter Redgrove is a celebrated British poet. In 1950, only 18 years old and having just completed secondary schooling (North American high school), Redgrove was called up for UK National Service. He joined the Royal Army Medical Corps. Within a week of basic training, he was hospitalized with a 'nervous disorder' diagnosed as obsessive-compulsive behaviour. He had already been labelled 'neurotic' by his family doctor before being called up. He was assigned to a young psychiatrist interested in psychoanalysis, who thought he might analyse Redgrove. The latter confessed to what this young psychiatrist would term a 'perversion'. Redgrove liked to dress up in a clean white shirt and then soil it by rolling in mud, followed by masturbation. Such compulsion was entirely free from exhibitionism, a purely private activity. In fact, this would be a lifelong practice for Redgrove, one that fed his imagination, giving him visions feeding directly into his poetry. We might say, generously, that what psychiatry termed a neurosis was in fact a well of inspiration for Redgrove's writing, a quirk spinning gold. The young psychiatrist, Peter Spaul, was seeing Redgrove daily for one-hour sessions, writing in Redgrove's notes that his 'perversion' had Oedipal origins (jealousy for his father and love of his mother) and could be 'cured' in around three months (Roberts 2012).

A psychiatrist diagnosed Redgrove with 'incipient schizophrenia' and recommended insulin shock therapy ('deep insulin treatment'). This was, along with psychosurgery and electroconvulsive shock therapy, the most invasive treatment available for severe mental illness, with no rigorous evidence base for success. Redgrove was discharged from the army while in hospital and subsequently took the entrance examination for Cambridge University, where he would later study natural sciences. In talking with his general practitioner in 1973, Redgrove was told that there was no such diagnosis as 'incipient schizophrenia' and that if he did not have symptoms of dissociations, delusions, lack of insight, and hallucinations, then he was not suffering from schizophrenia. Redgrove later wrote that he was relieved that he was not an 'accredited madman' (in *ibid.*). However, Redgrove's GP was partly mistaken – there is a diagnostic category of 'incipient schizophrenia', and he was certainly suffering from some dissociation. But he did not suffer from hallucinations. In fact, he welcomed the intrusion of the imagination as a gift, bringing poetic visions. Juvenile over-confidence might have been mistaken for narcissism, but there was certainly no lack of insight on the budding poet's part. In fact, Redgrove suffered from a surfeit of insight. His later prodigious poetry and prose output testified to this. If his early bane was mainstream psychiatrists eager to apply a psychopathological label to his creativity, his later bane would be frugal editors attempting to curb his extraordinary volume of output.

At the time of Redgrove's initial diagnosis, the diagnostic criteria for schizophrenia included ideas of reference (exaggerated belief that contingent circumstances and events refer to oneself and are not just coincidental), paranoid ideation, perceptual disturbances, magical thinking, and generally odd thinking and speech. Are these conditions not often attributed to an artistic temperament or seen as the valued sensitivities of a poet? Attribution of voices to nature, or animation, is sometimes added to this list. Here is an extract from Redgrove's (2012) 1979 poem 'Among the Whips and the Mud Baths':

How she was said to have learned to ease the slow blue
                                        lightning

Out of her skin and out of her lover's skin
So that they were sheathed in radiance, and the dark room
Flickered with their body-prints, like sand-dunes electrified

After a dry day.

. . .

All that sex populates my imagination and makes me happy.

The natural world's electrification of its skin, the gathering of unseen lightning, is the crucible for the cross-electrification of lovers' skins that might seem to glow in the dark, phosphorescent. (The enjambed 'lightning' is a beautiful touch, especially as it is 'slow' and 'blue' and then not dropped conventionally to the next line at left field but rather displaced far to the right of the field as if a literal step-down into the heart of the metaphorical electricity, again slow and blue. I say 'metaphorical', but for Redgrove, the electricity of the skin during sex was real, fully embodied). The deepest intimacy is poetry, itself a phosphorescent 'new skin'. What was said to be a madness treatable by induction of coma, a near-death experience, becomes the creative hub of Redgrove's vision as an opposite of coma, indeed as vigour. His eroticism probably alarmed his psychiatrists. Returning to his psychiatric journey, Redgrove was eventually diagnosed with 'schizophrenia in obsessional personality', placing him at the fringes of delusion. Psychiatrists again recommended deep insulin coma therapy to 'coalesce' a dissociative personality. In response, Redgrove wrote that he 'favours the abstruse, but now tries not to use a long word unless it expresses the exact shade of meaning' (*ibid.*: 46). This clearly doesn't signal *dissociation* but rather an exact *association*. Again, the skin really is electric, the metaphor fully embodied. It is a dis-embodied psychiatry numbed to such sensuousness that fails us. At this time, Redgrove had not written poetry, but it was stirring within him, and these are surely the words of a poet.

From 17 July 1950, deep insulin therapy was administered six days a week for nine weeks. In all, Redgrove had around 60 treatments, as sometimes the insulin coma would not ensue, and the process would be repeated. The coma brings one near to death, where glucose injections then revive the patient. Introduced in 1927 by an Austrian-American psychiatrist Manfred Sakel, insulin shock therapy was largely discontinued by the 1970s, replaced by use of neuroleptic drugs. As noted, there proved to be no evidence base supporting its use. Sakel's initial claims for its success have proven in retrospect to be wildly exaggerated.

Nearly a quarter of a century later, in the semi-autobiographical novel *In the Country of the Skin*, Redgrove's (1973) alter ego Jonas describes going through insulin shock therapy and its paradoxical benefits, where, as a consequence of the therapy,

> he was dead, truly dead, and dissolved into the soil. Later, when he began to write poetry, he didn't see why anything he had done in his life gave him the right to see things that were true in nature. Then he remembered that death had taken him to pieces, that he was conscious of being the mud and soil.

'Dissolved into the soil'. Redgrove later said that while the insulin therapy experiences had taken him many times to the edge of death, he felt in retrospect that no abiding vision had stayed with him. He needed some vehicle to give meaning to these mythological descents, where he met Charon the ferryman but could offer no gifts. Poetry later provided that medium and that gift. His 'symptoms', particularly his fetish for spoiling in mud, could be made sense of through poetry. Rather than just a cathartic experience, meaning emerged for Redgrove's variety of bodily, mental, emotional, and intuitive descents through the fertile matter of poetry or the messy 'field' of poetic form. Redgrove was now authentically 'dissolved in the soil' (*ibid.*). A vision emerged. A territory opened, where the electrical charge of the air could be pooled and grounded, reflected in 'the country of the skin' (*ibid.*). Redgrove had found his turf. More, his character could be stabilized through poetry. Poetry itself was not simply expression or catharsis but the medium through which his pact with death (as medically induced near-death) could be given meaning. Poetry was truly therapeutic. It became for Redgrove a curriculum, a lifelong course of learning, a primary process. Importantly, it eschewed the personal-confessional genre for a direct celebration of raw nature, in which nature became both subject and object of poetry:

> I am startled by comparisons.
> Ice melts from the thatches with the bare restraint
> With which the flesh disquantities.
> The sound of it beats back like small hearts in sheer spaces.
> Stars lie in pools black as pupils
> That return their stare, ice-irised
> > (from 'The Wizard's New Meeting' 2012)

Poetry here is both medicine and curriculum. Medicine in two senses: as specific treatment for symptom and as general restorative or life-course (*currere*): again, Olson's field – 'the HEAD by way of the EAR, to the SYLLABLE/the HEART by way of the BREATH to the LINE'. Redgrove himself might have added: the IMAGINATION by way of the SKIN to the WHOLE POEM. Curriculum is life-course, as is poetry: both ways of hearing and breathing.

Peter Redgrove was a mentor, friend, and colleague. He taught me how to write. I was in therapy with him while we shared collaborative educational ventures. I know how poetry acted as medicine and curriculum for him, sustaining him and constantly restoring his confidence. His early experiences of standard psychoanalysis did little for his aesthetic sensibility – that gap was plugged by his chance encounter with the rebel analyst John Layard. Layard was a celebrated anthropologist who had been in analysis with C.G. Jung. He came to Falmouth in Cornwall in the late 1960s and met Lionel Miskin, head of painting at Falmouth School of Art. (Co-incidentally, Miskin was my art teacher at grammar school [high school]). Miskin went into analysis with Layard, as did Redgrove later. Ironically, Layard told Redgrove to give up poetry (probably out of jealousy for his talent), but it was precisely because of this advice that Redgrove doubled down on his verse. In rejecting Layard, he threw off the father-figure and gained poetry. In my own therapy with Redgrove, poetry was the central medium for our conversations.

Before entering Cambridge (he never completed his degree, leaving after two years, disillusioned with academia), Redgrove had doubts about studying natural sciences. He believed that the formal curriculum might squash his spirit of inquiry. He was probably right. Again, poetry saved him by providing what he later called a 'science of the strange'. In his education at university level, even tinkering with studying medicine, Redgrove found formal science suffocating. There was so much more at the edges, an unseen world that science rejected but science fiction embraced. His student contemporary, colleague, and friend Ted Hughes – later UK poet laureate – agreed. They met frequently and corresponded often between 1966 and 1984. Redgrove also knew Hughes' wife Sylvia Plath, identifying with her depressive episodes and general mood swings. Hughes went to Cambridge in 1951 to study English but switched to an archaeology and anthropology degree in his third year, finding that the English course was stifling his creativity. While Hughes went on to describe the darker side of visible Nature (red in tooth and claw), Redgrove investigated the invisible world – the unseen and unacknowledged in Nature, available to anybody who cares to tune their senses. He called this 'the unseen real', referring to a 'sixth sense' that is our unconscious with its 'uncommon sense' or irrationalities (1988). With this book, Redgrove offered his riposte to the psychiatric establishment that he felt had abused him as a young man.

While he worked as a science journalist after leaving Cambridge, it was only through dedicating himself to creative writing as his primary concern (even while gaining a series of academic posts after his journalistic work) that Redgrove was able to work out just what a 'scientist of the strange' might study and how that study might be executed. Poetry was his laboratory, instrument, and medium for encapsulating an extraordinarily heightened sensuous appreciation of the natural world – particularly the weather, its electrical atmospheres, and sudden shifts in tone. In *The Black Goddess and the Sixth Sense*, Redgrove (1987) explores 'how we are surrounded by invisibles; forces which animals know but humans have come to ignore or only participate in unconsciously. These forces include electricity, magnetism and the deeper reaches of touch, smell, taste and sound'. Explaining such poetic sensitivities to a traditional psychiatrist, rooted in reductive biomedicine, is likely to lead to a diagnosis of derangement and, paradoxically, of limited capacity rather than poetic capability as unbounded capacity.

Coda

I have entwined three conversations to form what Bill Pinar, the 'father' of curriculum reconceptualization, calls a 'complicated conversation', introduced earlier. Here, as noted, I am calling this a 'complex conversation', including first, the poetics of 'anti-psychiatry', now termed 'mad studies'. Second, I include Pinar's own work that frames curriculum not as pedagogical techniques of teaching and learning but as a process of deepening experience akin to the use of the poetic imagination. This, like a mad recovery programme, through four steps: (1) the regressive or historical, the exercise of memory; (2) the progressive or future-facing, the exercise of deliberate anticipation; (3) the analytic moment in which reflection and insight occurs; and (4) the synthetic moment in which action follows that is innovative, generative, and generous. Such action moves from a deep sense of an evolving subjectivity to a collaborative or democratic gesture. Here, the poetic imagination is again core. Third is the contribution to the conversation of career poet and 'scientist of the strange' Peter Redgrove, who, naturally, finds forces such as the charge of thunderclouds a more potent healing medium than deep insulin coma therapy.

Pinar (2012: 190–91) says that,

> Curriculum as conversation . . . is a matter of attunement, an auditory rather than visual conception, in which the sound of music . . . jazz specifically – being improvised is an apt example . . . poetry provides another sound of complicated conversation.

Curriculum as jazz and poetry. At last, somebody who literally talks sense and sees the educational imperative in any subject area – here our concern is medicine and health care – as one of sensibility. Aesthetics is the core of *currere* – with beauty, the sublime, and quality as the chief concerns. Pinar draws on Michael Oakeshott's (1959) important work *The voice of poetry in the conversation of mankind* to suggest that the complex conversation that constitutes *currere* is in fact poetic innovation, the improvising poetic sensibility at work, the poetic voice projected in the classical Freudian sense as the forward-facing recovery of repressed memories and affect through catharsis and subsequent insight. Oakeshott (*ibid.*: 12) describes this as public conversation, where we attempt 'to restore to it some of its lost freedom of movement' – poetics at the heart of public discourse as a communal therapeutic gesture. Or medicine realized as conviviality.

Again, we bring agility and fragility, presence and persistence, rage and outrage to the table of evolving democracy and bargain eloquently with rhythm and form, care and consideration, and, above all, experimentation. The voice of poetry, suggests Pinar, moves plain speaking to allegory, something more complex, stimulating, and perhaps intimidating. Poetry is the wonder drug here. In 1951, Williams (1951/1967: 286–87, 289) said in his autobiography, 'When they ask me, as of late they frequently do, how I have for so many years continued an equal interest in medicine and the poem, I reply that *they amount for me to nearly the same thing*' (my emphasis). Writing, says Williams, relieved him from the dilemma of facing medicine's (and surgery's) ever-increasing demands for cures, where the human condition is inevitably so fragile, and we dance around the rim of death through risk and lifestyle yet simultaneously race into the arms of medicine for cures. Williams is echoing Edith Wharton's adage that the only cure for life's ills is to make something of life itself. Poetry, claims Williams, gives life, where the person treated

> as material for a work of art made him somehow come alive to me . . . in the permission I as a physician have had to be present at deaths and births, at the tormented battles between daughter and diabolic mother, shattered by a gone brain – just there – for a split second – from one side or the other, it has fluttered before me for a moment, a phrase which I can quickly write down on anything at hand, any piece of paper I can grab.

You don't have to be a physician to follow Williams' prescription: you can and have been present at deaths and births, at battles between mothers and daughters, and in the presence of shattered brains. Famously, Williams would use his prescription pads to capture such inspirational scraps of experience, of *currere* soaked in a kind of madness. What could be more fitting than the work of medicine as both witnessing and treating being channelled as scraps of poetry (and not poetry scrapped)?

Peter Redgrove's unique voice advertises the value of Pinar's formulation: the deeply subjective, idiosyncratic, and troubled voice steps into community through art. (Poetry again). And waits for the echo. Redgrove (personal communication) steps out of the confines of the personal into the world soul, into weathers and mud baths, where he 'hears voices', 'senses the extra-sensory' and has 'visions'. A rich and wonderful madness. Troubling for some, yes, but poetry promises trouble as it deals the richer hand of deep sensibility, close noticing, the intensive inhabitation called 'indwelling' by Martin Heidegger, and the recreational use of the natural pharmaceuticals that the brain produces at the extreme borders of everyday perception, in the animal realms of knowing, the bandwidths of extreme body and extreme mind. For Redgrove, the 'sixth sense' – all the senses combined and more. Or 'Imagination' – following Samuel Taylor Coleridge's guiding light.

In entangling these three minds or imaginations – David Cooper's, William Pinar's, and Peter Redgrove's – I turn a complicated conversation into one that is complex, open, adaptive, and at the edge of chaos but able to regroup at higher levels of complexity, avoiding chaos. We have, together, taken a mud bath in a poetic field. The specific brief narratives spun around these three figures hint at more general, wider, and more embracing meanings and hence are allegorical. They suggest that medicine's educational embrace – formal contemporary medical education – is limited and stiff, merely a formality. Yes, the basic knowledge and skills are attained, and, yes, an identity is achieved of both 'doctor' (the practical) and 'professional' (the ethical). But we need more: medicine must be aesthetically and politically attuned. It must strive for quality and authentic democracy, seeking beauty and poetic fervour. It must (narratively) revise its plot where it often loses the plot and (poetically) relocate and review its field. Medical education cries out for a new turf, a relocation. It will find hospitable mulch in the field of poetry.

References

Bateson G. 2000. *Steps to an Ecology of Mind: Collected Essays in Anthropology, Psychiatry, Evolution, and Epistemology*. Chicago, IL: University of Chicago Press.

Bleakley A, Neilson S. 2021. *Poetry in the Clinic: Towards a Lyrical Medicine*. Abingdon: Routledge.

Burstow B. 2017. *The Other Mrs Smith*. Toronto: Inanna Publications and Education.

Cooper D. 2001. *Psychiatry and Anti-Psychiatry*. London: Routledge.

Deleuze G, Guattari F. 2013. *Capitalism and Schizophrenia (2 vols: Anti-Oedipus and A Thousand Plateaus)*. London: Bloomsbury Academic.

Doll MA. (ed.) 2017. *The Reconceptualization of Curriculum Studies: A Festschrift in Honor of William F. Pinar*. Abingdon: Routledge.

Flexner A. 1925. *Medical Education: A Comparative Study*. New York, NY: Macmillan.

Flexner A. 1940. *I Remember: The Autobiography of Abraham Flexner*. New York, NY: Simon & Schuster.

Flexner A. 1973 (originally pub. 1910). *Medical Education in the United States and Canada*. New York, NY: Carnegie Foundation for the Advancement of Teaching, New York Heritage Press.

Goodman P. 1964. *Compulsory Mis-Education*. New York, NY: Horizon Press.

Illich I. 1973. *Deschooling Society*. Harmondsworth, UK: Penguin.

Laing RD. 1973. *Knots*. Harmondsworth: Penguin Books.

Montgomery S. 2005. *Islands*. Etruscan Books.

Oakeshott M. 1959. *The Voice of Poetry in the Conversation of Mankind: An Essay*. Cambridge: Bowes and Bowes.

Olson C. 1950. *Projective Verse*. Available at: www.poetryfoundation.org. Last accessed: 21/12/2013.

Pinar W. (ed.) 2000. *Curriculum Studies: The Reconceptualization*. Troy, NY: Educator's International Press.

Pinar W. 2012. *What is Curriculum Theory?* (2nd ed.). Abingdon: Routledge.

Redgrove P. 1973. *In the Country of the Skin*. London: Routledge and Kegan Paul.

Redgrove P. 1987. *The Black Goddess and the Sixth Sense*. London: Bloomsbury Publishing.

Redgrove P. 1988. *The Black Goddess and the Unseen Real: Our Unconscious Senses and Their Uncommon Sense*. London: Grove Press.

Redgrove P. 2012. *Collected Poems*. London: Jonathan Cape.

Roberts N. 2012. *A Lucid Dreamer: The Life of Peter Redgrove*. London: Jonathan Cape.

Russo J, Sweeney A. (eds.) 2016. *Searching for a Rose Garden: Challenging Psychiatry, Fostering Mad Studies*. Monmouth: PCCS Books.

Sass LA. 1994. *Madness and Modernism: Insanity in the Light of Modern Art, Literature, and Thought*. Cambridge, MA: Harvard University Press.

Singer J. 2017. *Neurodiversity: The Birth of an Idea*. Amazon: Judy Singer.

Williams WC. 1951/1967. *The Autobiography of William Carlos Williams*. New York, NY: WW Norton.

PART 5

The intimate soma

20

BODY-RELATED POETRY THERAPY IN PSYCHO-ONCOLOGY

Alfonso Santarpia

Introduction

Representation of a Metaphorical Body

We are embodied human beings open to the world, but this world is not an abstract world. It is characterized by the subjective interpretation of embodied experience embedded in a specific cultural and physical environment (Santarpia 2022). There is strong *scientific evidence* that cognitive processes (included the language and imagination) are grounded in our bodily experiences and that high-level cognitive processes cannot be detached from the peripheral brain systems that process input from the outside world (Barsalou 1999; Lakoff and Johnson 1999; Gallese and Lakoff 2005; Gibbs 2006; Marre et al. 2021; Santarpia 2022). For example, visual imagery relies on the manipulation of representations that share the same attributes as precepts (Shepard and Metzler 1971; Kosslyn 1994; Borst and Kosslyn 2008; Albers et al. 2013; Marre et al. 2021; Santarpia 2022) and requires the activation of the same brain systems that are involved in visual perception. Concerning language, experiments using fMRI (Hauk et al. 2004; Buccino et al. 2005; Tettamanti et al. 2005) have shown that a parieto-premotor circuit becomes active during the processing of action-related sentences. Data from these investigations have provided direct evidence that listening to action-related sentences engages the audio-motor circuits that initiate action, execution, and listening. Embodied simulation theory could explain the link between perception, language, and imagination where this theory states that the brain captures modal states during perception, action, and introspection and later simulates these states to represent knowledge (Gallese and Lakoff 2005). Being an embodied human means not only to experience physical reality but also to conceive possible worlds, to surrender to imagination and to fictional realms (Gallese 2017a, 2017b).

What are the characteristics of these possible embodied worlds? They could be composed of *embodied schemata* (Johnson 1987), these preconceptual schemata (containment, locomotion, etc. – see Lakoff and Johnson 1999) emerge as meaningful structures for us chiefly at the level of our bodily movement through space, our manipulation of objects, and our perceptual interactions. For

 DOI: 10.4324/9781003341796-27

example, the image schema CONTAINER results from our recurrent and ubiquitous experiences with containers, as Johnson (1987: 331) suggests:

> You wake *out of* a deep sleep and peer *out from* beneath the covers *into* your room. You gradually emerge *out of* your stupor, and pull yourself *out from* under the covers, climb *into* your robe, stretch *out* your limbs, and walk *in* a daze out of the bedroom and *into* the bathroom.

As this example reveals, by the recurrent use of the expressions *in* and *out*, a great number of everyday objects and experiences are categorized as specific instances of the schematic concept CONTAINER: not only obvious containers like bathroom cabinets and toothpaste tubes or less obvious 'containers' like bed-covers, clothing and rooms but also states like sleep, stupor, and daze (Tompkins and Lawley 2022).

These embodied schemas are organized and associated with a multitude of bodily experiences and generate imaginative scenarios (Lakoff and Johnson 1999) that can be told through linguistic metaphors of the body (Cavallo and Santarpia 2005; Santarpia et al. 2006, 2010; Santarpia 2022). These are body-related metaphorical scenarios composed of one or more sentences which have as *tenor* (Richards 1936) body elements (parts, functions, actions, perceptions of the body, such as *the body*, *the heart*, and *breathing*) and as *vehicle*[1] (*ibid.*):

- non-contextual bodily experiences (memories of past bodily experiences or possible bodily experiences, not present in the real context, e.g. *I feel like I'm drowning, suffocating, dancing, swimming, for me it's like a crushing weight on my chest*[2]*, etc.*)
- fictional/abstract elements (impossible, unrealistic actions/categories/properties, e.g. *heart of gold, heart of stone, hard-hearted, cold hearted, in your heart, my blood feels like it's a raging river coursing through the veins of my whole body* or *my head pounds like someone is using a jackhammer on it*[3]*, etc.*)

In the field of psychopathology and psychotherapeutic techniques, patient and therapist utterances frequently include metaphors of the body (Santarpia et al. 2006, 2010), in anomalous or normal embodiment (Cole et al. 2000). Normal embodiment relies intrinsically on the continuity of our sensitive, perceptive, and affective bodily experience, which gives us our body as being familiar; in contrast, anomalous embodiment refers to the experience and/or the activity of breaking or interrupting such a continuity (*ibid.*). More precisely, in the field of "anomalous embodiment," patients frequently include metaphors, similes, metonymies, and other figurative language focused on the body. We can find the following complex and articulated body metaphorizations in clinical practice (Schuster 2017) from patients suffering anxiety disorders such as panic attacks:

> For me it's like a crushing weight on my chest while my heart feels like it's going to jump right out of my body, my blood feels like it's a raging river coursing through the veins of my whole body, my head pounds like someone is using a jackhammer on it, I'm suffocating and all the while my brain won't shut off. – Monika S.

> Like my skeleton is trying to escape through my skin. – Jessica L.

> It feels like having an itch on your whole body while walking on a tight rope hundreds of feet up in the air. You want to explode out of your skin, but you don't want to move to

avoid losing the little balance point you have, and you can't get distracted scratching a spot because you need your entire focus to get across to the end. – Helen H.

From this embodied and imaginative perspective, a series of interdisciplinary studies on psycho-pathology, Freudian psychoanalysis, and Italian poetry (Cavallo and Santarpia 2005; Santarpia et al. 2006, 2010) described different metaphorical categories of body schemata that refer to the general (superordinate level) or specific properties (Rosch 1975; Rosch et al. 1976) in an attempt to articulate the uniqueness of the bodily experience in a dynamic representation termed *metaphorical body* (Cavallo and Santarpia 2005; Santarpia et al. 2006, 2010; Santarpia 2022). This dynamic representation of the body is composed of several body-related metaphorical categories:

- BODY-CONTAINER, a ubiquitous and ontological category in Western culture that refers to the general or specific properties of spatiality (interior–exterior, closed–open, over–under), boundary, protection, safety, filter, containment, constraint, cover. From poetry: 'Losing himself in his body' (Merini 1993) or 'The body is the shelter of the soul' (Tasso 1581/1999). From psychoanalysis: 'The sexual urge had a sexual object outside the body proper' or 'The incorporation process refers explicitly to this bodily envelope' (Laplanche and Pontalis 1998). From psychiatry: 'Destructive impulses of objects on the body' (Brusset 1987) or 'The body is perceived as inhabited by a bad object of maternal introjection' (Gabbard 1995).
- BODY-SUBSTANCE, a category that refers to the general or specific properties (see Rosch 1975; Rosch et al. 1976) of concrete substances (natural or artificial elements in their pure state), created by natural physical and chemical reactions, and the same used in cultural symbolism (earth, air, fire, water). From poetry: 'A heart of marble would have taken pity on him' or 'Love wrote in my heart' (Petrarca 1336/1988). These examples express the idea of an impenetrable heart and a body that one can write upon and read. From a psychiatric work: 'Refusing food means making the body evanescent, which signifies the negation of one's identification with the mother' (Lalli 1991). In psychoanalysis, we have metaphoric imagery such as water–uterus, genital organs–landscapes, penis–mountain, penis–rock, and excrement–gold. From Freudian works: 'In its form and movements, a flame evokes the phallus in action' or 'the representation of the penis as a weapon, a sharp knife, a sword . . . underlies many phobias' and other examples, penis–silver, mug–penis, vagina–bud, vagina–lock (Delrieu 2001).
- BODY-ORGANISM, a category that refers to linguistic representations of the body, body parts, actions, gestures, movements, specific perceptions, and physiological functions depicted as general attributes (adjectives or verbs), general or specific properties (Rosch 1975; Rosch et al. 1976) that represent the body in the form of general biological systems (animal or plant world). From poetry: 'This submissive wildcat, heart of a tiger or bear' (Petrarca 1336/1988) or 'The body falls frozen, deprived of fire/Like the dying of a listless crimson flower' (Ariosto 1516/2000). From psychoanalysis, several kinds of associations: penis–bird, penis–snake, vagina–snail and vagina–shell, penis–tree, breast–fruit, penis–mushroom, vagina–flower, vagina–garden, pubic hair–forest (Delrieu 2001).
- METONYMICAL BODY refers to the body or its parts that are associated metonymically with specific functions such as hearing or sight or to parts of the body. From poetry: 'Here, in life's last light, your body still breathes' (Pasolini 1996). From psychoanalysis: 'The foot fetish relates to the woman's absent penis' or 'The concepts of excrement and penis are easily interchangeable' (Delrieu 2001).
- METAMORPHICAL BODY, a category that refers to the body, or parts of the body, objectively transformed into substances, animals, or new creatures (for example in the emotion icons,

cartoon, science fiction movies) or experienced by the patient as perceptual bodily transformations and/or bodily hallucinations in modified states of consciousness (for example, hypnosis, meditation) or a psychotic state. From poetry: 'See Tiréslas,/who changed from male to female,/bit by bit' (Ariosto 1516/2000) and 'in the eyes where my heart had made its home' (Petrarca 1336/1988). From Freudian works: 'He thinks that the two sexes have the same genital organ, the male organ' (Delrieu 2001) and 'Incorporation, a process in which the subject places and keeps an object inside the body in a more or less fantastical manner' (Laplanche et Pontalis 1998). From psychiatric texts: 'the fantasy of incorporation' (Brusset 1987) and 'the bulimic patient symbolically destroys and incorporates people' (Gabbard 1995).

- MYTHICAL BODY, a category that refers to the general or specific properties (Rosch 1975; Rosch et al. 1976), where the body or its parts are associated with attributes (verbs, adjectives) of supernatural, divine, mythical, sacred creatures/personages/characters or objects (for example lightness, brightness, clearness, immortality). From poetry: 'She showed who, in all his grace,/Resembled the god Mars, except for his face' (Ariosto 1516/2000), 'May your heart conquer, in its great triumph,/extraordinary angel' (Petrarca 1336/1988), and 'Your flesh is bread, your blood is wine' (Pascoli 1999). From psychiatry: 'Anorexics want a subtle body, without flesh' (Trattato italiano di Psichiatria 1992) and 'In a perverse relationship, the body becomes a sacred fetish offered to another to deny the laws of nature'; from psychoanalysis: 'her immortal body', 'the ideal body', and 'a body without flesh' (Semi 1989).

- ABSTRACT BODY, a category that refers to the body or bodily parts associated with abstract concepts, characterized by the absence of figurative properties related to natural or biological elements. These figurative utterances require in-depth interpretation. From poetry: 'I offered you my body as a movement of happy sadness' (Merini 1993) and 'Freedom returns/and the flesh is a pure sound' (Pasolini 1996). From psychoanalysis, the idea of a body-source or body-zone: 'In anorexia, the negation of the body's representation as a source of pleasure' (Semi 1988) and 'Every part of the body can become an erogenous zone' (Delrieu 2001). From psychiatry, ideas of a body-place: 'The subject's relationship with his/her own body . . . the preferred place for conflicts' (Brusset 1987).

BODY-CONTAINER, BODY-SUBSTANCE, BODY-ORGANISM, METONYMICAL BODY, METAMORPHICAL BODY, MYTHICAL BODY, ABSTRACT BODY are categories that, integrated with *non-contextual bodily experiences*, can provide an alternative to the anatomical description of the body. This metaphorical body (Cavallo and Santarpia 2005; Santarpia et al. 2006, 2010; Santarpia 2022) is characterized by a bodily narrative based on figurative utterances that can represent and describe stable (trait metaphorizations) or transient (state metaphorizations) human bodily experiences.

Cancer and metaphors of the body

Cancer generates physical, psychological, or spiritual issues and provokes questions regarding existence and finitude. An existential central conflict can be found in the tension between one's immediate consciousness of real or phantasmatic death and the deep desire to exist and stay alive (Frankl 1959; Yalom 1980, 2009). Cancer confronts the patient with the fragility of life, forcing him or her to mourn the loss of immortality (Hurbault and Imbert 2007) or a possible loss of parts of oneself. In discussing spiritual care of patients with terminal cancer, Murata (Murata 2003: 17) defined 'psycho-existential suffering' as 'pain caused by extinction of the being and the meaning of the self' (see also Murata and Morita 2006). Psycho-existential suffering is caused by loss of essential components composing both being and the meaning for human beings, either of relationships with others, autonomy, or temporality.

In an embodied perspective, metaphorically (Lakoff and Johnson 1999) the body becomes the object of external forces. In this passive metaphorical representation of the body (Murphy 1996; Santarpia et al. 2006, 2010), Menzel (1954) depicts cancer as a battle or a war in which cancer cells attack the body, following a long historical tradition. Stolberg (2014) found that metaphors of war were frequently used to describe cancer in early modern Europe, with references to armies of hostile cells attacking the body and needing to be fought off. Such war metaphors continue; for example, Jasen (2009) describes cancer as a 'silent killer'.

The use of metaphors of the body is particularly helpful in allowing patients to express in depth the experience of death and dying in an oncology context (remission phase, palliative care, chemotherapy). In breast cancer experience, the suffering can take the form of distressing body metaphors, as expressed below by a patient who was asked about her femininity. Mrs. V used the metaphor 'I am an alien' in order to describe herself (Santarpia et al. 2013; Santarpia 2021: 34) using a stable metaphorization from the category MYTHICAL BODY:

I put on a bikini, I put on a prosthesis, I never go out without my prosthesis. This is me. On the contrary. It's me who . . . who looks at everyone and says yeah, well she's a woman and I'm not . . . I 'm not a woman and . . . I . . . I am maybe an extra . . . well in my head, **I am an alien**. I'm missing something. My femininity has been damaged that's for sure.

From the METAMORPHICAL BODY category, a late-stage breast cancer patient expressed the following (Cannone et al. 2008: 191):

They took my heart when they took my breast, they took everything. . . . I am dirty, my insides are rotten, I want to scrub and scrub myself with bleach to get rid of this filth, take out my organs and put them back when they are clean, wash away the **dark blood**, do you think that's possible?

This narrative includes perceptual experience of a 'dirty body', 'dark blood', and a sort of 'containing body' (Santarpia et al. 2006, 2010; Santarpia 2022) from which things can be taken out and put back. The patient continued, expressing her desire for healing and freedom using a body metaphor of a bird (Cannone et al. 2008: 191): 'Of course, I know it isn't . . . I wish I could fly away like a bird, be free, I would be a raven'. From a clinical and pragmatic perspective of therapy in this tragic context where there is a strong identification with a sick body or with tragic body-related metaphors, many questions emerge. How can we help these oncology patients to disidentify from their sick bodies? How can we help them to generate new body metaphors? How can we stimulate them to seek in themselves metaphors evoking experiences of transcendence or vitality?

A body-related poetry therapy, a literary form that privileges figurative language associated with bodily experiences, could be well suited to this kind of transformative work. Generally, poetry therapy is an artistic and therapeutic approach that explores the effects of poetic reading/writing on psychological processes from a multidisciplinary point of view (Mazza 1996, 1999). The field has already developed a significant literature (Shrodes 1949; Blanton 1960; Leedy 1969; Prescott 1970). Mazza (1996, 1999) and Reiter (1997) have identified the therapeutic processes specific to poetry therapy, for example symbolizing experience with metaphor and improving communication skills through a more figurative use of language. Others have identified additional therapeutic aspects, stimulating the imagination and developing awareness of harmony, symmetry, and aesthetics in general (Gergen 2000), while outlining and synthesizing a productive imagination (Ricoeur 1982).

In a psychoanalytical model, writing poems centred on bodily sensations generates bodily metaphors that evoke archaic experiences of the child with the mother: finding lost and forgotten psychic objects (Clancier 2001). Poetry therapy shows how working with poetic forms can help patients deal with the drastic life changes that accompany serious medical conditions and illness. It has been recognized in the psychiatric (Langosch 1987; Houlding and Holland 1988; Shelton 1999) and psychotherapeutic (McLoughlin 2000) literatures. Recent research is based on specific protocols, for example SANTEL, associated with a sensual poetry in the context of breast cancer (Santarpia et al. 2013; Santarpia 2022). This is aimed at transforming the cancer patient's anxiety-ridden experiences by means of new metaphors and creative imagery.

The creative use of the haiku

Of particular interest to me and my colleagues is the possible use of a specific poetic form, the haiku, in psycho-oncology. A haiku is a very short form of Japanese poetry written in three phrases, each of which traditionally has a set number of syllables: a short phrase of five syllables followed by a long phrase of seven syllables and then another short phrase of five syllables (Santarpia et al. 2015b). Haiku usually include a word that ties the poem to the real world and, in general, to nature. Haiku contain a caesura, or cutting, which punctuates the movement from one image to another. These poems try to express the evanescence of the world and things, containing a reference to the seasons and including a caesura that divides the verse into several parts (*ibid.*). One of the best-known Japanese haiku was written by Basho Matsuo (translated by Aitken 1978: 25): *The old pond/a frog jumps in/the sound of the water*).

Haiku poetry has already been used both in therapeutic work with schizophrenic patients (Collins et al. 2006) and as a pedagogical tool in the neurosciences (Pollack and Korol 2013). Stibbe (2007) described several aspects of haiku poetry that could evoke new bodily experiences of transcendence or vitality to disidentify patients from their sick bodies. Haiku use language to go beyond language, beyond the world of intellectual abstractions, and to reconnect directly with bodily perceptions. The way haiku do this is to describe actual encounters with everyday nature in straight present tense, using a minimal amount of metaphor and abstraction, placing poetic emphasis on individual animals and plants, representing them 'as agents of their own lives living according to their natures, with implicit assumptions of empathy and positive regard built into the discourse' (Stibbe 2007: 110). The focus on the everyday is important because it encourages direct encounters with living plants and animals in natural settings rather than encounters mediated by linguistic abstractions. This characteristic could stimulate bodily experiences and metaphors from the BODY-ORGANISM category. Indeed, haiku represent animals as sentient beings with mental lives, who know, feel, and have desires. These representations can generate processes of identification in persons. This poetical perspective can bring new therapeutic horizons to psycho-oncological treatment.

These scientific and literary premises gave birth to a constantly evolving protocol termed SAD-UPA (Santarpia et al. 2015a, 2015b). SADUPA consists of four processes at separate times: a) a preliminary exploratory interview; b) 15 haiku proposed without a part of the poem for the patient to complete; c) a free form haiku composed by the patient; and d) a final interview. The interviews for the protocol were conducted by mental health professionals (clinical psychologist, therapist, psychiatric nurse, etc.) as facilitators. The style of the interviews was inspired by Rogerian psychotherapeutic principles: empathy, congruence, non-directivity, and positive unconditional regard (Rogers 1951, 1975; Santarpia 2020).

In a specific session, 15 haiku were read to the participant by the mental health professional, for example: 'As we grow older/even the length of the days/is a source of tears' or 'Beat of butterfly wings/as if in desperation/of this world' (cited in Santarpia et al. 2015a, 2015b). The patients were in a posture focused on all the bodily sensations of the moment, closing their eyes to contact the sensations of the body and any associated images. After this, haiku were read again, and the middle line of each was omitted. The patients slowly opened their eyes, read the list of haiku without the middle line, and again closed their eyes to stimulate imagination and bodily perception. Finally, they opened their eyes and filled in the missing middle lines of the haiku to give them a personal meaning.

This personal meaning can be focused on the bodily sensations/actions of the present, past, or future and associated with possible mental images. Next, the professional read the haiku with the newly added lines aloud to the participant. This process can be repeated several times according to the state of health of the patient, with the presence of the professional or without. The protocol can be done comfortably in the hospital bed or in home. After this process, termed *poetic impregnation*, in another session, the patients would first encounter their own bodies with their eyes closed, then gradually open their eyes, and then write a series of haiku to best describe their bodily sensations, their 'being there in the world'.

Presentation of the case

Below, I describe the transformations of the metaphors of the body with cancer patients before and after the SADUPA protocol (Santarpia et al. 2015a, 2015b), focused on several haiku poems. The first case study was conducted in a French oncology unit by a psychologist. The patient, Mr A, was a male age 70, widowed, who had retired from the French national education system. He had a malignant tumour of the thigh that had metastasized to his lungs; the cancer was in terminal phase. In the preliminary interview, he expressed his stable bodily experience through the abstract metaphorization (see ABSTRACT BODY category in the paragraph *Introduction: the representation of a Metaphorical Body*) of "I'm in parentheses" (Santarpia et al. 2015b: 185):

I'm in parentheses. And I've been cut off from others. Because I can't, look I'm stuck. That quadriceps muscle won't move. I can't get dressed by myself: no, not for that, she tries not to hurt me.

Mr A filled in the missing middle lines of the haiku (underlined), giving a personal meaning centred on bodily sensations, for example (*ibid.*: 184):

As we grow older/<u>and each of our weaknesses</u>/is a source of tears
In the young grasses/<u>the old man lying stretched out</u>/forgets his roots.
All in this world/<u>would become more beautiful</u>/to consider the flowers

Here, Mr A filled in the missing line with his own body-related poetry. After this work of sensory openness to images and to the world of nature, Mr A (in another session) wrote the last free haiku (*ibid.*: 184):

The hundred-year-old olive tree before me
Unfurls its branches and its hues
I feel, standing there, my ephemeral existence

When my cat on my lap lets go and purrs
I feel that he is so trusting, happy
That my own soul is calmed
The scent of fresh-cut grass,
Is the spring which returns
And the time which each year has passed is forgotten.

His free haiku included a new body metaphor from the BODY-ORGANISM category – the 'hundred-year-old olive tree' – accompanied by a somewhat spiritual reflection on time and existence.

In another clinical situation, Mr D, aged 25 years old, suffering from Ewing's sarcoma (in treatment), living as a couple, childless, web designer by profession, initially used the body metaphor of 'the fall' in order to describe his loss of an existential direction (Santarpia et al. 2015a: 133). Later, evoking his hope, he recounted the bodily pleasure of going out into the streets, at the arrival of summer, and of identifying himself metonymically with the taste of the fresh fruits he ate at the arrival of summer.

Towards a poetry therapy-related corporeal elevation

The purpose of this chapter is to describe healing work in the oncology context through the mobilization of metaphors of the body in patients' narratives after a poetic experience. My hypothesis is that psychological work with haiku poetry, in the presence of the therapist, could not only distance patients from a medicalized narrative of illness (symptoms, complaints and physical pains) but also generate revitalizing metaphors of the body from a figurative categorization termed metaphorical body (Cavallo and Santarpia 2005; Santarpia et al. 2006, 2010; Santarpia 2022), useful in the elaboration of death anguish.

In keeping with the literature on the effects of poetry therapy (Shrodes 1949; Blanton 1960; Leedy 1969; Prescott 1970; Mazza 1996; Reiter 1997; Mazza 1999), I described the body-related metaphorical variations in Mr A's narrative of his illness before and after his haiku writing. The patient's experience of death anxiety was contained in the metaphorization of *I'm in parentheses*, i.e. in his body metaphor, Mr A told me about his loss of autonomy, about a body that had lost the pleasure of moving: the patient was totally identified with his sick body. At the end of the protocol, Mr A told me about a body that seems to have freed itself for a moment. We are faced with a poem and a rich body experience composed by all elements of haiku poetry (Santarpia et al. 2015b: 184), where the plant world is a place of transcendence and existential questions, represented in poetic verses:

The hundred-year-old olive tree before me
Unfurls its branches and its hues
I feel, standing there, my ephemeral existence
. . .
The scent of fresh-cut grass,
Is the spring which returns
And the time which each year has passed is forgotten.

While the world of animals welcome us and reassure us, in the poetic verses:

When my cat on my lap lets go and purrs
I feel that he is so trusting, happy
That my own soul is calmed

In this chapter, the question has arisen: 'how can we help oncology patients to disidentify from their sick bodies?' I have proposed a body-related poetry therapy, and in particular a poetic protocol inspired by haiku poetry. I believe that this type of poetic work can influence the way cancer is experienced and represented. Poetry writing workshops based on short, structured forms such as haiku can allow for a poetic bodily elevation. It is a process of disidentification from the disease towards new experiences of being using metaphors of the body. The mobilization of new body metaphors can offer a new form of *spiritual presence*, offering hope to the patient and to the medical providers. In addition, if death sadly comes, the effective heirs (parents, children, friends) – those who remain on earth – will bring the memory of a poetic presence of their loved one and not just traces of his or her physical pain.

The body-related poetry therapy approach is a first step in a larger research programme within a humanistic/existential framework (Santarpia et al. 2013, 2015a, 2015b; Santarpia 2020, 2021, 2022) that will include additional studies involving larger numbers of cancer patients in group and individual poetry-writing workshop sessions. Specifically, I believe that the protocol termed SADUPA, based on haiku poetry, can be a useful tool in the context of supportive interventions in palliative care and/or as preparatory work for engagement in psychotherapeutic intervention. The formal structure of haiku can create conditions for a specific poetic work composed of poetic evocation, synthesis, and mapping of the most intimate experiences in an oncology environment towards a poetic corporeal elevation.

Acknowledgment

The author and colleagues would like to share their warmest appreciation of Mr A, who has passed away from cancer; his poetic sensibility and acuity brought much compassion.

Notes

1 These terms are taken from the famous rhetorician Richards (1936): the *tenor* is the thing being described. The *vehicle* is the figurative language you use to describe it. According to Richards, the co-presence of the vehicle and tenor results in a meaning which is not attainable without their interaction.
2 See the examples in Schuster 2017.
3 See the examples in Schuster 2017.

References

Aitken R. 1978. *A Zen Wave: Basho's Haiku and Zen*. Berkeley, CA: Weatherhill.
Albers AM, Kok P, Toni I, et al. Shared Representations for Working Memory and Mental Imagery in Early Visual Cortex. *Current Biology*. 2013; 23: 1427–31.
Ariosto L. 2000 (originally pub. 1516). *Roland Furieux. Traduction de Michel Orcel*. Paris: Le Seuil.
Barsalou L. Perceptual symbol systems. *Behavioral and Brain Science*. 1999; 22: 577-660.
Blanton S. 1960. *The Healing Power of Poetry*. New York, NY: Thomas Crowell.
Borst G, Kosslyn SM. Visual Mental Imagery and Visual Perception: Structural Equivalence Revealed by Scanning Processes. *Memory & Cognition*. 2008; 36: 849–62.
Brusset B. 1987. *Encyclopédie Médico-Chirurgicale: Valeur sémiologique des anomalies des conduites alimentaires*. Vol. 37–144-A. Paris: Elsevier.
Buccino GL, Riggio G, Melli F, et al. Listening to Action-Related Sentences Modulates the Activity of the Motor System: A Combined TMS and Behavioral Study. *Cognitive Brain Research*. 2005; 24: 355–63.
Cannone P, Marie D, Dudoit E. 2008. *Cancer du sein avancé*. Paris: Springer Paris.
Cavallo M, Santarpia A. Le corpo metaforico. *Attualità In Psicologia*. 2005; 20: 205–14.
Clancier A. Poetry work: Poetry and Representation. *Revue française de psychanalyse*. 2001; 65: 1283–90.

Cole J, Depraz N, Gallagher S. 2000. Unity and Disunity in Bodily Awareness: Phenomenology and Neuro-science. *Association for the Scientific Study of Consciousness Workshop*. Available at: https://philpapers.org. Last accessed: 31/12/2023.

Collins KS, Furman R, Langer CL. Poetry Therapy as a Tool of Cognitively Based Practice. *The Arts in Psychotherapy*. 2006; 33: 180–87.

Delrieu A. 2001. *Sigmund Freud. Index Thématique* (2nd ed.). Paris: Anthropos.

Frankl V. 1959. *Man's Search for Meaning*. New York, NY: Washington Square.

Gabbard GO. 1995. *Psichiatria Psicodinamica*. Milano: Raffaele Cortina Editore.

Gallese V. 2017a. Mirroring, a Liberated Embodied Simulation and Aesthetic Experience. In: H Hirsch, A Pace (eds.) *Mirror Images: Spiegelbilder in Kunst und Medizin: Reflections in Art and Medicine*. Wien: Verlag für Moderne Kunst, 27–37.

Gallese V. 2017b. The Empathic Body in Experimental Aesthetics – Embodied Simulation and Art. In: V Lux, S Weigel (eds.) *Empathy*. London: Palgrave Macmillan UK, 181–99.

Gallese V, Lakoff G. The Brain's Concept: The Role of the Sensorimotor System in Conceptual Knowledge. *Cognitive Neuropsychology*. 2005; 22: 455-79.

Gergen KJ. 2000. The Poetic Dimension: Therapeutic Options. In: KG Deissler, S McNamee (eds.) *Phil und Sophie im Dialog Die soziale Poesie therapeutischer Gespräche*. Heidelberg: Carl-Auer Verlag, 97–108.

Gibbs RW. 2006. *Embodiment and Cognitive Science*. Cambridge: Cambridge University Press.

Hauk O, Johnsrude I, Pulvermüller F. Somatotopic Representation of Action Words in Human Motor and Premotor Cortex. *Neuron*. 2004; 41: 301–7.

Houlding S, Holland P. Contributions of a Poetry Writing Group to the Treatment of Severely Disturbed Psychiatric Inpatients. *Clinical Social Work Journal*. 1988; 16: 194–200.

Hurbault A, Imbert A. From Medical Consultation to Psychological Consultation, Reflections in Oncological Medicine. *Psycho-Oncologie*. 2007; 4: 26.

Jasen P. From the 'Silent Killer' to the 'Whispering Disease'. Ovarian Cancer and the Uses of Metaphor. *Medical History*. 2009; 53: 489–512.

Johnson M. 1987. *The Body in the Mind*. Chicago, IL: The University of Chicago Press.

Kosslyn S. 1994. *Image and Brain: The Resolution of the Imagery Debate*. Cambridge, MA: MIT Press.

Lakoff G, Johnson M. 1999. *Philosophy in the Flesh: The Embodied Mind and Its Challenge to Western Thought*. New York, NY: Basic Books.

Lalli N. 1991. *Manuale di Psichiatria e Psicoterapia*. Napoli: Liguori.

Langosch DS. The Use of Poetry Therapy With Emotionally Disturbed Children. *The American Journal of Social Psychiatry*. 1987; 7: 97–100.

Laplanche J, Pontalis, J-B. 1998. *Vocabulaire de la psychanalyse*. Paris: Presses universitaires de France.

Leedy JJ. 1969. *Poetry Therapy: The Use of Poetry in the Treatment of Emotional Disorders*. Philadelphia, PA: Lippincott.

Marre Q, Huet N, Labeye E. EXPRESS: Embodied Mental Imagery Improves Memory. *Quarterly Journal of Experimental Psychology*. mars 2021; 174702182110092.

Mazza N. Poetry Therapy: A Framework and Synthesis of Techniques for Family Social Work. *Journal of Family Social Work*. 1996; 1: 3–18.

Mazza N. 1999. *Poetry Therapy: Interface of the Arts and Psychology*. Boca Raton, FL: CRC Press.

McLoughlin D. Transition, transformation, and the Art of Losing: Some Uses of Poetry in Hospice Care for the Terminally Ill. *Psychodynamic Counseling*. 2000; 6: 215–34.

Menzel R. 1954. *Countering Cancer: Worldwide Scientific Research and Discoveries* (A Henry, Traduit.) Paris, France: Éditions Pierre Horay.

Merini A. 1993. *La Presenza di Orfeo*. Milano: Libri Scheiwiller.

Murata H. Spiritual Pain and Its Care in Patients with Terminal Cancer: Construction of a Conceptual Framework by Philosophical Approach. *Palliative and Supportive Care*. 2003; 1: 15–21.

Murata H, Morita T. Conceptualization of Psycho-Existential Suffering by the Japanese Task Force: The First Step of a Nationwide Project. *Palliative and Supportive Care*. 2006; 4: 279–85.

Murphy GL. On Metaphoric Representation. *Cognition*. 1996; 60: 173–204.

Pascoli G. 1999. Nuovi Poemetti. In: P Stoppelli, E Picchi (eds.) *Letteratura Italiana Zanichelli in 6 CD. ROM*. Bologna: Zanichelli.

Pasolini P. 1996. *Bestemmia (Sonetto Primaverile. I Pianti. Il canto Popolare)*. Vol. III–IV. Milano: Garzanti.

Petrarca F. 1988 (originally pub. 1336). *Le Chansonnier. Traduction de Pierre Blanc et Gérard Genot*. Paris: Bordas.

Pollack AE, Korol DL. The Use of Haiku to Convey Complex Concepts in Neuroscience. *Journal of Undergraduate Neuroscience Education: JUNE: A Publication of FUN, Faculty for Undergraduate Neuroscience*. 2013; 12: A42–A48.

Prescott JW. 1970. Early Somatosensory Deprivation as an Ontogenetic Process in the Abnormal Development of the Brain and Behavior. In: IE Goldsmith, J Moor-Jankowski (eds.) *Medical Primatology*. New York, NY: Karger Basel, 356–75.

Reiter S. Poetry Therapy: Testimony on Capitol Hill. *Journal of Poetry Therapy*. 1997; 10: 169–78.

Richards IA. 1936. *The Philosophy of Rhetoric*. London: Oxford University Press.

Ricoeur P. Imagination and Metaphor. *Psychologie Medicale*. 1982; 14: 1883–87.

Rogers C. 1951. *Client-Centered Therapy: Its Current Practice, Implications and Theory*. London: Constable.

Rogers C. Empathic: An Unappreciated Way of Being. *The Counseling Psychologist*. 1975; 5: 2–10.

Rosch E. Cognitive Representations of Semantic Categories. *Journal of Experimental Psychology*. 1975; 104: 192–233.

Rosch E, Mervis CB, Gray WD, et al. Basic Objects in Natural Categories. *Cognitive Psychology*. 1976; 8: 382–439.

Santarpia A. 2020. *Introduction aux Psychothérapie Humanistes: Deuxième Edition*. Malakoff: Dunod.

Santarpia A. Healing Cancer Through Body Metaphors. *Cancer(s) et psy(s)*. 2021; 5: 33–43.

Santarpia A. 2022. An Arts-Informed Idiographic Perspective in the Oncological Context : A Humanistic-Existential View. In: S Salvatore, J Valsiner (eds.) *Yearbook of idiographic science*. Charlotte, NC: Infoage Publishing, 141–55.

Santarpia A, Blanchet A, Venturini R, et al. The Categorization of Conceptual Metaphors of the Body. *Les Annales Medico-Psicologiques*. 2006; 164: 476–85.

Santarpia A, Dudoit E, Paul M. The Discursive Effects of the Haiku-Based SADUPA Poetry Technique in Palliative Care. *Journal of Poetry Therapy*. 2015b; 28: 179–94.

Santarpia A, Paul M, Dudoit E. The Use of Haiku Poetry in psycho-Oncology. *Psycho-Oncologie*. 2015a; 9: 127–34.

Santarpia A, Tellène J, Carrier M. The Effects of Poetry-Writing SANTEL on Erotic Body Image in Remission of Cancer in Women: A Pilot Study. *Psycho-Oncologie*. 2013; 7: 156-62.

Santarpia A, Venturini R, Blanchet A, Cavallo M. Metaphorical Conceptualizations of the Body in Psychopathology and Poetry. *DELTA: Documentação de estudos em lingüística teórica e aplicada*. 2010; 26: 435–51.

Schuster S. 2017. 23 Metaphors That Might Help You Explain What a Panic Attack Feels Like. *The Mighty*.

Semi A. 1988. *Trattato di Psicoanalisi: Clinica*. Vol. 2. Milano: Raffaele Cortina Editore.

Semi A. 1989. *Trattato di Psicoanalisi: Clinica*. Vol. 2. Milano: Raffaele Cortina Editore.

Shelton DL. 1999. *Healing Words*. Washington, DC: AMA Staff News. Available at: http://amaassn. org/scipubs/amnews/pick 99/feat0517.htm. Last accessed: 5/1/2023.

Shepard RN, Metzler J. Mental Rotation of Three-Dimensional Objects. *Science*. 1971; 171: 701-3.

Shrodes C. 1949. Bibliotherapy: A Theoretical and Clinical Experimental Study (Unpublished Doctoral Dissertation). Berkeley, CA: University of California.

Stibbe A. Haiku and Beyond: Language, Ecology, and Reconnection with the Natural World. *Anthrozoos: A Multidisciplinary Journal of the Interactions of People & Animals*. 2007; 20: 101–12.

Stolberg M. Metaphors and Images of Cancer in Early Modern Europe. *Bulletin of the History of Medicine*. 2014; 88: 48-74.

Tasso T. 1999 (originally pub. 1581). *Aminta At.3. Gerusalemme Liberata. Dans Letteratura Italiana Zanichelli in 6 CD ROM* (P Stoppelli et E Picchi, édité.) Bologna: Zanichelli.

Tettamanti M, Buccino G, Saccuman MC, et al. Listening to Action-Related Sentences Activates Fronto-Parietal Motor Circuits. *Journal of Cognitive Neuroscience*. 2005; 17: 273–81.

Tompkins P, Lawley J. 2022. Embodied Schema: The Basis of Embodied Cognition. *The Clean Collection*. Available at: www.cleanlanguage.co.uk/articles/articles/245/1/Embodied-Schema-The-basis-of-Embodied-Cognition/Page1.html. Last accessed: 5/1/2023.

Trattato italiano di Psichiatria. 1992. *Trattato Italiano di Psichiatria [Italian Treaty of Psychiatry]*. Vols. 1–3. Milano-Parigi-Bonn: Masson.

Yalom ID. 1980. *Existential Psychotherapy*. New York, NY: Basic Books.

Yalom ID. 2009. *Staring at the Sun: Overcoming the Terror of the Death*. San Francisco, CA: Jossey-Bass.

21

ONCOLOGY AND POETRY

The case of Patrick Kavanagh

Martin Dyar

In March 1955, under the care of the young surgeon Keith Shaw, the poet Patrick Kavanagh had his left lung removed at the Rialto Chest Hospital in Dublin. Multiple tests, including a bronchoscopy, had not revealed the large tumour that Shaw discovered when he commenced what was at first intended as exploratory surgery. The life-saving resection was carried out without reviving the famous patient and without the gamble of scheduling a second surgery, a pressurized decision that was allowed by Kavanagh's consenting signature. Prior to this, Kavanagh was in the Rialto for more than a month with an uncertain diagnosis of tuberculosis, a possibility which, when compared to cancer, had been viewed by the poet and his doctors as more hopeful (Quinn 2001).

The speciality of thoracic surgery was in its infancy, but Shaw, a former member of the Royal Army Medical Corp, might have been the ideal surgeon. Not long before he began to work at the Rialto, he was mentored by Clements Price Thomas, who is remembered for the fact that he removed the left lung of George VI in an improvised theatre in Buckingham Palace in 1951.[1] In 1960 Shaw would carry out Ireland's first successful open-heart operation.

By the mid-1950s, the Rialto Chest Hospital itself was a progressive facility (Coakley and Coakley 2018). It had been boosted in the previous decade by a young Minister for Health by the name of Noel Browne. Five of Browne's siblings and both of his parents had died of TB, and he took a personal interest in the Rialto's development, its infrastructure, staffing, and clinical methods. For the Rialto's sake, Browne insisted that the Irish Sweepstakes, a national health care fund linked to horse racing, should begin spending from its total annual profits and not just its interest earnings, as had been the practice since its inception in 1930. Browne, who had studied medicine, was a maverick, but he was not a lone figure. The Rialto's first medical superintendent, Frank Duffy, was himself a TB survivor. He also had an interest in the philosophical writings of the Canadian physician William Osler, whose literary versions of the principles of medical altruism, care, and communication he had a jovial tendency to share with his juniors. Duffy had international experience, and he thought in terms of international standards, the therapeutic impact of hospital ethos, and the importance of nurturing interdisciplinary teams; physiotherapy and nursing in Ireland were key beneficiaries of his leadership, and it is no surprise that a rising star like Keith Shaw was appointed during his tenure.

By the time Patrick Kavanagh needed to be admitted, the Rialto had momentum, a diverse and highly regarded staff, and a touch of prestige. The choice of the title 'chest hospital' pertained to

DOI: 10.4324/9781003341796-28

the growing ambition of thoracic surgery, and it was also meant to assist in making the hospital less synonymous with the fearful and depressing history of TB in that particular Dublin neighbourhood. In 1955, the last remnants of the notorious South Dublin Union Foundling Hospital were being demolished nearby. It was felt that the Rialto Chest Hospital had a ring to it, and some were willing to imagine it promised an escape from ingrained stigma and poverty.

When Kavanagh (2004) first published his poem 'The Hospital' in 1956, many readers would have caught a connotation of progress in its jaunty first line: 'A year ago I fell in love with the functional ward/Of a chest hospital'. Here the poet was incorporating a morbid Dublin-specific meaning of consumption, 'the scourge of the tenements', something that is further evoked later in the poem with the image of the old Rialto gate. But Kavanagh was also suggesting an exotic health care excursion.

Kavanagh's time in the Rialto Chest Hospital holds a fascinating medicine and poetry story that has not yet been fully set down. It includes at least one outlandish anecdote: the surgeon met the poet in a Dublin pub almost a year after his being discharged and in exchange for a signed copy of his banned novel *Tarry Flynn* presented him with a parcel that contained one of his own ribs, which had been retained at the hospital after the surgery. Kavanagh, in his colourful and cantankerous way, had made a moral point of its being returned.

With this opening account of the Rialto, I hope to indicate a foundation for Kavanagh's vision of the setting of his convalescence as offered in 'The Hospital'. It is also a means to begin to gloss the poet's ambiguous approach to autopathography. I will return to Keith Shaw, who has something to tell us about Kavanagh's discrete 'cancer world' (Kirklin et al. 2000). But my primary intention in this essay is to read 'The Hospital' in more technical than contextual terms and, with that emphasis, to attempt to explain what the poem can offer to students of creative writing and poetry who are also medical students.

To go in that direction, I require of the reader an indulgence from the outset. If is not already true, let us imagine, for the purposes of this exploration of medicine and poetry, that both of these ancient fields have a personal and professional claim upon us and that we are duty-bound to strive to meet the various hurdles of apprenticeship and advancement that are synonymous with learning to write poetry and training to be a doctor. Ultimately, it is my intention to try to show that a careful reading and interpretation of 'The Hospital', one that approaches it as a text worth emulating, can yield significant insight into the craft of poetry while also facilitating a special depth of reflection on the lived realities of cancer and cancer care.

'The Hospital' can be viewed as a kind of diary entry, something close to personal truth. It takes a memory of painful illness and hospitalization as its starting point, and it presents a particular clinical space in beguilingly concrete detail. But the poem remains enigmatic for the fact that it does not mention the care that the poet received. Rather, Kavanagh is inclined to give the credit for the process of healing, and the stores of fortitude and perceptiveness that underlie it, to poetry, or, more specifically, to his own poethood. His prospects had been poor, but Kavanagh's surgery was a success. He lived until 1967, and following on from his time in the Rialto, he entered a profound poetic rebirth. Late career poems such as 'Canal Bank Walk', 'Lines Written on a Seat on the Grand Canal, Dublin', and the 'The Hospital', each defined by ardent and beatific modes, have a canonical place in Irish literature.

For Kavanagh's biographer. Antoinette Quinn (2001: 343), the 'insistence on love and cherishing' in much of the post-cancer work represents a happy 'discontinuity' with his long-term experience of being an alcohol-dependent and impoverished writer, one who tended to be overcritical of the work of others and who found Dublin too small for artistic growth. Darcy O'Brien (O'Brien 1975) has made a related point very memorably: 'Barely eluding death had a serious and positive effect on [Kavanagh's] poetry . . . His sickness deprived him of a lung and much hatred . . . '. Kavanagh's own words from the chilling autobiographical sonnet 'Nineteen Fifty-Four' indicate something of the struggle that marked his existence before his diagnosis. Embodying the year as a departing aggressor on New Year's Eve, and fearing the loss of his will to attain poetry, Kavanagh (2004) wrote, 'My lamp of contemplation you sought to shatter.'

Manifestly, the rebirth poems stem from the relief and optimism that followed from Kavanagh's experience of surgery, care, and convalescence. At the same time, they frame poetry and life itself with a 'rhapsodic insistence' that involves not only a beautiful transcendence of illness but a seeming obliteration of it in memory (Quinn 2001). As Kavanagh (2004) wrote in another later poem, 'That Garage', which mirrors 'The Hospital' in interesting ways, 'This is not longevity/But infinity'.

When Kavanagh refers to his cancer in his poetry of the late 1950s, he does so only obliquely. He appears to have been in some way compelled to signal that the real story, the proper illness narrative, was the fact that he gained a new lease on life. For the student of creative writing, this seeming discrepancy could stand as an introduction to the generative mercuriality of poets' imaginations. It could also provide a reminder of the role of fiction in the writing of lyric poetry; there is of course no rule that dictates that personal experience ought to be faithfully rendered. 'The Hospital' might be viewed as the best possible literary fruit of a fertile but tricky source material.

A number of poems that Kavanagh wrote during and in the years after his recovery reflect a reprocessing and playing down of his struggles. The loose epistolary poem 'Dear Folks', addressed to a generalized audience of inquisitive Dublin literati, begins as follows: 'Just a line to remind my friends that after much trouble/Of one kind or another I am back in circulation'. These are euphemistic lines. While they do not lead to something more candid with respect to the poet's health, Kavanagh (2004) does rise to an uneasy reflection on literary reputation at the end of 'Dear Folks' before signing off with a touch of complicated good will. It is notable here that the word 'love' is again used idiosyncratically: 'The main thing is to continue,/To walk Parnassus right into the sunset/Detached in love where pygmies cannot pin you/to the ground like Gulliver. So good luck and cheers'.

'The Hospital', in its absorbing and elliptical way, is Kavanagh's most direct poetic account of his time in the Rialto. It is also one of his best and most enduring poems. For the ways that it communicates a humane knowledge of illness and hospitalization, together with an intense philosophy of resilience, it has proven to have a broad appeal. The aura of universality is partly achieved through a powerful concentration on an individual place, a locality that yields a sense of the world, a sense perhaps of everyplace, and potentially every hospital (McGahern 2009).[2] But the relevance and applicability of the poem also appear to be connected to the poet's effort to sublimate the more difficult particulars of his circumstances. In turning away from what he has been through and some of what he recalls, by being averse to the subject of cancer, he arguably arrives at a more convincing argument about the human need to face suffering. The opening line of 'The Hospital' can be read as an example of Kavanagh's revisionist approach to his condition. He fell in love, he tells us, with the functional ward of a chest hospital. That is, his medical need, if we paraphrase it faithfully, was a matter of ardour and affinity and communion, not pain, not loss, and not loneliness.

Not all readers, of course, will come to the poem primed with the background details of the poet's illness and hospitalisation. And this fact is relevant for students who wish to learn to write poetry well and who find themselves reading 'The Hospital'. A poem, in order to reach readers and to satisfy them, must not be too dependent on uncertain associations or allusions. Nor should it be so bound up with its source material that it requires an uncommon authority from the reader. A poet is free to write obscurely if they wish, and poetry can be powerful and ambiguous at once.

Poets and readers of poems have differing ideas about where the threshold of the interpretive challenge offered by a poem ought to be set. But for the purposes of taking a serious beginner's approach to the genre of poetry, let's pretend here to sign ourselves up provisionally as students in the poetry school of reasonable clarity and relatability.

If we are to achieve some form of poetic strength and originality in our writing, and the personal creative fulfilment associated with that, and if we are to grant our reader an experience of poetry and an interpretation of the world that is worth re-reading, it will be necessary to pursue some classic technical goals. We will have to become committed to such things as verbal freshness and control, compression, acoustic variety, and narrative and tonal and rhythmic interest, together with emotional and conceptual power. It is best, however, to begin by establishing a framework of down-to-earth and even prose-like writing, and in this respect, Kavanagh's 'The Hospital', while also being a perfect text for speculations about what poetic strength and originality might mean, can act as a good teacher.

As a poet and a creative writing instructor in medical education, one who emphasizes the close reading, analysis, and emulation of poems as a core dimension of the craft, I try to facilitate my students in getting into the driving seat of a given exemplary text.[3] It amounts perhaps to an aesthetic doctrine, one that requires reflection and experimental application: when you begin to develop an empathic and immediate sense of what a poet is trying to do and what they have achieved in an individual poem, you yourself are progressing as a poet.

In my analysis of 'The Hospital' here, I will have the abstract goal of an empathic and immediate understanding of that poem in mind. I will, in short, be trying to convey some of what I have learned through approaching and re-reading that poem, both as a writer of poetry and as a teacher of medical students who are learning to write creatively. In that light, it seems appropriate to elaborate briefly on those two terms: *empathic* and *immediate*.

The idea of an empathic understanding is connected to the poetry student's growing sense of themselves as a writer, someone who works imaginatively in the medium of words, who perseveres in trial and error while pursuing ideal effects through deliberate decisions. An early-stage poetry writing process might be said to be promising when it has acquainted the student with an endemic messiness and pressure, together with a counterbalancing sense of the craft of poetry as rational, technical, and informed by traditional and contemporary models and ideas. The sense of power and finish in an exemplary poem (ideally a poem that speaks to the student personally and matches their deeper personal and artistic gravitations) inspires an empathic response to the extent that the student can discern and identify with the reality of work and process, the verbal and affective digging deep that the poem represents.

The idea of immediacy involves a student's growing sensitivity and eagerness as a reader of poetry and the quasi-professional habit of contemplating the dynamic relationship between the poet, the poem, and the reader (Lea 2012).[4] At issue here is the pursuit of a combined literacy of poetic process and poetic quality and a necessary curiosity with respect to how good poems are made and how they tend to engage and stimulate their readers. An awareness of immediacy in one's own recognition of the deliberate effects of a good poem, and the dimensions of craft and intention that lie behind its technical features, is a further sign of progress for the student poet.

I'd like to proceed now on the basis that the fascinating literary biographical details of Kavanagh's experience in 1955 are beyond the reader. If 'The Hospital' (which I will present in full shortly) is not relying on the poet's fame, what then is the opening line doing? Or what is it trying to do? Let's imagine that Kavanagh is, like ourselves, a beginner.

If this poem has to truly earn the reader's interest, it seems to be rising to the task very well indeed. Curiously, when we suspend the idea that we know or that we ought to know who Patrick Kavanagh is, one of the first things that emerges is the sense that Kavanagh the craftsman knows who we are. I mean to suggest here that the quality of the writing is to a great degree based on the poet's own imaginative (and even empathic) sense of the reader and their word-for-word experience of reading the poem.

'The Hospital' is a lyric poem. It works with ideas related to personal and subjective experience, and it includes a concept of poethood that is defined by special sensitivity and special sensory and linguistic capacity. The idea of naming things well and passionately and thereby creating deeper understandings is central. If there is a risk of insularity associated with this approach, the legends of Kavanagh's alcoholism and egotism, what John McGahern (2009) referred to as the 'violent energy' of his stature in literary Dublin, and his 'messianic' sense of himself as a true poet ('Gods make their own importance,' Homer tells Kavanagh in the sonnet 'Epic') will be relevant, as will the fact that his Rialto is doctorless. But we have undertaken not to judge the poem so much by the life of the poet. And Kavanagh can also be defended from a charge of insularity if we consider the manifest outward-looking quality of his regard for the reader and the manifest thematic expansiveness he achieves through writing about hospitalization from, as it were, a poetry perspective.

Here is 'The Hospital' in its entirety:

A year ago I fell in love with the functional ward
Of a chest hospital: square cubicles in a row,
Plain concrete, wash basins – an art lover's woe,
Not counting how the fellow in the next bed snored.
But nothing whatever is by love debarred,
The common and banal her heat can know.
The corridor led to a stairway and below
Was the inexhaustible adventure of a gravelled yard.

This is what love does to things: the Rialto Bridge,
The main gate that was bent by a heavy lorry,
The seat at the back of a shed that was a suntrap.
Naming these things is the love act and its pledge;
For we must record love's mystery without claptrap,
Snatch out of time the passionate transitory.

There are two ostensible joking moments in this poem. The second occurs in the final line when Kavanagh ingeniously and even a little shamelessly rhymes 'heavy lorry' with the word 'transitory'.[5] The first is in the opening line, which is exemplary for the way it sparks attentiveness. A poem's opening line is never without a certain risk, and Kavanagh has banked on us wanting more. To get the poem, and to get into it, a reader needs to recognize the humour at the start of 'The Hospital'. They also need to scoff a little. What is being said, for all its factual-sounding spokenness, is knowingly extreme. As readers we ask an amused and sceptical question here. Who in their right mind could fall in love with a hospital? Then we read on in the expectation of an answer. And if we do, we are of course caught by Kavanagh's hook.

I have suggested that the words 'chest hospital' propose a kind of modernization, along with a winnowing of old associations of suffering, but Kavanagh does not intend that subtle quotient of positivity to diminish the ironic quality of his opening lines. The word love, in order to be meaningful, requires that the assertion be understood as preposterous, and this understanding is based on a universal idea of illness. If hospitalization, and such things as serious disease and major surgery, were not difficult things to face, if they were not associated with true personal and societal challenges related to a loss of habitual freedom, movement, and even creativity (Carel 2010), to say nothing of physical pain, then this line would have no proper function within the semantic circuitry of the poem.

In order to fittingly commence the poem's progress towards its meaningful and delightful conclusion, this opener must provoke, as I've said, a common-sense question along the lines of, 'Who in their right mind could fall in love with a hospital?' In response to which Kavanagh begins to present the poem proper, relying as he does on a second implicit response from his reader. It's as if we have said, 'All right, you fell in love with a hospital. This sounds a little unnatural. What kind of love are we talking about? What do you mean by suggesting hospitalization can inspire love?'

There is a powerful sense of a physical setting in 'The Hospital'. If we are to interpret the word 'love', we might begin by considering the place in question, the apparent object of the poet's affections. There is a poetry lesson to be derived from Kavanagh's consistently unadorned descriptions, his naked nouns: square cubicles, plain concrete, wash basins, a stairway. Such things are 'common and banal', and yet they are also transfigured things. But even without their being bound up with a revelatory effort, they possess on the page a distinctive quality of vision that belongs to their being so easy to visualize. By evoking the adventurous dream world of the hospital and its grounds as he knew them, Kavanagh proves that there is such a thing as a poetry of restraint, a perceptual minimalism that intersects with forms of passion and wisdom while leaving space for the reader's mind's eye. In considering this quality of un-showiness in 'The Hospital', we might reach for a working principle, one to explore in our own writing: good poems are not made up entirely of poetry or overt poetic effects.

There are at least two other important technical functions associated with Kavanagh's use of restraint in 'The Hospital'. The first of these relates to the challenge of fulfilling the title of the poem. As Kavanagh's readers, we subliminally expect, and possibly require, a significant portrait of a clinical space. We've been given in the title, functioning as it does as the first part of the poem, coequal with the first line, a promise of detail and an implicit promise of scenes and characters. The same title would suit well for a work of fiction, but how will the relatively tight frame of a sonnet grant the reader this sense of a world? In figuring this out, Kavanagh seems to have concluded that truncated lists are the basis of a necessary illusion of scope. Twice he enumerates aspects of the Rialto, creating a sense of photographic or cinematic observation and, very cannily too, a sense that his lists might not end, that they might indeed be 'inexhaustible'. The dash after 'wash basins' in the third line signals an interrupting thought but not an ultimate end to the roll of perceptions that precedes it. We naturally infer more than we are told here, and again universality is at play. Kavanagh anticipates this irrepressible narrative tendency in his reader, and he trusts that our archetypal understanding of the word 'hospital' will furnish and populate and perhaps even in some way supplant his own discrete clinical setting.

In his essay 'Poetry and Happiness', Richard Wilbur (1966) theorized that when a poet deploys a catalogue mode, the reader is made to feel the pleasure of being 'vicariously alert'. Wilbur believed that this alertness was dependent on the poet's gift of 'instant designation', their 'ability to pin things down with names'. As such, the poem that contains a list invites a reader 'to share in an articulate relishing and mastery of phenomena in general' (Wilbur 2000).

In 'The Hospital', at the beginning of the second verse, the sestet, there's a similar sleight of hand, and a related appeal to phenomena beyond the poem, whose general plurality is conjured.

Kavanagh's declaration 'This is what love does to things' connects back to the clever bathos at the beginning of the poem. The reader's initial doubt has been marshalled and carried forward. There is a note of argumentation too, a sternness in the presenting of evidence. The bridge, the gate, and the seat are expressed with a fine and characteristic restraint. Mere nouns, Kavanagh seems to be saying, are sufficient to truly convey presences. And furthermore, in the light of love, they have a symbolic property.

In the context of the technical problem of transcending the brevity of the sonnet form, and the problem of needing to present a real hospital to his reader, Kavanagh has a further strategy here. The colon that precedes the words 'the Rialto Bridge' adds succinctness in the commencement of the list: 'This is what love does to things: the Rialto bridge,/The main gate . . .'. This is unobtrusive and standard punctuation, but it also serves to qualify the beginning of the line, so that the words 'This is what love does to things' can also be read as 'The following is representative of what love does to things'. There is deep craft in that suggestion of representativeness, supporting as it does the invocation of the world established by the poem's title.

The second technical purpose of Kavanagh's use of a more restrained diction relates to the way the poem balances at least two modes of writing: that which appears to be spoken and that which aspires to lyricism. The former has a basic poetry of its own: it allows, as has been explained, nouns to be asserted. The sense of the character of the poem's speaker, the poet as an 'expressive entity' (Bugan 2021)[6] with his feet firmly on the ground, is also involved in this oral sounding register.

The unfussy and demotic detail of a 'A year ago' in the first line prompts the impression of a mind being cast back, as if in the middle of a personal conversation. It could be said that it is an arbitrary detail and, in aesthetic terms, a not quite necessary situating of the poem in 1956. But in the context of the ironical opening, it adds intriguing intimacy and an important measure of non-literary assurance. 'The Hospital' can be read as a virtuosic balancing of conversational phrasing with a language that pertains to deep feeling and philosophical daring. In order for that balancing to attain a true fusion in the reading experience, and for the reader to be transported convincingly and satisfyingly from the lower to the upper levels of the poem, from the grounds of the hospital to the poet's inexhaustibly subtle speculations on love, suffering, resilience, and time, the stylistic sense of thinking out loud is pivotal.

Ultimately, 'The Hospital' arrives at theoretical richness. The poem can be read as a vision of acceptance in the face of chronic illness. Switching from the 'I' that provides a spine for the poem to the dramatic 'we' at its conclusive threshold, Kavanagh seems to be determined to turn that vision into a lesson. He's not unwilling, amid his lyrical pirouetting, to sound didactic. The phrasing 'we must' is a ramifying one. We must stay afloat, he seems to say, we must hold fast to the world, we must defend our will to live, we must graft ourselves to the basic beauty of the world, and we must square up to illness as we must square up to the shared facts of our mortal condition. In the face of built-in adversity, Kavanagh suggests, keeping going is our primary art.

The image 'snatch out of time' is another telling one, and a dramatic close to the poem. It's as if Kavanagh is saying love is the ultimate shield, the ultimate standpoint, and yet, nonetheless, we have a battle on our hands if we would preserve meaning and authenticity in our mortal lives, but in that battle against time, we can win now and then. To paraphrase his coiled wisdom: we tend to pursue permanent things, but we ought to seize upon the transitory, that which is fleeting in our minds and in our lives. There's a higher experience of life, a form of fulfilment, and even a form of invulnerability, that we can know, and it amounts to a kind of wholeness of presence for Kavanagh, one that is supported by the pointed artistic acts of seeing and naming. In 'The Hospital', in order to get to this approximate point, and to orient his readers in the same direction, he has made a kind of monastic scene out of the grounds of the Rialto Chest Hospital, within which he presents himself in a convalescent guise, but more than that, more radically, he presents himself in an act of purification.

Returning to the subject of cancer, are we expected to live up to this? And, to borrow a phrase from 'Nineteen Fifty-Four', could Kavanagh himself live up to this 'mystical patter'? These might be appropriate questions to conclude with in the hope that I have led the reader to interesting points of departure for their own re-reading of the poem, and their own journey in poetry.

I have suggested that Kavanagh was a man of contradictions, and I began by saying that there was a fuller medicine and poetry story behind 'The Hospital'. The broader context, for the reader who has engaged with the philosophy of resilience at the heart of the poem, can lead to a hospital portrait that not only retains elusive elements but also might help to connect the poem's humanity, such as it is, with the emotional challenges faced by doctors, patients, and medical students alike in real cancer worlds.

More than 30 years after Kavanagh's death, Keith Shaw, in correspondence with the geriatrician and historian Davis Coakley (Coakley and Coakley 2018), recalled his patient as follows:

> He felt he had a lot to write before his operation, therefore he asked for a room and a typewriter. These were gladly provided, but never used, as his spare time was spent in the local pub, and short of confiscating his clothes, he could not be kept in the hospital. . . . He made a good recovery after successful surgery despite his refusal to stop smoking. However he was frightened and insecure, and needed a lot of support and reassurance.

The argument that Kavanagh sought to escape this reality through the brilliant formal and thematic strategies of 'The Hospital' is worth making. And if we read the poem in that way, we arrive potentially at the image of a conventionally distressed and conventionally reticent cancer patient, one that should be embraced in any discourse of oncological training. And yet the poem undeniably also expresses a refusal of fear and despair that is based at once on a vivid accommodation of mortality and a humane sense of affinity with the reader. As such, without presuming to tell doctors how to do their jobs, this great and contradictory sonnet appears to sketch out the very essence of medicine.

Notes

1 The retired cardiac surgeon David Luke, who trained under Keith Shaw at the Royal City of Dublin Hospital, commonly known as Baggot Street, generously shared his memories with me in a recorded interview in May 2023. Shaw's insider perspective on the political and professional intensity of the Buckingham Palace surgery fascinated and amused his Irish colleagues decades later and added to his reputation as an exceptional medical talent. Luke remembers Shaw as being deeply attentive to his patients up to the end of his career.

2 John McGahern commented on similar qualities throughout Kavanagh's later poetry: '[t]hese later poems are steeped in space in time, while still happening in one dear, specific place. What they have in common with the early poems is the genius that restores the dramatic to the common and the banal'. 'Journey Along the Canal', in McGahern (2009).

3 Rita Charon has theorized about the importance of quality in medical training initiatives that focus on or incorporate literature. The question of standards is a slippery one, and it is dogged by bias and other limitations. Charon has suggested that the appropriate standard can in part come from the authority of the teacher and in part from a process of finding out what a given class or medical cohort can get their teeth into and enjoy. There is a distinct sense of pedagogical idealism in Charon's thinking that suggests the importance of emotion and subjectivity in the field of narrative medicine:

The fiction, poem, play, visual image, or musical composition has to support repeated visits, surprising the reader not only with aspects that were hidden upon former readings but also exposing to the reader how he or she has changed since that last reading.

'A Framework for Teaching Close Reading' (in Charon 2017[0])

There may be a parallel here with Seamus Heaney's description of an ambivalent group of students gaining something from one of his classes through the essentially indefinable power of poetry: 'For a concentrated moment the words they were attending to made sense and went home as only poetry can'. 'On Poetry and Professing', in Heaney (2002).

4 In her excellent essay 'Poetics and Poetry', Bronwyn Lea (2012) used the word 'contemplating' in a candid instructor's summary of the needs of the poetry student: 'Contemplating these ideas, along with a lot of reading and practice writing poetry, can help you to develop your own sense of what you think a poem should be and do. It will help you to develop your own poetics'.

5 The first published version of 'The Hospital' concluded with an inferior but intriguing final line which Kavanagh later revised: 'Experience so light-hearted appears transitory'. Cited in Quinn (2001).

6 This wording is taken from Carmen Bugan's (2021) essay 'The Lyric I: Private and Public Narratives'. Bugan writes, 'The "lyric I" is the expressive entity located between the poet's biographical self and the world of readers. In some sense it represents the poet's essential connection with language'.

References

Bugan C. 2021. *Poetry and the Language of Oppression: Essays on Politics and Poetics*. Oxford: Oxford University Press.

Carel H. 2010. *Illness: The Cry of the Flesh*. Durham: Acumen.

Charon R. 2017. A Framework for Teaching Close Reading. In: R Charon, S Dasgupta (eds.) *The Principles and Practice of Narrative Medicine*. Oxford: Oxford University Press.

Coakley D, Coakley M. 2018. *The History and Heritage of St James's Hospital, Dublin*. Dublin: Four Courts Press.

Heaney S. 2002. *Finders Keepers: Selected Prose, 1971–2001*. London: Faber and Faber.

Kavanagh P. 2004. *Collected Poems*. London: Penguin Books.

Kirklin D, Meakin R, Singh, S, et al. Living and Dying From Cancer: A Humanities Special Studies Module. *Medical Humanities*. 2000; 26: 51–54.

Lea B. 2012. Poetics and Poetry. In: D Morley, P Neilsen (eds.) *The Cambridge Companion to Creative Writing*. Cambridge: Cambridge University Press.

McGahern J. 2009. *Love of the World: Essays*. London: Faber and Faber.

O'Brien D. 1975. *Patrick Kavanagh*. Lewisburg: Bucknell University Press.

Quinn A. 2001. *Patrick Kavanagh: A Biography*. Dublin: Gill and MacMillan.

Wilbur R. 1982 (originally pub. 1966). Poetry and Happiness. In: D Hall (ed.) *Claims for Poetry*. Ann Arbor, MI: University of Michigan Press.

Wilbur R. 2000. *Responses: Prose Pieces, 1953–1976*. Ashland, OR: Story Line Press.

Acknowledgement

The quotations from poems by Patrick Kavanagh are reprinted from *Collected Poems*, edited by Antoinette Quinn (Kavanagh 2004), by kind permission of the Trustees of the Estate of the late Katherine B. Kavanagh through the Jonathan Williams Literary Agency.

22

CLINICAL TIME AND THE POETRY COLLECTION

Alastair Morrison

Gnosis and narrative

What can be known, we often feel, is what can be narrated. Sometimes this is not much. 'But now', reads the last line of Ian McEwan's *Atonement*, 'I must sleep' (2001: 372). Briony Tallis, a celebrated novelist whose narration is still eloquent and lucid, peers into the abyss of oncoming vascular dementia. The edge of Briony's lucidity is the limit of her story; wherever she is going after this, she won't be taking us with her.

In its plot as well as its narrative frame, *Atonement* takes a tragic view of what stories transmit. Making up stories about what she can't properly know has led Briony to ruin the lives of people dear to her. The only reparation she has found is to make up more stories, which now, as the novel closes, are likely to strike the reader as painfully inadequate. In her somnolent final demurral, we may fault Briony with showing herself more kindness than she has shown others, or we may credit her with a new flinty integrity. Either way, the fictive novelist's refusal enfolds that of the real-life novelist writing her. Having sketched at length the disastrous effects of claiming knowledge we don't possess about other people's lives, McEwan is not about to offer conjectures on what it is like to live with dementia. Like Briony, the novel gestures and falls silent.

For more optimistic writers, dementia is precisely *not* the end of the story. In the last sequence of Lisa Genova's (2007: 292) bestseller *Still Alice*, the title character watches her daughter practice a monologue for a theatre class:

> Her voice and body created an energy that filled Alice and moved her to tears. She squeezed
> the beautiful baby in her lap and kissed his sweet-smelling head.
> The actress stopped and came back into herself. She looked at Alice and waited.
> 'Okay, what do you feel?'
> 'I feel love. It's about love'.

Alice's experience here flows seamlessly from her earlier life in the novel, and readers are meant to appreciate this continuity even if Alice cannot. Stylistically, everything is done to minimize that distinction. The diffident omniscience of free-indirect style spares the reader from wondering

 DOI: 10.4324/9781003341796-29

whether Alice could frame this episode as it has been framed for us. Obligingly, the names of people Alice cannot remember are dropped, but the reader knows perfectly well who they are and can comfortably forget how *not* knowing who they are could change a moment like this one.

These two writers do not afford an equitable comparison. McEwan is a prizewinning literary celebrity, and his scepticism about storytelling is a recognizable prestige stance in fiction. Genova's book, which one anonymous reviewer describes as 'worthy', pursues less rarified objectives of destigmatization and empathy recruitment. Despite the different publics they imply, however, these twin endings are profoundly similar. In McEwan, when narratives fail, nothing more can be said; in Genova, for anything to be said, narrative continuity must be preserved: these are only positive and negative versions of the same epistemology.

Epistemologies so naturalized that we do not notice them: this is a common complaint about medical training, one to which attention to narrative is sometimes offered as antidote. Often, however, narrative has been a new implement for an old kind of discovery. Genova is a neuroscientist; her claim that there is still a coherent singular Alice, whom we can find and know through narrative, amounts to scientific positivism by other means. In one of the most influential sources of humanistic pedagogy for medical students in recent decades, Rita Charon (1990: 106) writes of 'the heart of the story' as an object of knowledge that through rigorous reading and interpretation the student can reach and possess, with clear clinical corollaries. Reading *The Wings of the Dove* properly will tell us what's wrong with its heroine, Milly Theale, and reading our patients' stories properly will tell us what they need, or at least how they feel, as well. Little wonder then that dementia, which so often frustrates the determination of what the patient really wants, has found so much attention in the detective genre. In Emma Healey's *Elizabeth Is Missing*, the protagonist sorts her fragmentary memories to solve a long-buried murder. In the McEwan camp, meanwhile, are the stories where dementia makes detection impossible: Mankell's *Den Orolige Mannen, True Detective*, or *Memento*.

In his essay 'What is it like to be a bat?', the philosopher Thomas Nagel (1974) takes a position of pragmatism with regard to knowing other minds. No one ever possesses the bat's experience except the bat, but if we accept that bats have experience at all, much of the ethical situation is already clear: we should not harm bats, destroy their habitat or food supply, and so forth. Some medical scenarios are much like this: when the patient without contraindications asks for a flu shot, the provider should give a flu shot, not an overdose of potassium chloride. Certain conditions, however, make a patient's feelings or desires particularly difficult to assess and therefore particularly pressing. And yet the stratifying epistemology suggested by 'the heart of the story' – the deep truth occulted beneath opacity and illusion, waiting to be dug out – may not be the best guide for these moments. As with Nagel's bat, we never definitively possess the interiority of any patient, but our senses of partiality and fallibility cannot become an embargo on inference. As in all interpersonal situations, as well as all intertextual ones, inference is what we have.

In the context of this *Handbook of Medicine and Poetry*, it is a foregone conclusion that my gesture beyond these antimonies will have to do with poetry. In an era when most poems are not narrative, poetry is sometimes credited with utopian alterity, with catching something ignored by more prosaic and quotidian registers. In the medical context, it is easy to imagine the argument that poetic attention to a single moment will relieve us of the impulse to package patients of different neurologies and memories into time-bound models of experience that do not suit them, allowing for a more utopian recognition of people as they really are, here and now. This is more utopian than I propose to be. When we promote poetry in terms of access along these lines, it inherits the same revelatory claim of which narrative is thereby divested; instead of a 'real story', we now have a synchrony with its own pretention to realness. The touchstone among modern short poems in English, Ezra Pound's 'In The Station of the Metro' (1990: 111), was already announcing itself in precisely this way in 1914:

> The apparition of these faces in the crowd:
> Petals on a wet, black bough.

On Hugh Kenner's (1974: 184) reading, Pound's famous variation on Japanese haiku is also an instance of katabasis. Stepping down into the Paris underground, the speaker meets the thronging Hadean 'apparitions' of classical epic. The past – literary, historical, and spiritual – is not past at all for those who recognize the full presence of a single moment. Pound was always claiming to bypass time-bound forms of understanding, to spontaneously 'get' things in their essence. In *Canto XX*, he recounts meeting as a student with the philologist Emil Levy for help in interpreting a poem from old Provencal. Despite (or perhaps because of) his erudition in textual *history*, Levy cannot see the text in front of him, and it is the young Pound (1993: 89) whose sudden insight cracks the case.

Medicine, for better or for worse, must be with Levy in this matter. This is not only a question of epistemic humility but also of historicity, of the dusty work of piecing together uncertain fragments separated by time.[1] We cannot, as Genova's passage invites us to pretend we can, simply forget chronology[2] or know what it is like not to know it. The idea that such a forgetting would help us understand anyone, were it possible, is already a mistake. It is sometimes thought that because they have issues with memory, people with certain illnesses do not experience story. This is a crushing simplification, dealing in impossible absolutes: even the briefest lyric may have implicit elements of duration and sequence, and people of all neurologies have many ways of living in time, any of which may be opaque to others.

How does a physician encounter the state of mind of a patient? Very often, in tightly bounded interchanges which are both semantically rich and frustratingly inconclusive. Much can be learned from the choice of anecdote or accompanying family member, the excited movement of the hands, the repeated phrase, the avoidance of certain words, the loaded pause, but much also refuses resolution, into either a single story or a single synchronic frame. The short, vivid poem can be profoundly useful in conceptualizing aspects of this encounter, by virtue of the same immersive focus that makes single poems such popular pedagogic set pieces in literary studies, but patient encounters are not *only* singular. They are also episodic, taking place across time, as portals onto a longer *durée* which they can only partly illuminate. Even as doctors must be alive to the singularity of each encounter, they must also remember the course of past encounters, which may take them away from what the patient is presently disclosing.

As Rita Felski (2000: 3) writes, apropos of Ernst Bloch, 'we inhabit both the same time and different times: individuals coexist in the same moment, but often make sense of this moment in strikingly disparate ways'. The irresoluble tension here, between sharing *this* encounter, with *this* patient, *now* and reading her against the patient you saw six weeks ago, is a cousin to the tension one inhabits in reading a short poem in sequence. Its natural medium is the collection, the single volume of 60 poems, the chapbook of 15, the selected works plucked from adjoining decades of productivity.

Serial forms

Most writing on serial forms deals with television. Anita Wohlmann and Madaline Harrison (2019), for instance, draw on John Fiske's reading of serial television as an open medium to illuminate the experience of life with Parkinson's disease. Traditional narrative structure, they suggest, often governs the way prognoses are given for this illness, with the expected relations of beginning, middle, and end generating a presumptive closure: you'll be able to work for ten more years. They contrast this structure with Fiske's (2003: 180) idea an 'infinitely extended middle' in the multi-episode television series. Wohlmann and Harrison argue that this form offers patients something both less grand and less final than traditional narrative; episodic repetition honours the ordinariness of life, not all of which is lived in the shadow of prognosticated decline.

Poems in a collection are episodic in a very different sense. They do not, in most cases, perpetually reestablish the backdrop against which they unfold – the beginning always in place so that the middle can always extend – in the way that episodes of situation comedy do. They *can* do this, of course, as perhaps in Zbigniew Herbert's *Mr. Cogito* or John Berryman's *Dream Songs*. They can even relate longer continuous stories, as in amatory sequences from Dante forward. In the contemporary default, however, poems in a collection often share no references at all. Rather than diegetic sequence, their common temporality is the read series in which they appear, where one colours another in terms of theme, rhythm, timbre, or mood by appearing before or after.

These inferred and sometimes mysterious connections probably overshoot Wohlmann and Harrison's purpose. David Herman (1997) offers a distinction pertinent here between scripts and frames, where a script is a set of linked expectations arranged in time (first X then Y), while a frame links associations synchronically (where X, there also Y). If we follow these distinctions, serial television could be said to demote script by privileging frame, the presumed baseline each episode departs and then returns to. Poems in a collection, meanwhile, often have opaque relations to both script and frame. If episodic television shifts the *grands récits* of illness towards something homelier and more livable, a collection of bounded lyrics may be disjunctive to a degree surpassing what would be tolerable in life, plunging its reader into a constant struggle to integrate one impression with the next. (Again we may imagine the essentialist argument that this is "what it is like" to live with certain illnesses, and again we should resist it). Rather than the patient's life itself, what the poetic collection best dramatizes is the physician's experience in trying to understand that life through clinical encounters. Here, the work of inference across time, the perplexing relationship of one presentation to the next, the new dynamic that emerges silently and can only be seen in motion, are all inescapable.

Pia Tafdrup's extroverted lyric

This dynamic of collected poetry becomes all the more clear when we consider it in a case which also *does* have a clear diegetic frame, a case where tension between instance and sequence is not only a consequence of publication formats but also an explicit thematic preoccupation.

In the 'Intro' to her collection *Tarkovskijs heste* (quoted below in David MacDuff's translation for Bloodaxe Books), the Danish poet and Nordic Prize winner Pia Tafdrup (2010: 94) stages a troubling responsibility:

> Will Eurydice fetch
>   Her dead father –
> like Orpheus sing
> of what's lost?

The poems that follow, 50 short lyrics and a coda, detail the progress of illness, from the onset of the father figure's dementia through stages of increasing dependence to the speaker's reflections after his eventual death. In a comment in English on the biographical origins of the collection, Tafdrup (*ibid.*) underscores this sequential quality: 'his loss of his faculties and then my loss of a father'. The double invocation of loss speaks to how his experience is and is not hers, the rough road between her experiences of him and his of himself, and the uncomfortable degree to which thinking about his subjectivity in the third person also involves thinking about him as an object. The 'and then' is particularly suggestive, raising the subject of sequence which – like the conjunctive adverb itself – both links and separates the daughter's painfully clear memory from the father's unpredictable powers of recall. This same duality is essential to how the book works as a sequence. In distinction to many collections of short verse, these poems are linked by a comprehensive narrative framework; readers are aware of a continuous backdrop of changing circumstance that places an earlier poem in relation to a later one, and the speaker's own awareness of these changes is part of caring for her father. But the poems themselves remain steadfastly focused on what is present in given moments, fixing that presence outside of chronology in unplotted excurses between 20 and 75 lines.[3] Overwhelmingly, the poems concern themselves with the content of the father's experience, with the never-quite-answered question of what a quiet moment or painful transition feels like as it happens. In these caregiving scenarios, the poems stage reading as an ethical imperative, but the reader never has a secure temporal footing for this reading, always shuffling back and forth between time signatures.

In contemporary Danish poetry, Tafdrup's work represents the romantic lyric as revised by deconstruction. From the starting point of romantic introversion, her poems often move towards uncertain encounters between perspectives or investigate relationships between speaking subjecthood and the materiality of language and print. From her 1998 collection *Droningeporten* (*My Mother's Hand*, translated by John Irons 2011):

> my mother's cool hand round mine, which was hot.
> – And then we wrote
> in and out of coral reefs,
> an underwater alphabet of curves and points,
> of snail spirals, of starfish arms

In the dash as much as anywhere, its simultaneous thrust forward and effect of separation, we see a kind of extroverted lyric. On the one hand, the dash represents a still point, an organizing vacuum between subject and subject, or subject and act. On the other it is a departure, a direction forward in the line spatially as well as in the diegetic act of writing. The hot hand and the cool do not become one, but there is no falling back into the self as in the Kantian sublime or the Freudian abject consolation. Instead, there is work to be done.

In *Tarkovskijs heste* (Tafdrup 2010: 97), the speaker is now caring for a parent rather than vice versa, and the vision of *écriture* as an extroversion of lyric selfhood takes on the explicitly ethical dimension particularly relevant to medical care. 'The Wheel', the first lyric, directly succeeding the 'Intro' poem, offers a very imperfect instance of perspective-taking. The speaker and her father are in his stable, observing a setting sun, and she is suddenly, literally compelled into an effort to see things from his position:

> Round and round,
>   my father
> holds my head tight
> with both hands, no answer,

>   makes me
> stare in
> at the stone wing's sharply illuminated windows

As in the poem from *Dronningeporten*, the spatial configuration of the lines adds sensual and kinetic purchase to an idea of intersubjective distance. 'My father' is a concept more abstract than the grasping hand which, in folding across the margin of the printed line, also crosses into the speaker's immediate phenomenal experience. Then, as she sees herself as object, as something 'made' to do things by him, another indented start enacts a moment of self-distance or alienation. Crucially, what the speaker sees is never what her father describes, and his diegetic speech is kept meticulously separate from her poetic speech (*ibid.*: 97):

> – Look!
> Says my father.
> – Look, the sun!
> It isn't the courtyard
> going up in flames but me
> Who's dazzled by the light in the glass.

As elsewhere, dashes signal direction, the prompt to look, and by looking to see what the father sees.[4] But again they also represent separation, the impossibility of joining with his perspective. The epiphany that results is not, as it might be in Pound, an escape from isolated selfhood or a dissolution of the boundaries of experience between people. Rather it is self-produced, the speaker recognizing that apparent changes in the world, even apocalyptic ones, are always partly a function of self: looking through the windows of the stone barn, the speaker sees her own reflection.

She is pulled from the possible solipsism of this moment not by access but rather by obligation (*ibid.*):

> All of a sudden I'm certain:
> My father doesn't know
>   What he's doing.

The sense of separation or loss here, whose effect is again compounded by spacing in the indentation of the last line, is then echoed in the return to external description which closes the poem (*ibid.*):

>   The horses
> have torn themselves free.
> Long-legged flight
>   Towards a black horizon.

Abject consolations

Horses reappear throughout this collection. The father has been a horse farmer, and in their association with him, the horses' repeated scenes of escape point to his increasing distance from the speaker. The title, *Tarkovskijs heste*, links them to the horses of Andrei Tarkovsky's 1969 film *Andrei Rublev*, where they appear as luminously intransigent objects of the Russian icon-painter's artistic attention and figures of idyllic contrast to the frantic human innovations that make up the film's plot. In this binary, the film participates in an extended romantic tradition, where an untroubled animal nature sits always beyond our intellectualist grasp.

This tradition is an important backdrop to Tafdrup's animal scenes: it serves to link these scenes to dementia via its concern with memory and foreknowledge. The speaker of Robert Burns's (2006: 268) 'To A Mouse', for instance, tells the creature of his address that 'thou art blest, compar'd wi' me!/The present only toucheth thee/But Och! I backward cast my e'e'. In 'At Grass', Philip Larkin (2003: 75) writes of bucolically retired racehorses, 'Do memories plague their ears like flies?/They shake their heads . . . they/have slipped their names, and stand at ease'. The idiom Larkin does not need to name is that of being put out to pasture: the spectre of death, invisible to the horses, is inevitable for the reader. As well as animals, this has been a way of looking at neurologically different people. Two years before Burns' poem, Charlotte Smith (2018: 58) wrote in 'The Lunatic' that,

I see him more with envy than with fear;
He has no nice felicities that shrink
From giant horrors; wildly wandering here,
He seems (uncursed with reason) not to know
The depth or the duration of his woe . . .

These longings do not in the end serve their neurodivergent objects at all well. In another poem, 'The Old Fools', Larkin (2003: 132) contemplates the residents of a care home 'crouching below/ Extinction's alp, the old fools, never perceiving/How near it is'. As in psychoanalytic abjection, the object of fantasy – life without chronology, or without existential dread – has become an object of repulsion, as Larkin's speaker walls up the same boundaries between human and animal, sane and insane, past and present that other poems in this tradition dream of crossing. His abject consolation is a stoic knowledge of his own solidity, his limitations, his death. People with dementia serve him as something like the memento mori of European medieval and early modern art, precisely because they themselves have forgotten death. It is tempting to call this pernicious conceit 'Demento Mori'.

Tafdrup's book plays on this tradition – which is to say, departs from it – in a key respect. First, though, the similarities are significant. In the image of the runaway horses, we have once again the idea of a gulf between minds that the lyric speaker cannot cross and possibly even the idea of a loss of self-consciousness in the other before whom the speaker is abject: 'my father's loss of his faculties, and then my loss of a father'. But Tafdrup's speaker is not pursuing her father's mind for her own aesthetic or spiritual edification, like the jealous voices in the poems just mentioned. Nor can she console herself by withdrawing into Kantian self-knowledge, like the Larkin speaker in the care home. In *Tarkovskijs heste*, perspective-taking is an ethical, almost fiduciary, act which cannot be abdicated even while it is never satisfactorily discharged: the horses are always getting away. The duty of their pursuit, in contrast to the self-resolving temporalities of these other poems, is an open sequence, unfolding across time.

The long and short of collection time

The poem following 'The Wheel', 'Trees are Read', is the first to fully mobilize the disjunctive temporality of the collection form. 'Trees are Read' is itself about whether calendar time, as perceptible to the daughter, is also apprehended by the father. In a small metonym for the double-time signature of the collection, the speaker's attitude towards this question seems to shift over the poem, her consciousness departing and returning to the static tableau she shares with her father diegetically.

The opening lines announce a condition of security in that the father can always determine the time of year by observing his physical surroundings: 'there are always trees that can tell my father/ what season we're in, they glow/in his brain' (Tafdrup 2010: 98). Thirteen lines in, however, after bucolic descriptions of the cycles of the foliage, the poem's tone makes an unmarked shift:

> Whether it's today,
> or fifty years ago,
> >   what is the difference?

The grammatical inversion, which allows the dependent clause to precede and to some extent camouflage the question itself, keeps the moment deadpan, and it is almost possible to read the revelation which follows this point as continuing in the same pastoral tone as the opening. That revelation is that while he can tell the time of year, the father doesn't know the year, or his own age, and believes that the much younger woman sitting with him is his wife. We learn this entirely through rhetorical questions like the one above (*ibid.*):

> Whether it's me or my mother
> sitting in the chair,
> >   what does it matter?

Inasmuch as we take the questions to be rhetorical, the speaker's tone seems even and positive: the father remains aware of his immediate surroundings and receptive to their beauty, so the fact that he does not know the year is no cause for worry. That happy thought is suggested again in another turn, back towards declarative statement (*ibid.*):

> The climbing shadows
> are so far away that they can't be perceived.
> The shadows don't mean a thing,
> For at this moment a squirrel is darting
> From branch to branch in a cherry tree,
> >   And *that* we can see
> The birch trees' branches flail newly-sprung,
> It is *now* that matters
> *Now*

The italicized *Now* is a rather blunt reference to the same epiphanic presentism found in short poems like 'In the Station of the Metro'. In the squirrel, there is once again the figure of an animal contentment, sensually conscious of the immanent present and indifferent to larger scales of time. The speaker even includes herself in this present: 'we're alive . . .' (*ibid.*: 99). The poem's ending then banishes this idyll with an apparently unforeseen alarm:

> But what happens
> when the trees are pulled up
> >   by the roots –
> when they drift slowly out
> >   where stars are asphalted over?

It might be tempting to read this conclusion as the poem's definitive turn, like the closing couplet of an English sonnet: having thus far participated contentedly in the scene of the father's contentment, the speaker then finds herself separated from him by the volta of more precipitous cognitive changes. This would be a version of the romantic abjection discussed above, where, having once been free to share an untroubled moment with her father, she is now pulled into worry and solitude, but in fact the separation has been present for the entire length of the poem. The questions quoted above were never purely rhetorical. They *are* rhetorical, in a performative sense ('it doesn't matter'), and they could furthermore suggest denial in their speaker ('it actually *does* matter'), but they are nevertheless also genuine questions, and they evoke conflicting obligations for both their reader and their speaker as they situate this moment in time.

The speaker, to begin with, has an obligation to be present in this particular moment with her father, to consider and respond to his experience of it. The uncertainty of this effort, as in the previous poem, furnishes one sense of the questions: *Does this matter?* and *Do I need to think about it to understand his experience right now?* But then she must also consider a sequence of events which is different from the one he is experiencing, and from this second obligation comes the more troubling, less binary sense of the questions: *How does this matter? Where is it going to take us in the future?* and *How should my plans take it into account?*

The reader must face these questions too. We notice that things have changed with the father between the previous poem and this one. But by how much? Is the diegetic figure who speaks the poem aware of this degree of change? Can we properly treat the poem's singularity while also plotting the arc it forms with its predecessor? The fact that we may only recognize the darker sense of the speaker's questions once we reach the end of the poem adds to this urgency in sequence. They are like the 'climbing shadows' that Tafdrup plants with apparent innocence in the poem's first section, signifying differently from different vantages in time. Readers will feel compelled, as the speaker does, to interpret according to two temporalities at once.

The stakes of this paradox become directly clinical in a late poem, 'My Brother's Eye', when decisions around goals of care pit one interpretive stance against another (*ibid.*: 134):

Should we follow my father's will
From a proud moment?
Avoid life-prolonging treatment?
– It's not difficult, says the doctor,
he's already decided for you . . .

The long view, taken in this resolute fashion (note again the distancing dash), means overruling the present moment, in which the father, frightened, asks 'you're not going to kill me, are you?' (*ibid.*). The point is not that this present should totally overrule prior directives either. The family does decide to withdraw life support, and the speaker includes herself in this decision. What she refuses is the offer of certainty that one position is right, an offer expressed in the poem with the euphemistic banality of a mathematical equation (*ibid.*):

Total kidney failure combined
with more or less
total memory loss
                produces an astronomical sum
which does not offer the best prospects.

For the speaker, past wishes and present fears continue to pull in opposite directions. Neither can be dismissed, and no single decisional scheme can contain them. Appropriately, the poem ends in another future-facing question: 'isn't that going to kill him?' (*ibid.*: 135).

Narrative and synchrony often represent contrasting visions of certainty as furnished by stable relations to time. My goal here has been to show how collections of poems deny us this certainty by forcing us between temporalities. On the one hand, by reading individual poems as arranged one after another, we inevitably append the individual poems with some concept of sequence. As Wilhelm Dilthey (1996) points out, that most basic unit of linguistic meaning, the sentence, relies already on sequence, with beginning and end intelligible only in reference to one another. But the singular, sometimes opaque encounter of the short poem leaves the terms of this sequence inchoate, multiple, perpetually up for grabs. In books of poems as in clinical encounters, instance and sequence remake each other continuously such that there is not, as medical uses of the humanities have sometimes suggested, *a* story, which one has, has some of, has wrong. Cognizance of this unstable relation of now to later is particularly important when we consider how different clinical time is likely to feel for doctors than it feels for patients, with dementia or otherwise. To be present with people but also to think about their larger lives is to be pulled, as Tafdrup's speaker is pulled, towards two interpretive problems at once.

Notes

1 As Volker Hess and J Andrew Mendelsohn (2010: 287) remind us, the arrangement of instances is the modern era's 'basic operation of medical knowing'.
2 *Forget Memory* is the memorable title of Ann Basting's book on dementia stigma. As an exclusionary criterion for the value of human life, memory is indeed something we should forget. This is, rather obviously, different from asking people to forget that they have memories.
3 In this respect, the individual poems coincide with what Sharon Cameron calls 'lyric time' even as the larger frame of the collection transgresses it.
4 The Danish word which David McDuff translates as 'look' is *se*, which is also used in the sense of the English 'see'. 'Look' is obviously the more idiomatic translation for an imperative use like the father's here, but the different implications of *seeing* – of not only searching for but of *finding* access or understanding – also belong to the line. The father is not only telling her where to point her eyes but requiring an act of insight which she is then, a few lines down, able to perform only through the imperfect membrane of her own perception.

References

Burns R. 2006. To a Mouse. In: D Wu (ed.) *Romanticism: An Anthology*. Oxford: Blackwell, 268.
Cameron S. 1979. *Lyric Time: Dickinson and the Limits of Genre*. Baltimore, MD: Johns Hopkins UP.
Charon R. The Great Empty Cup of Attention: The Doctor and the Illness in The Wings of the Dove. *Literature and Medicine*. 1990; 9: 105–24.
Dilthey W. 1996. Hermeneutics and the Study of History. In: RA Makkreel, F Rodi (eds.) *Selected Works*. Princeton, NJ: Princeton University Press.
Felski R. 2000. *Doing Time*. New York, NY: New York University Press.
Fiske J. 2003. *Television Culture*. London: Routledge.
Genova L. 2007. *Still Alice*. New York, NY: Pocket.
Herman D. Scripts, Sequences, and Stories: Elements of a Postclassical Narratology. *PMLA*. 1997; 112: 1046–59.
Hess V, Mendelsohn JA. Case and Series: Medical Knowledge and Paper Technology, 1600–1900. *History of Science*. 2010; 48: 3–4.
Irons J. 2011. *Today's Translation is of a Poem by the Danish Writer Pia Tafdrup*, Monday September 19. Available at: johnirons.blogspot.com. Last accessed: 27/1/2023.

Kenner H. 1974. *The Pound Era*. Los Angeles, CA: University of California Press.

Larkin P. 2003. *Collected Poems* (A Thwaite, ed.). New York, NY: Farrar, Strauss and Giroux, 75, 132.

McEwan I. 2001. *Atonement*. Toronto: Knopf.

Nagel T. What is It Like to Be a Bat? *The Philosophical Review*. 1974; 83: 435–50.

Pound E. 1990. In the Station of the Metro. In: L Baechler, W Litz (eds.) *Personae*. New York, NY: New Directions, 111.

Pound E. 1993. *The Cantos*. New York, NY: New Directions.

Smith C. 2018. On Being Cautioned Against Walking on a Headland Overlooking the Sea, Because it was Frequented by a Lunatic. In: DS Lynch (ed.) *The Norton Anthology of English Literature – The Romantic Period*. New York, NY: Norton, 58.

Tafdrup P. 2010. *Tarkovsky's Horses and Other Poems* (D MacDuff, trans.). Tarset, Northumberland: Bloodaxe, 94, 97, 98–99, 134–35. Available at: www.bloodaxebooks.com/ecs/product/tarkovsky-s-horses-and-other-poems-932.

Wohlmann A, Harrison M. To Be Continued: Serial Narration, Chronic Disease, and Disability. *Literature and Medicine*. 2019; 37: 67–95.

23

TIMECREVASSES AND BREATHCRYSTALS

How poetry and philosophy can refresh an instrumental medicine to re-engage patients

Martina Ann Kelly and Megan EL Brown

Introduction: the trajectory of our chapter

The poet Paul Celan, in the collection 'Breathturn' (Celan 2014: 19), writes,

ERODED by
The beamwind of your speech

. . .

Deep
in the timecrevasse,
in the
honeycomb-ice,
waits a breathcrystal,
your unalterable
testimony

Poetry brings neologism, elision, portmanteau, metaphor, and the challenge of trying to understand. Isn't this what every physician faces in a differential diagnosis or an impossible-to-diagnose condition? Simultaneously intrigued and captivated by Paul Celan's poetry, we, the authors of this chapter, are drawn into its spell as both physicians and poetry lovers. Through its intricacy, his poetry creates a pause – a 'breathturn' in a 'timecrevasse'. Celan's elisions bring together two concrete experiences that create a third, more expansive, experience (breathturn) or an abstract and concrete experience fused in order to nail the abstraction or give it body (timecrevasse). Do physicians not regularly meet patients whose symptoms exactly match 'breathturn' (respiratory disorders) or 'timecrevasse' (depressive disorders)? We are reminded that the poet Samuel Taylor Coleridge offered us elided neologisms such as 'psychosomatic'.

In this chapter, we respond to Paul Celan's eloquent metaphor of 'breathcrystal', drawing parallels between how we experience poetry as physicians and how doctors and patients encounter

DOI: 10.4324/9781003341796-30

each other in health care as forms of poetic diction. To highlight our mutual experiences of poetry, we engage with ideas from philosophy, particularly the writings of Heidegger and Gadamer. As physicians, we find that poetry enhances our understanding of the worlds of our patients, as we are enchanted through language, sound, and multiplicity of meanings. Poetry causes us to pause time, yet the experience of a poem is long-lasting, as a history. When we take a history from a patient, are we not reading a poem? When we revisit a poem, it continues to fascinate, and new meanings are revealed. Reading a poem is also like taking a breath or as the 18th century English poet Thomas Gray says, 'Poetry is thoughts that breathe, and words that burn'. At a time when the world recovers (we hope) from the COVID-19 pandemic, or at least finds forms of adaptation from when breath itself felt poisonous, we propose that poetry as pedagogy can breathe new life into an otherwise suffocating medical education sadly enchanted by the instrumental, or 'what works'.

We start by reflecting on our experiences of poetry as a gateway to exploring language – where 'Language Speaks' (Heidegger 1986) to us, engaging with the thinking of Heidegggger and Gadamer. We acknowledge much day-to-day language, including that of the patient encounter, as instrumental. This promotes a transactional type of medicine, an economics, unfulfilling for patient and physician alike, where we must be economic with our time and our words. We wonder how close attention to language might reveal new interpretations of those seeking health care as persons, in contrast to the distancing and anonymous language of 'patients,' or worse, 'symptoms'.

We turn to Celan's metaphor 'breathcrystal' as inspiration, allowing us to experience the beauty of a more poetic doctor–patient encounter where time, language, and the experience of a single breath are lived rather than mechanically enacted. Finally, we reflect on our ideas, relevant to present day health professions education, of how poetry and pedagogy feed one another. We do this in conversational style.

Poetry and philosophy, poetry and medicine: parallel histories

We were surprised to discover, given the connections we made in our personal experiences between poetry and philosophy, that (in the West) the two historically have a troubled relationship. For Plato, poetry, as something 'made', was an influence to be avoided for risk of moral corruption (Pappas 2012). Philosophy, as a field of inquiry, is concerned with logic and explanation. Philosophers should strive to answer existential questions such as 'what is silence?' using careful deduction and reasoning. The pursuit of philosophy is often an answer to such questions that allows us to better know concepts such as 'silence'. Poetry, on the other hand, is exploratory. Poetic knowing is a process – rather than trying to reason one's way to knowledge on the concept of silence, poets probe and use language to journey towards, through, and around concepts like silence and their meaning. We could say that philosophy and poetry are then epistemologically different territories (Leighton 2015). Whereas in philosophy knowledge can be possessed, in poetry the process of knowing is a journey that allows only temporary recognition of meaning (Scruton 2015). Poetry and poetic language are also deeply concerned with ontology – with being and becoming. We have both experienced poetry as a medium that intensifies reflection on our relationships with past, present, and future selves.

We see this uneasy tension in the use of poetry within the health humanities. Often, health care professionals see benefits in engaging with poetry (such as empathy development) and so wish to instrumentalize the use of poetry within medical pedagogy. Poems and poetry become tools in achieving some end or other. This conflicts with the fundamental epistemology of poetry, as we have outlined above. Engaging with poetry should not be done in the pursuit of knowledge (like philosophy), of skills, or of some truth about medicine and health care. Instead, poetry encourages us to consider multiple and partial meanings, often reflecting on *how* we know (through emotional engagement and language) rather than *what* we can know (Zamir 2015).

Although poetry and philosophy have a long and complicated history of engagement, this relationship altered in the nineteenth century through the dominance of lyrical poetry. The philosopher Hegel called poetry 'the universal art of the mind', and hermeneutic philosophers such as Heidegger, Gadamer and Merleau-Ponty reflected in depth about the significance of poetry in human experience. We anticipate that a similar turn in medical education might move us away from instrumental approaches to both medicine and poetry for a deep and multi-layered engagement between the two, a productive conversation. In the writings of prominent existential and phenomenological philosophers who focus on humanity's lived experience in the world are considerations of the possibly symbiotic relationship of poetry and philosophy (Heidegger 1971; Gadamer 1993). Phenomenology presents a way to consider poetry's existential character, in other words, what it is to *experience* poetry bodily and affectively rather than to abstract poetry into ideas. Below, we explore what we see as medicine's existential crisis and how phenomenology's relationship with poetry may be one way to address this crisis.

Medicine in existential crisis

We see both poetry and medicine as living in perpetual existential crisis, where relevance, meaning, and purpose are the foci of continuous public scrutiny; in other words, the world is first and foremost instrumentalized in terms of means–end trajectories. In a post-pandemic world, as physicians and educators, we join our colleagues to reflect on the meaning of medicine in contemporary society. Tensions in medicine pervade at present; medical practice is predominantly portrayed as technological, transactional, and tired, with burned-out doctors and disillusioned patients. The art of medicine has been infected by the tainted breath of the COVID-19 pandemic, crystallized by these stressors. Ironically, this coincides with a time of exciting innovation in health professions education, including a revitalized attention to learner experience within collectives, addressing structural inequities, and the imperative of aligning medical education and social accountability.

Poetry as resuscitation: thoughts that breathe

Perhaps medicine, like philosophy, could benefit from exploring new epistemologies beyond the philosophy of science to embrace a phenomenological turn, from logic and truth as 'measured' to truth as co-constructed, emergent, and ephemeral. As we read a poem, we become absorbed in the text, closeted to the noise of the everyday business. The best expression of the meaning of the poem is the poem itself (Vessey 2013). As a poem stands alone as an aesthetic entity, to be interpreted in its uniqueness, so too a patient presents to a physician. In medicine, the interpersonal encounter of one human being with another is perhaps never fully 'understood' but is best appreciated as ambiguous and stirringly beautiful. Like experiencing a poem, the physician–reader *experiences* a patient as unique.

Poetry as a breathing space

Phenomenology is a call to consciousness – to re-experience the taken-for-granted-ness of daily experience: to listen, see, and feel the familiarity of the mundane with new awareness. Language is central to how our awareness is awakened. This is illustrated in phenomenological writing through the invention of new terms, calling our consciousness to presence as we 'readers' tussle with and puzzle over the meaning of the text (reminding ourselves here that every patient is a text). For Heidegger and Gadamer, language is not merely a tool of expression, a means of communication, but is fundamental to human experience. Our attempts to objectify, define, and conceptualize language and almost trap it defy the nature of language, and we risk losing its essence. Heidegger, as is typical, turns the tables on our day-to-day thinking. Rather than acknowledging that the human speaks, Heidegger proclaims, *Language speaks*. In an essay on language, Heidegger (1986) develops his position by using an example of a poem as one of '*pure language*'. He analyses the poem to demonstrate that in everyday language we fail to listen to the 'call' of meaning. He inquires into how we can break free of the shackles of language as expression: 'can the spell this idea has cast over language be broken? . . . In its essence, language is neither the expression nor the activity of man. Language speaks'. Language speaks the human into Being.

Language 'bid[s] things and world to come'

The call, as issued by Heidegger and reinforced by Gadamer (Risser 2019), is to realize the power of language not as representation (statement and sign) but as always sedimented in meaning – historical, figurative, cultural, and creative. Words, by virtue of their disclosive power, grant the interpenetrative existence of man and world; words bid thing and world 'to come'. Here is a close connection between poetry and the truth of the world. Language not only represents the content of the world, or of minds, but reveals or unconceals the world, creating a space in which truth can be encountered and reckoned with. For these philosophers, everyday language has regrettably become almost meaningless – as a society we fail to attend to language and stop listening to its creative possibilities for understanding.

Poetry, like a 'breathcrystal' exhaled on a frosty morning, unconceals meaning, billowing with each breath. Heidegger and Gadamer turn to poetry, then, as pure language that maintains the meaning lost in everyday talk – its reliance on intense contraction, metaphor, syntax, image, and ambiguity make us pause. Voice, metaphor, symbols and images, and ambiguity (sometimes as a conscious contradiction) ferment the poetic imagination as they are present in medical encounters (Bleakley and Neilson 2022). Creation brings further into consciousness something that exists in unconscious life. Pure language, per Gadamer, presents a 'hold on nearness' (Gadamer, cited in Risser 2019: 113) as 'one of the ways through which we experience being moved within ourselves' (Gadamer 1992: 91). Language speaks – where poetry as a pure language moves us beyond language as a Castle of Logic', to allow the kiss of metaphor to awaken fresh life (Barfield 1973).

The use of metaphor as a figurative form of language within poetry adds meaning and moves us beyond the everyday use of language to the pursuit of understanding. If language is a fundamental way of being in the world for Heidegger, then metaphor is a path to revealing the hidden structures and layers of our understanding (Heidegger 2017). Metaphor is not about artistic embellishment or effect but about drawing rich parallels between language and the world around us. Metaphor educates close noticing and witnessing. By describing a phenomenon through expansive likeness, we explore its essence, going beyond the ordinary understanding of a thing to illuminate it in a new light. This is the paradox of seeing the familiar anew. Just as when light hits a crystal and is refracted in a dazzling display of colour, so too the use of metaphor within poetry reveals the spectrum of human existence. As poems are particularly rich in metaphors, they hold truths about being, the world, and being in the world that we cannot arrive at through other forms of communication (Leach 1997). Poems are not just ways of expressing our understanding of the connections in the world; they are ways of arriving at this understanding, and as we play with language and metaphor, we re-experience the world and create meaning in it (Leach 1997; Bleakley 2017).

Structure and meaning

The structure of a poem has a significant bearing on meaning. Form is the technical term for how we can describe the overall structure of a poem. Some poems are tightly structured and adhere to established and well-used forms. Other, 'free verse', poems do not adhere to a strict form, but this does not mean that their structure is without intent or meaning, for they may be rhythmic or tonally tuned. Form can invite meaning making in diverse ways. Writers, such as students invited to partake in creative enquiry, may use form to reflect on their relationship with a topic. Italian sonnets, for example, typically introduce a problem or conflict in the first four lines of the opening octave, move to explain this conflict in the second four lines, and then provide resolution in the sestet, marked by a change in rhyme scheme and form.

Such structures can invite students to consider conflicts and possible resolutions within their own lived experiences, while they can also relate structures to formulaic means of clinical reasoning such as semantic qualifiers (sharp/dull, acute/chronic, tender/non-tender, insidious/abrupt, proximal/distal) where the very descriptors are metaphors arranged symmetrically and oppositionally. Poems that do not rely on a strict form (free-verse poems) encourage writer and reader engagement with infinite possibilities and layered meaning through phrasing, breaks in phasing or in language, silence, and space. Consideration of how structure is employed and influences the meaning of a poem can open readers to the creative possibilities of language, the process of knowing, and the act of interpretation. Are these not also the stages of medical diagnosis?

Listening with the inner ear

Let us now reflect on the oral tradition – poems, often read in the silence of our bedrooms, or in transit, take on new meaning when spoken. Gadamer suggests that the poetic text must not only be read but also listened to, with what he calls the 'inner ear'. There is an internal resonance, an embodied experience where language speaks as she is spoken. The lips, tongue, mouth, shape the experience of poetry, as they often do in the vernacular ('coughing up blood', 'spitting venom'). Spoken, poetry reveals the interplay between meaning and sound, as well as the biding character of the poem's assertion that imposes its own temporality on the reader (Risser 2019: 90). The presenting of meaning in poetry is inseparable from this quality of sonority, where the melody of the sound is also used to augment what is said through the words.

The movement of sounds, what Hölderlin called the tone, balances with the movement of meaning as an 'extended metaphor' (Gosetti-Ferencei 2004) – gives the text its 'volume'. In writing this chapter for example, we were struck by our response to poems written and read aloud in their original languages, including the poem by Paul Celan that opens the chapter. Here, it was possible to understand at some intangible level even though the richness of meaning was sometimes more difficult to convey when translated. Poetry, then, has the ability to establish meaning on its own by the way language is bound back to its own resonances.

Poetry and the doctor–patient encounter – helping words burn

A poem then has its 'saying' in nobody's name but within its own terms (Risser 2019). It makes itself believable from itself and becomes *binding* in the reading and saying, in readiness to allow something to be said in response. Here, we draw an analogy between the epistemological possibilities of poetry for medicine and the doctor–patient relationship, which we posit is also binding.

This similarly calls out to a physician's commitment to allow something to be said, to listen, to hear, to dialogue, and to understand. In day-to-day clinical practice, could it be that everyday language, translated in the consultation, has become virtually meaningless? Words spoken are not heard. Sounds reverberate but do not elicit a sensory awareness of the embodied possibilities to heal. We breathe the same air but no words burn. Or we are left with cold cinders, burned out on failed words. We are then deaf to each other. This, we propose, is a problem of communication shackled by language as concrete, clarified, and cleansed. Language lost. Is this the curse of instrumentalism, where 'means–end' language is stripped of metaphor, or is literal rather than figurative?

Fundamental to phenomenological understanding is the world as already given and how we are called to it. Or, we walk into 'presence'. As we are called by poetry, we are called to our patients. Both are vocations. Our patients speak, and we long to hear. Words woo us, and we fall in love with them. In a poetic dialogue, where the physician permits language to speak, she may encounter the poem–patient on her own terms. Through the interpretive process of the consultation, doctor–patient can establish what it is that needs to be addressed. To draw on Paul Celan (2001) once more,

> a poem, being a form of appearing of language, may be a letter in a bottle thrown out to sea with the hope that it may somehow wash up somewhere. . . . In this way too, poems are en route: they are headed toward. Toward what? Toward something open, inhabitable, an approachable you, perhaps, an approachable reality.

In a poetic consultation, there is an interdependence between doctor and patient. If a consultation is considered to be an experience of poetry, it becomes one of the ways through which we experience being moved within ourselves (Gadamer 1992). This, we suggest, is an aesthetic experience as a revelation of beauty, when physician and patient connect as fundamental to the healing spirit of medicine. The instrumental is raised in value and quality to embrace the aesthetic. Healing is now not simply cure but humility: a humility to be human and share the interconnectedness central to our being in the world. Poetry then is an invitation to unplug our ears, to revel in discomfort and not only listen but also dwell in ambiguity to acknowledge the patient as person known and unknown.

In an era of efficiency, where time is currency and economic values are paramount, engaging poetically encourages us to take time. To draw again on Gadamer: to tarry, where tarrying is an experience of time that 'does not last long, nor does it pass away' (Risser 2019: 92). Gadamer (2007: 210) ties this movement to the basic character of living language as dialogue, where

> being in the mode of tarrying is like an intensive back-and-forth conversation that is not cut off but lasts until it is ended. The whole of it is a conversation in which for a time one is completely absorbed in conversation.

As a poem fills us, and lingers with us, we sit and breathe. Breathing in the words, exhaling meaning, each breath bringing us closer to understanding. In-between each breath more meaning is possible; as our breath turns, language and the poetic word originate, fuse, and fill us with life. In this whisper-like transition that consists of a thousand silent imperceptibilities, the 'breathcrystal' of the poem, like our experiences of patients, emerges in pure form like a single snowflake: irreproducible, unique, an encounter of transformative beauty.

The Greek concepts of *chronos*, *kairos*, and *scholê* can help us to reconceptualize our experiences of time when reading or contemplating a poem or when sitting with a patient. Our traditional conceptions of time within medical education and clinical practice are chronistic; that is, we follow a linear understanding of time that passes in an orderly and logical fashion. Most patients we see in primary care contexts have chronic or longstanding conditions, yet our time with them is brief. Consultation time must be measured, divided to maximize efficiency (Brown 2022). It is not taking time, as Gadamer describes tarrying – this is a different understanding of time akin to *kairos*.

Kairos is a more qualitative understanding of time that is about moments of meaning, or *opportunities* to make a difference and do the right thing. In *kairos*, time is unique – like our 'breathcrystal' – and fleeting or transient, as Gadamer describes it, as crystals of ice which are liable to quickly melt. In poetry (recalling that lyric poetry is essentially concerned with space rather than time), moments of meaning manifest and change our experiences of time, allowing the space for 'breathcrystals' to grow and develop. This can also be the case within patient encounters, though the ticking of the clock and relentless onslaught of appointment calendars can make kariotic moments rare. But the opportune moment is worth all the time in the world.

The poetic notion of *scholê* challenges us to think radically about clinical encounters and about medical education. *Scholê* is leisure, or free time, though it was used differently by the ancient Greeks from how we understand free time, as recreation. It is leisure not as a means to an end but as an end in itself. It is not resting on a weekend so you are refreshed (means) for work (the end) but rest for rest's sake (aesthetic forming of time). Through rest comes contemplation, deep reflection, and happiness. Within crowded medical curricula and pressurized clinical practice, no time is left for *scholê* in a professional sense; everything we do is a means to some end or other, is in pursuit of a goal. Even 'time off' is instrumentalized, as a 'break'. This goal-drivenness is the enemy of the space required for meaning, and for the 'breathcrystal' to form. In the presence of this crystallization of time as living in the 'moment', time paradoxically becomes irrepressible.

Lessons for pedagogy: crystallizing understanding by rejuvenating medical education

In 'Twelve Questions' Glenn Colquhoun (2015) says,

> Early on as a doctor there can be a lot of pressure to get everything right. There's a lot of noise in your head. 'What am I going to do? Do I give them drugs? Do they need to go to hospital? Shit, could they die!' I started to realize that at the center of the consultation were all these stories. If you just sit and let the story unfold you start to see the shape in things and you use intuition to ask the right questions. All of a sudden medicine went from being this thing that frightened me to something full of beauty and poetry.

Many of us physicians may not enjoy the same depth of poetic sensibility as Colquhoun, but let us assume that the potential is there – not in 'us' but in the language that shapes us. Let us now turn away from philosophical considerations to the practical world of health professions education without plunging habitually into the instrumental, functional, or literal. We consider how this dive into the philosophy of poetry has relevance to those studying, teaching, or practicing medicine.

Drawing on our own experience, with one of us (Martina) describes a patient presentation to the other (Megan):

> My heart would deflate somewhat when I saw Maggie's name on my schedule. I felt I could never quite give her the care she was hoping for. Consultations were perplexing: Maggie's symptoms were hard to grasp and I was frequently unable to come up with any diagnosis or care-plan that satisfied her. Often the visit ended with the need for a follow-up. I struggled sometimes to know why she even returned.

A chance comment one day about poetry as something I (Martina) enjoyed opened a new phase of relationship. At Maggie's next visit, she proudly shared that she wrote poetry and offered to read some of her poetry to me. 'Sure', I said, 'I'd love to hear it'. Maggie read aloud two poems. Her voice was clear, and despite a metaphorical language loaded with emotion, I could for the first time 'understand' her. Bizarrely, although I cannot recall the poem itself, she made reference to a swan . . . and it was a 'lightbulb' moment. Suddenly, instead of seeing an older, worn-out woman, my imagination conjured the image of something elegant, beautiful, and stately. I 're-saw', 're-heard' Maggie, in all her beauty; it was like seeing a new person. Although Maggie never read her poems out loud to me again, that experience created a deep bond between us. I never had trouble figuring out her symptoms going forward, and we had many content consultations over the subsequent years. Surely this is what literary theorists, drawing on the Russian Formalists, call 'making the stone stony', 'seeing' the stone as if for the first time (Bleakley and Neilson 2022).

In this encounter with a patient, I (Martina) put aside the day-to-day, literal, instrumental, functional, and – in the context of this encounter – 'meaningless' language of medicine to really listen to what the patient said. It was not that the poem was a Pulitzer Prize winner, but it held its own and opened a space to reveal Maggie – a space where physician and patient could encounter each other in language and time. It took mere moments for Maggie to read her poems, but 'tarrying' created a sense of *kairos* as the moment of 'opportunity' and sense-making for both Maggie and me, not just as her physician but as a fellow human being. We do not know what each took from the interpretation of the poem, but it was sufficient to establish a clearer way forward. While, of course, we are not suggesting that physicians and patients should routinely read poetry to each other (although one wonders what might change if we did), the call of language, when a person is allowed to speak, has the power to transform how we experience each other and the world we share together. Perhaps what we are saying with this example is that consultations can happen in registers other than the technical.

Concluding thoughts

There is discord between the time and space required for students and physicians to hear and respond to the call of language from poems and from patients and the foundation and structure of medical curricula. A phenomenological approach to education might help us to create spaces in which 'breathcrystals' can grow and flourish. Here, focus is shifted from the memorization of biomedical and clinical facts, relentless rotation through clinical teams and blocks of content, to exploring and understanding experience through close consideration of meanings in language. More, we may learn to tarry as an exercise in close noticing, in taking a breath, in forming a unique multifaceted crystal.

On reflection, as we co-wrote this chapter, we were struck by our own development of thinking on this topic. We suspect that each reader will take something unique from encountering the concepts in this chapter through a philosophical lens, creating their own 'breathcrystal' of meaning between the words herein and their own experiences. For us, new insight into the ways in which language speaks, especially through the melodic experience of a spoken poem, and our own experience of time, were prominent as transformative concepts in our conversations with one another. As we discussed this chapter and our learning, our common 'breathcrystal' enveloped our experiences of language in everyday life, clinical practice, educational experiences, and qualitative research. This has helped us to reflect on the various contexts in which we use language technically and instrumentally and how, through poetry, we can experience language differently, as value registers embrace the ethical and aesthetic for example.

Although we have always enjoyed poetry and appreciated that our experience of a poem is different from our experience of standard clinical language, the concepts in this chapter helped us to understand how and why the language registers of biomedicine and poetry can differ. More, we have dwelt on ways in which we may better attend to the call of patients' languages, their vernaculars. While all language is potentially metaphor rich and inventive, it is interesting that clinical registers work so hard to reduce language to the dry and technical. Poetry of course has an opposite taxis. Thinking about time added an additional dimension to our 'breathcrystal', highlighting to us a narrowness of how we conceptualize time not just within medicine but also medical education that can stifle experience through extreme goal-directedness ('objectives', 'outcomes', 'aims').

The relationships between poetry and philosophy are complex and impossible to synthesize succinctly. We have chosen to focus on how the ways in which poetry and philosophy can view the world may help us to think differently (or anew) about patient consultations. Moving on from Celan's 'breathcrystal' as our guiding metaphor, we close with a reminder to readers to regularly draw on another of Celan's neologisms, the 'breathturn'.

References

Barfield O. 1973. *Poetic Diction: A Study in Meaning.* Vol. 626. Hanover, NH: Wesleyan University Press.
Bleakley A. 2017. *Thinking With Metaphors in Medicine: The State of the Art.* Abingdon: Routledge.
Bleakley A, Neilson S. 2022. *Poetry in the Clinic: Towards a Lyrical Medicine.* Abingdon: Routledge.
Brown MEL. 2022. *Applied Philosophy for Health Professions Education: A Journey Towards Mutual Understanding.* Singapore: Springer Nature.
Celan P. 2001. *Selected Poems and Prose of Paul Celan.* New York, NY: WW Norton.
Celan P. 2014. *Breathturn into Timestead: The Collected Later Poetry: A Bilingual Edition.* New York, NY: Farrar, Straus and Giroux.
Colquhoun G. 2015. Twelve Questions: Glenn Colquhoun. *NZ Herald*, September 10. Available at: https://www.nzherald.co.nz/lifestyle/twelve-questions-glenn-colquhoun/H6LJUPRI5XDGXWOTIO77ITH4FM/. Last accessed: 21/12/2023.
Gadamer H-G. 1992. *Hans-Georg Gadamer on Education, Poetry, and History: Applied Hermeneutics.* Albany, NY: Suny Press.
Gadamer H-G. 1993. Gesammelte Werke. In *Aesthetik und Poetik I and II.* Tübingen: Mohr Siebeck.
Gadamer H-G. 2007. The Artwork in Word and Image: So True, So Full of Being. In: RE Palmer (ed.) *The Gadamer Reader: A Bouquet of Later Writings.* Evanston, IL: Northwestern University Press.
Gosetti-Ferencei JA. 2004. *Heidegger, Hölderlin, and the Subject of Poetic Language: Toward a New Poetics of Dasein.* New York, NY: Fordham University Press.
Heidegger M. 1971. *Poetry, Language, Thought.* New York, NY: Harper Perennial.
Heidegger M. 1986. Language. In: D Klemm (ed.) *Hermeneutical Inquiry: The Interpretation of Texts.* New York, NY: Oxford University Press.
Heidegger M. 2017. The Origin of the Work of Art. In: *Aesthetics.* London: Routledge, 40–45.

Leach N. 1997. *Rethinking Architecture*. London: Routledge.

Leighton A. 2015. Poetry's Knowing: So What Do We Know? In: J Gibson (ed.) *The Philosophy of Poetry*. Oxford: Oxford University Press, 162–82.

Pappas N. Plato on Poetry: Imitation or Inspiration? *Philosophy Compass*. 2012; 7: 669–78.

Risser J. 2019. 6. Language and the Poetic Word in Gadamer's Hermeneutics. In: R Ghosh (ed.) *Philosophy and Poetry: A Continental Perspective*. New York, NY: Columbia University Press, 84–96.

Scruton R. 2015. Poetry and Truth. In: J Gibson (ed.) *The Philosophy of Poetry*. Oxford: Oxford University Press, 149–61.

Vessey D. 2013. Dewey, Gadamer, and the Statue of Poetry among the Arts. In: P Fairfield (ed.) *Dewey and Continental Philosophy*. Carbondale, IL: Southern Illinois University Press.

Zamir T. 2015. The Inner Paradise. In: J Gibson (ed.) *The Philosophy of Poetry*. Oxford: Oxford University Press, 205–31.

PART 6

Unsettling poetry and pedagogy

24

MEDICINE, POETRY, AND IRIS MURDOCH'S INVITATION TOWARDS UNSELFING

Monica Kidd

Medical apprenticeship and enculturation place a heavy emphasis on behaviour, with its focus on 'entrustable professional activities; these are the overt skills of the trade, such as performing a vaginal delivery or reducing a tibia fracture. So-called soft skills of medicine are also included here: marks are assigned for one's ability to break bad news, work respectfully in teams, or demonstrate empathetic behaviour. Teachers appraise learners on their ability to enact medicine, and graduates entering practice are reassured that enactment equates with competence: medicine saves lives and prevents suffering. However, the danger with simple performance is that it can maintain historic power structures and undermine attempts to make human relationships – including those involved in providing health care – more just.

In such a cultural milieu of performance, poetry has been largely employed as consolation, adding a touch of sophistication to the work of medicine or offering entertainment and distraction. As a poet and a physician, I feel a wretched emptiness in this. 'Poetry', as Black American poet and scholar Audre Lorde writes (Lorde 1984), 'is not a luxury'. Instead, she argues, it is about sustained scrutiny and cultivating the habits of mind and spiritual strength required for change:

> When we view living, in the European mode, only as a problem to be solved, we then rely solely upon our ideas to make us free, for these were what the white fathers told us were precious. . . . [Poetry] forms the quality of the light within which we predicate our hopes and dreams toward survival and change, first made into language, then into idea, then into more tangible action.

Lorde convinced me as a young undergraduate that poetry held real power in the world – the power to watch, to remember, to integrate, to shapeshift, to unsettle, to speak up, to talk back, to reimagine. Though in recent centuries, poetry had been sidelined to a minor decorative role; if given an ear, poetry could organize and liberate. Decades later, after journeys through science, journalism, and medicine, I encountered another, gentler way of saying this:

> When we are attentive to the language of poetry, to the words we see before us in the poem, we start to get a glimmer of the actuality, the paradox and complexity and uncertainty, that

 DOI: 10.4324/9781003341796-32

lies behind the way we usually perceive the world. Words and ideas can loosen and break free for a moment, so we can experience them anew.

(Zapruder 2017)

Because of the intimate space it occupies, poetic scrutiny can dismantle walls between poet and reader. It can ask the poet to say more precisely and with more conviction what he means. It can ask the reader to see things she would otherwise miss, to reflect on alternate endings and world-views. It can ask to question what we think we know. Poetry is a sustained exercise in metaphor, and as essayist and scholar Robert Finley says, 'Metaphor opens a field of attention without naming it' (personal communication 2022).

Here, poetry draws us within whispering distance of transformational education, the learning that goes beyond performance[1] and changes perspectives. Authenticity for both teacher and learner is critical for this work, and authenticity requires grappling with discomfort. This can be particularly difficult for those asked to give up power, such as a physician who is asked to change a diagnosis or alter her perspective on a patient. In general terms, transformational education may be thought of as that which helps individuals understand the dynamics between their inner and outer worlds (Boyd and Gordon Myers 1988).

Behaviour is influenced by socialization patterns, including historical and cultural imagery; changing one's behaviour therefore requires seeing oneself in the context of one's social relationships. Medicine has its archetypes: the worried generalist at the bedside of a critically ill child in Luke Fildes's 1891 painting *The Doctor*; the white-gowned surgeons of Thomas Eakins's 1889 painting *The Agnew Clinic*, performing a dramatically lit mastectomy for a crowd of onlookers; the aloofness of the brilliant but misanthropic diagnostician Dr Gregory House in the Fox television series *House* of the early 2000s. Physicians (practising and learning alike) approach patients while both are inhabited by archetypes such as these. One could deny them and claim that the clinical encounter is only ever just two people in a room with a clear, if contested, course of action. Ironically, to do so grants those images licence to have their way with us.

What both sides need is to be able to see the archetypes, nod to them, and then to form with them, in Boyd and Gordon Myers's (1988) words, 'a disciplined alliance'. The first step, they say, begins in mystery and silence, when a person 'assumes the posture of listener, open to receive the symbols, images, and alternative expressions of meaning'. This is followed by recognition and grieving that occur 'as the self argues with the extrarational'. Transformation finally happens with discernment: the creation of personal meaning and an enhanced capacity for imagining what it is to be human.[2]

A good poem can achieve this in a single page of text, and metabolizing poetry in an excited level of engagement can train a reader in the habit of being alert for surprise, silences, and new fields of meaning. Irish philosopher and writer Iris Murdoch calls this 'unselfing' (Murdoch 1970). I will borrow from her to try to show how an unselfed approach to text (here a proxy for other minds and bodies) offers the kind of generosity required to approach a medical encounter with justice, compassion, and humility. I believe that medicine should not treat poetry as consolation or a place of retreat but as a low stake destabilizing opportunity, therapeutically shifting our attention or point of view.

In her examination of German Enlightenment philosopher Immanuel Kant's 'ideal man' – and recalling the image (one could say archetype) of the heroic, solitary physician – Murdoch writes, 'How recognizable, how familiar to us, is the man [who is] free, independent, lonely, powerful, rational, responsible, brave, the hero of so many novels and books of moral philosophy' (Murdoch 1970). She contrasts this primacy of will with the virtue of attention, which she calls 'the attempt to join the world as it really is'. She employs art – and privileges here literature – as the place of humanity's most fundamental insight because

> Great art, especially literature . . . carries a built-in self-critical recognition of its incomplete-ness. It accepts and celebrates jumble, and the bafflement of the mind by the world.[3] . . . Great art, then . . . inspires truthfulness and humility.

Furthermore, Murdoch argues, art is not a 'quasi-play activity, gratuitous, "for its own sake" (the familiar Kantian–Bloomsbury slogan), a sort of by-product of our failure to be entirely rational'. Rather, the responsibilities of the artist and viewer/reader are 'exactness and good vision: unsenti-mental, detached, unselfish, objective attention'. In other words, art (including poetry) is the place of humanity's most fundamental insight and can be employed in cognitive projects: it requires mental flexibility and alertness while presenting opportunities for insight not available elsewhere.

Yet poetry has had little place in the formal education of most physicians who have entered medical school from a traditional science background and whose close reading skills are less likely to have been put to work in ferreting out symbols and allegories than in memorizing steps along the coagulation cascade or the course of the sciatic nerve. So, if poetry is to be used in the education of doctors, it should probably begin with plainspoken words that are most accessible to readers across a vocational fence. Polish poet Wisława Szymborska wrote such unadorned poetry. Szymborska was awarded the 1996 Nobel Prize in Literature for 'poetry that with ironic preci-sion allows the historical and biological context to come to light in fragments of human reality' (Wisława Szymborska n.d.), and I think provides an excellent working collection to watch unself-ing in action.

'Exactness and good vision: unsentimental, detached, unselfish, objective attention'

One of the last collections published before Szymborska's death in 2012, *Here* (2010), is a slim volume of 27 poems that address a range of topics from the marvel of microscopic organisms to one's minuscule life in the time-space continuum. In her review for the *Los Angeles Times*, Dana Goodyear called Szymborska 'a poet of looking, and looking askance. Her voice, expressed through simple, wry declarations and observations . . . is defined by the perspective she adopts more than by flourishes of language, form or syntax' (Goodyear 2010). Goodyear was somewhat peeved by the poet's 'insouciance', griping that '[so] deliberate a lack of style is its own form of pretension. Not to mention that it feels a bit lazy coming from a writer of Szymborska's acuity and perceptiveness'. My guess is that Iris Murdoch, like I, would disagree and see the poet's lan-guage as her deliberate choice to allow provocative images and ideas to lead out front of stylistic showmanship.

In the titular poem, the narrator argues with an unspecified other the merit of 'here', Earth, where 'we've got a fair supply of everything', compared with elsewhere, where 'they lack paint-ings,//picture tubes, pierogies, handkerchiefs for tears'. She gives no clue as to who or where 'they' might be; neither does she invite us to question, only carrying us along in the argument. She is not overly proud of Earth, since here we have wars, then peace, then wars again, and

> Ignorance works overtime here,
> something is always being counted, compared, measured,
> from which roots and conclusions are then drawn.

I know, I know what you're thinking.
Nothing here can last

And yet it does, and life on Earth is a bargain. 'Dreams, for one, don't charge admission'. There are tables to sit at, sheets of paper to spread, and open windows where occasional breaths of air enter. In all, she tells us, one must not be too uppity in one's assessment of the planet – or anywhere or anyone, really, for every place and every person is a jumble of beautiful imperfection.

It follows, as she tells us in 'Before a Journey', that imperfect and conflicted you will have to find a way to be in the great staggering space of the universe that is 'inflated beyond all limits' and yet 'empty and full of everything at once'. She grounds us by telling us we can't hope to understand or even experience very much of it at all, but that is not our job. Our job is to live our small individual lives in the fullest way we can:

Well, all fine and good. But go to sleep now.
It's night, tomorrow you've got more pressing matters
made to measure for you:
touching objects placed close at hand,
casting glances at the intended distance.
Listening to voices within earshot.

Because as all great storytellers know, the more specific a story is, the more universal it becomes.

But Szymborska is not all matronly reassurance: she has lived long enough to know that darkness resides everywhere. In 'Assassins', she reflects coolly on those who plot for days about how to kill and how '[a]part from this they eat their meals with gusto,//pray, wash their feet,//feed the birds'. In her simple rendering of the daily habits of trained killers, she refuses to set them apart from us, and we are invited to perhaps see ourselves as assassins, to wonder whether we are all not capable of bland goodness and great malice. To set evil apart from goodness gives it the power of shadows; it's best to keep evil in view so it doesn't run amok. Seeing that we are all capable of good and evil is an exercise in both humility and vigilance: best not to get too comfortable in our own perceived benevolence. *Primum non nocere.*

However, this does not mean we will always be hospitable towards truth. Szymborska's poem 'Identification' depicts a wife receiving a guest after she has seen her husband's remains pulled from the wreckage of a plane crash. She denies the remains are his despite all evidence to the contrary: a scrap of his shirt ('The stores are bursting with those shirts'), his watch ('just a regular old watch'); even her own names on his wedding ring ('they're only the most ordinary names'). We know she is bargaining. We see her friend allowing it as the widow bustles about to get their tea. Her preposterous rationale ('I got furious, that can't be him.//He wouldn't do that to me, look like that'.) shows her level of shock, and we readers wait patiently on the couch with her guest for the moment she might settle into the armchair and meet our gaze. We are not too harsh with her for we have done the same thing in similar moments. And besides, the whole of the world resists trauma. A tragedy has occurred in 'Highway Accident', 'afternoonish, Thursdayish, September', and while the townsfolk are cooking supper, raking the leaves, returning a borrowed frying pan, ignoring a ringing phone, the sky swirls silently on:

If someone were to stand at the window
and look out at the sky,
he might catch the sight of clouds

drifting over from the accident.
Torn and tattered, to be sure,
but that's business as usual for them.

The sense here is a familiar one: that of time stopping at a before-and-after moment with a flash of perceived omniscience that allows us to glimpse the quotidian brushing up against the monumental. Often the moment carries a strong compulsion to keep living.

Szymborska does not place the narrator at the solitary, authoritarian centre of a story; instead, she shows that others' centres are as real as our own, a further act of humility. This is demonstrated best in the poem 'In Fact Every Poem', where one phrase is

. . . enough so that everything
borne on words
begins to rustle, sparkle,
flutter, float,
while seeming
to stay changeless
but with a shifting shadow

One phrase is enough to make the world rustle and sparkle.[4] Or, my phrase is not better than yours, but each contains the way we have, in a Whorfian sense, worlded our respective lives. Your words may awaken new realities for me. I need only listen and watch for mystery and trust it can be powerful medicine.

Conclusion

To show how an excited engagement with text can move poetry's role in medicine past consolation or luxury and in fact provide a map for approaching others in a just and compassionate medical encounter, I have tried to bring Iris Murdoch's concept of 'unselfing' to the work of Polish poet Wisława Szymborska. Murdoch defined unselfing as 'exactness and good vision: unsentimental, detached, unselfish, objective attention'. Szymborska's work itself I would describe as unsentimental, detached, and unselfish. She reveals our hubris, and she grounds us by entreating us to live our small individual lives in our jumbles of imperfection in the fullest way we can. She shows how evil accompanies goodness and that others occupy worlds as real as our own. Her work demonstrates how poetry's invitation to metaphor, its requirement to accept paradox and uncertainty, can be important habits of mind for anyone striving for authenticity within relationships strained with power imbalance and historical injustices, such as the practice of medicine.

Notes

1 There is a danger in 'medical humanities' education insofar as it seeks to *demonstrate* transformation as the result of an encounter – educational or clinical – especially when curricular buy-in requires proof. Conjuring the appearance of transformation by asking loaded reflective questions or assigning mandatory reflective assignments can elicit inauthentic performative empathy from trainees and practitioners well-practised in divining correct (sanctioned) answers.

2 I am purposely not using the word 'empathy' here as it has been so heavily commoditized in medical education.

3 John Keats termed this 'negative capability'.

4 Or, in Emily Dickinson's words, 'tell[ing] all the truth, but tell[ing] it slant' (Dickinson n.d.)

References

Boyd RD, Gordon Myers J. Transformative Education. *International Journal of Lifelong Education*. 1988; 7: 261–84.

Dickinson E. n.d. *Tell All the Truth, But Tell It Slant*. Available at: www.poetryfoundation.org/poems/56824/tell-all-the-truth-but-tell-it-slant-1263. Last accessed: 16/12/2022.

Finley R. 2022. *E-mail Message to Author*, December 22.

Goodyear D. 2010. Book Review: W Szymborska. *Here*. Translated from the Polish by Clare Cavanagh and Stanislaw Baranczak. Houghton Mifflin Harcourt. *Los Angeles Times*, November 28. Available at: www.latimes.com/archives/la-xpm-2010-nov-28-la-ca-wislawa-szymborska-20101128-story.html. Last accessed: 16/12/2022.

Lorde A. 1984. Poetry is Not a Luxury. In: *Sister Outsider*. Feasterville Trevose: The Crossing Press, 36–39.

Murdoch I. 1970. *The Sovereignty of Good*. London: Routledge.

Wisława Szymborska. n.d. Accessed December 15, 2022. Available at: www.poetryfoundation.org/poets/wisaawa-szymborska. Last accessed: 16/12/2022.

Zapruder M. 2017. *Why Poetry?* New York, NY: Harper Collins.

25

CAN POETRY BE USED AS A TOOL TO ENHANCE OR MAINTAIN FINE MOTOR SURGICAL SKILLS?

Sarah Fraser and Jessica Chaytor

Introduction

The integration of the humanities into medical education is gaining prominence (AAMC 2020). Within this movement, increasing attention has been given to the use of literature, more specifically poetry, in medical education and clinical contexts (Bleakley and Neilson 2021). Studies have shown that poetry can be used to help medical trainees improve in areas of communication and empathy (Wolters and Wijnen-Meijer 2012; Joshi et al. 2022). But can poetry help build procedural competence? Here, as a thought experiment, we explore the theoretical basis for using poetry with complex syntax to improve or maintain the fine motor skills required in surgical disciplines.

Language and fine motor skills: the connection

Children have been the primary focus of research on the link between language and fine motor skills development. Beginning in infancy, motor abilities have been shown to predict language emergence, and within preschool populations, motor skills and speech develop concurrently (Libertus and Violi 2016; Alcock and Connor 2021). Brozzoli and colleagues (2019) explored the relationship between language and fine motor skills in adults, finding a functional link between linguistic production and tool use.

Thibault and colleagues (2021) took this finding one step further by incorporating functional magnetic resonance imaging (fMRI) testing into their work and focusing on syntax comprehension more specifically. The fMRIs were used to track participants' neural activity while they performed manual and linguistic tasks. The individuals were asked to carry out a task using 30 cm pliers to transfer pegs across a board. For the linguistic task, the same individuals read sentences with complex syntax (specifically, centre-embedded object-relative clauses such as, 'The poet [that the scientist admires] reads the research paper'). Though the activated regions of the brain were not identical between the tool use and language comprehension activities, there were significantly overlapping regions of brain activation in the fMRI results, predominantly in the basal ganglia. The subsequent portion of this study involved different participants and examined whether training in fine motor skills improved syntactic abilities and vice versa. We found that those who completed the tool-use activity in advance were more likely to correctly interpret the complex syntax

 DOI: 10.4324/9781003341796-33

sentences than those who did not complete the tool use activity. Similarly, when study participants took part in an exercise to improve syntax comprehension, their tool use ability improved significantly compared with their baseline test.

Using a tool requires one to incorporate an object as a body part, changing the relationship of interdependent subcomponents in the brain. The functional structure of the tool becomes embedded in the user's motor function (Cardinali et al. 2009). Thibault and colleagues (2021: 6569) reason that similar cognitive hierarchies exist in syntax comprehension. They conclude that training in syntax improves abilities in fine motor control and vice versa, referring to this coupling phenomenon as 'cross-domain learning transfer', where

> these findings reveal the existence of a supramodal syntactic function that is shared between language and motor processes. As a consequence, training tool-use abilities improves linguistic syntax and, reciprocally, training linguistic syntax abilities improves tool use. The neural mechanisms allowing for boosting performance in one domain by training syntax in the other may involve priming processes through preactivation of common neural resources, as well as short-term plasticity within the shared network. Our findings point to the basal ganglia as the neural site of supramodal syntax that handles embedded structures in either domain and also support longstanding theories of the coevolution of tool use and language in humans.

The authors then emphasized the findings as important in the understanding of the co-emergence of language and fine motor skills from an evolutionary perspective, but they did not discuss the medical implications of their work. However, the most obvious potential use that comes to mind is for direct patient care. For example, if a patient has had a basal ganglia stroke resulting in impaired fine motor abilities, could language exercises involving syntax comprehension be used as an adjunctive treatment along with physiotherapy and occupational therapy? Conversely, could patients with receptive aphasia improve their linguistic comprehension by training their fine motor abilities? These are areas that warrant further attention through modelling and research. Our suggestion in this chapter is that application to surgical training is another important area of potential use, and here we suggest that poetry has value.

Poetry as a surrogate for surgical skills training

A major focus of surgical training programmes is technical mastery, and rightly so: not surprisingly, technical competence in surgery saves lives (Stulberg et al. 2020). At the same time, there are many reasons why surgeons may not have access to the technical training they need to build or maintain their skills. Surgeons, after all, are human. They get sick. They get injured. They have children and may take extended time away from work for parental leave or other reasons; during the coronavirus pandemic, for instance, many non-urgent surgeries were cancelled. In public systems with already stretched resources, operation room (OR) time is often limited, even in non-pandemic times. During circumstances such as these, surgeons or trainees are vulnerable to experiencing 'surgical decay' – the worsening of surgical abilities during a period of absence (Kelc et al. 2020). Some studies have shown that this can be prevented through training initiatives that do not involve the OR. For example, surgeons may train using virtual reality (Common and Thomas 2021). Other non-surgical activities requiring manual dexterity have been associated with improved surgical performance, including playing the piano or even video games (Glauser 2019; Comeau et al. 2020).

Yet technical surgical training need not always be tactile in nature; rather, cognitive training may be used. Kohls-Gatzoulis and colleagues (2004) examined the effect of increasing cognitive training time in orthopaedic residents, comparing surgery performance and error analysis abilities across two groups of residents. In the technical group, residents each completed five to six total knee arthroplasties (TKAs), while in the 'cognitive group', they each completed three to four TKAs. The cognitive group was also given special cognitive training focused on error analysis. After the training, both groups showed a similar level of procedural competence, but the cognitive group had superior error detection.

Mental imagery (MI) is another effective cognitive training process. Rehearsing an activity in one's mind is the premise of MI, a practice that has been validated in fields such as the arts, sports, and aviation (Stulberg et al. 2020; Souiki et al. 2021). MI is now gaining traction in medicine: Tarik Souiki and colleagues (2021) found that general surgery residents who took part in MI completed surgeries with greater competence than those who did not take part in the intervention.

But why poetry?

If engaging in fine motor activities improves syntactic abilities and vice versa, why focus on poetry? Why not simply use syntactically complex sentences? First, poetry does not always conform to rules of grammar, lending itself well to complex syntax. For example, in Kahlil Gibran's 1923 poem *On Marriage*, the poet uses phrases such as 'Love one another but make not a bond of love' and 'Fill each other's cup but drink not from one cup'. E.E. Cummings (1923) was famous for syntactic inversions, evident in the title 'All in Green Went my Love Riding'. In the same poem, in reference to the deer, he says, 'fleeter be they than dappled dreams'. As noted earlier, the study of poetry has been associated with increased empathy and better communication. So, the study of poetry may facilitate multiple competencies that are necessary to be a doctor. And finally, perhaps the most important point of using poetry rather than non-descript sentences is simply for fun.

Limitations

That studying syntactically complex poetry could enhance or maintain surgical skills is both a thought experiment and a hypothesis based on the findings of selected papers. Though the findings were significant and published in reputable journals, the sample sizes in the papers were small. In addition, in the primary study inspiring this essay, participants used pliers when conducting the fine motor skills activities. This is not necessarily generalizable to all surgical instruments. Even if future research finds that linguistic training improves surgical skills, implementation could be difficult since the biomedical model still dominates in the world of medicine and surgery already leans this way.

Conclusion

Given the strong need to optimize surgical skills, especially with the risk of potential surgical decay, alternative training techniques not requiring an OR are needed. Using poetry with complex syntax as a tool for enhancing or maintaining surgical skills is a humanities-based training intervention that deserves to be explored.

References

Alcock K, Connor S. Oral Motor and Gesture Abilities Independently Associated with Preschool Language Skill: Longitudinal and Concurrent Relationships at 21 Months and 3–4 Years. *Journal of Speech, Language, and Hearing Research*. 2021; 64: 1–1963.

American Association of Medical Colleges. 2020. *The Fundamental Role of Arts and Humanities in Medical Education*. Available at: www.aamc.org/about-us/mission-areas/medical-education/frahme. Last accessed: 4/1/2023.

Bleakley A, Neilsen S. 2021. *Poetry in the Clinic: Towards a Lyrical Medicine*. Abingdon: Routledge.

Brozzoli C, Roy AC, Lidborg LH, Lövden M. Language as a Tool: Motor Proficiency Using a Tool Predicts Individual Linguistic Abilities. *Frontiers in Psychology*. 2019; 10: 1639.

Cardinali L, Frassinetti F, Brozzoli C, et al. Tool-Use Induces Morphological Updating of the Body Schema. *Current Biology*. 2009; 19: R478–R79.

Comeau G, Chen K-CJ, Swirp M, et al. From Music to Medicine: Are Pianists at an Advantage When Learning Surgical Skills? *Music and Medicine: An Interdisciplinary Journal*. 2020; 12: 1.

Common D, Thomas C. 2021. How a Canadian Invention is Keeping Surgical Skills Sharp While COVID-19 Idles Many ORs. *CBC*, February 10. Available at: www.cbc.ca/news/health/virtual-reality-surgical-simulator-precisionos-1.5895914. Last accessed: 20/4/2023.

Cummings EE. 1923. *Tulips and Chimneys*. New York, NY: Thomas Seltzer.

Gibran K. 1923. *The Prophet*. New York, NY: Alfred Knopf.

Glauser W. Concerns About Surgical Skills Slipping in Younger Doctors Unfounded, Say Canadian Surgeons. *Canadian Medical Association Journal*. 2019; 191: E24–E25.

Joshi A, Paralikar S, Kataria S, et al. Poetry in Medicine: A Pedagogical Tool to Foster Empathy Among Medical Students and Health Care Professionals. *Journal of Poetry Therapy*. 2022; 35: 1–13.

Kelc R, Vogrin M, Kelc J. Cognitive Training for the Prevention of Skill Decay in Temporarily Non-Performing Orthopedic Surgeons. *Acta Orthopaedica*. 2020; 91: 523–26.

Kohls-Gatzoulis JA, Regehr G, Hutchison C. Teaching Cognitive Skills Improves Learning in Surgical Skills Courses: A Blinded, Prospective, Randomized Study. *Canadian Journal of Surgery*. 2004; 47: 277–83.

Libertus K, Violi DA. Sit to Talk: Relation Between Motor Skills and Language Development in Infancy. *Frontiers in Psychology*. 2016; 7: 475–75.

Souiki T, Benzagmout M, Alami B, et al. Impact of Mental Imagery on Enhancing Surgical Skills Learning in Novice's Surgeons: A Pilot Study. *BMC Medical Education*. 2021; 21: 545.

Stulberg JJ, Huang R, Kreutzer L, et al. Association Between Surgeon Technical Skills and Patient Outcomes. *JAMA Surgery*. 2020; 155: 960–68.

Thibault S, Py R, Gervasi AM, et al. Tool Use and Language Share Syntactic Processes and Neural Patterns in the Basal Ganglia. *Science (New York, NY)*. 2021; 374: 6569.

Wolters FJ, Wijnen-Meijer M. The Role of Poetry and Prose in Medical Education: The Pen as Mighty as the Scalpel? *Perspectives on Medical Education*. 2012; 1: 43–50.

26

UNSETTLING MEDICINE'S COLONIALITY

Poetry's (missed?) anticolonial potential in medical education and practice

Sarah de Leeuw

Introduction

How shall we address the concerns of the writer and activist Chrystos (1988: 101) when they say

> I will not wear dancing clothes to read poetry or
> explain hardly anything at all
> I don't think your attempts to understand us are going to work so
> I'd rather you left us in whatever peace we can still
> scramble up after all you continue to do

The University of British Columbia's (UBC) Undergraduate Medical Education (UGME) programme is called[1] 'Canada's' second largest. The programme is delivered at four autonomous, geographically diverse university sites over four years, in more than 80 clinical settings, to ~288 students in each year. UBC's Faculty of Medicine mission, boldly announced on its main homepage (https://mdprogram.med.ubc.ca/about/), is to prepare

> future physicians to collaborate with patients and their circle of support in providing culturally safe, high-quality healthcare for the diverse and changing populations in BC and beyond, including Indigenous Peoples, people living in rural and remote communities, and those who disproportionately experience adverse outcomes in health care.

In line with this mission, in 2017, UBC's UGME launched the UBC 23 24 Indigenous Cultural Safety Program (https://ubc2324.med.ubc.ca/about-ubc-23-24/). The name of the programme deliberately signals a response to Action Calls #23 and #24 released in 2015 by Canada's Truth and Reconciliation Commission (TRC), which called the country to account for a long history of cultural genocide and a contemporary landscape rife with anti-Indigenous racism (Allan and Smylie 2015; Turpel-Lafond and Johnson 2021;[2] Browne et al. 2022). The goals of UBC's '23/24' (as it is colloquially referred to) curriculum include increasing the number of Aboriginal professionals working in the health care field; ensuring the retention of Aboriginal health-care

 DOI: 10.4324/9781003341796-34

providers in Aboriginal communities; and providing cultural competency training for all health care professionals.

The 23/24 curriculum is characterized by strong attention to detail. Every person who delivers the curriculum must undergo between 12 and 18 hours of orientation and training, for which completion must be proven in the form of user-authenticated downloaded certification, making false completion of the training impossible. The curriculum is, mandatorily, delivered across the province by dozens of Indigenous and non-Indigenous settler facilitator-pairs, to small groups of approximately 15–20 undergraduate medical students. There are compulsory debriefing sessions. At several key intervals during their training, facilitators are informed that they are not allowed to (re)use the curriculum for teaching purposes, or what they learned from the curriculum, outside the confines of authorized 23/24 sessions.

According to its website, which features a video of UBC's 2019 president praising and endorsing 23/24, the curriculum was designed in consultation with 'an advisory committee representing UBC faculties and health professional programs, the First Nations Health Authority, Indigenous leaders, community members, and organizations' (https://ubc2324.med.ubc.ca/about-ubc-23-24/). The curriculum website goes on to note that The Centre for Excellence in Indigenous Health, where the curriculum is housed and staffed,

> worked collaboratively with many departments at UBC in the development and implementation of the curriculum, such as UBC Health, the Centre for Teaching, Learning and Technology, UBC Studios, UBC Student Services (Health and Wellness and Counseling Services), Copyright and Permissions, and UBC First Nations House of Learning.

So, what does any of this have to do with poetry? Or poetry in medicine? A department of copyright and permissions at UBC was consulted in the development of 23/24, clearly evidenced in the firm regulations about the curriculum's delivery and usage, and (very laudably) multiple Indigenous and health care leaders, communities, and organizations guided the curriculum's development. Yet nowhere is there evidence that in designing, testing, or implementing 23/24 was there any consultation, or even cursory conversation, with literary programmes, departments of creative writing, or poets. This offers no big surprise.

As this chapter explores, faculties of medicine across Canada and around the world are not well-known for their sustained or particularly engaged partnership with poetry, poets, or departments of literary arts and writing (Peterkin et al. 2020; Axelrod et al. 2023). What is somewhat beguiling, however, is how prominently poetry is featured in both facilitator-training around the 23/24 curriculum and in student activities. 'Poetics' (lacking any clear definition) are actively cited, called upon, and used to enliven the curriculum. During introductions and at various intervals in the training sessions, facilitators are asked to compose 'poems' about themselves and their positionality. They are given 'poetic prompts' in the form of opening lines that they are asked to build off and wrap up as completed 'poems'. Facilitators-in-training are invited to 'poetically' sketch details about their families, cultural backgrounds, and identities. Resultant 'poems' are read aloud, complemented, and used for conversational prompts. Subsequently, post training and during lectures to medical students, undergraduate students are invited, in small groups, to become 'poets' during and in the space of the 23/24 classes by composing group poems on large sheets of newsprint.

Pedagogically, this is touted as ensuring that the curriculum enacts small group independent and 'hearts-based' (as opposed to 'heads-based') learning. The students are encouraged to share, read aloud, and discuss their poetic creations, as are their facilitators. It is worth noting, however, that poetry as poetry, that poems as poems, both with long-standing and well-established disciplinary contours (just like medicine – see Bleakley and Neilson 2021) are not actually anywhere discussed. Poems are never engaged as *specific practices and expressions* informed by very well-established protocols, publication records, conventions, debates, and social functions. Poems and poetry, in UBC's 23/24 medical education and learning environment, are dished out to learners and facilitators in disembodied, de-historicized, uncontextualized, uncritical fashions so that they (the poems) can be somewhat mindlessly used and extracted from to perfunctorily move participants from one learning objective to the next. Poetry in the 23/24 curriculum becomes a site for teachers, facilitators, and medical students to, somewhat transactionally, perform Brené Brown-esque authentic vulnerability (Brown 2015). Medicine, via medical education, becomes a perfunctory agent regarding poetry and poetics. This is surely a kind of slippery colonizing.

This chapter's primary concern is medicine's wider and ongoing state of coloniality, unequivocally concurring with much needed and fast-growing demands about the necessity to unsettle and decolonize well-evidenced colonial anti-Indigenous racism. This, along with multiple other biases and 'isms' (Raycraft 2021) remain rampant within, and foundational to, almost every aspect of clinical medicine and health care, health and medical education, and health care scholarship. The use of poetry then, as it is currently and oft being deployed in at least some health and medical education contexts, might be yet another colonial conceit, another way to, perhaps counterintuitively or even unconsciously, buttress coloniality. Is there a missed potential of poetry to do some unsettling anti-colonial work? Can poetry be used in conscious anticolonial ways that might realistically disrupt the deeply seeded anti-Indigenous racism held by so many non-Indigenous settler peoples across Turtle Island and beyond? In the poem 'Colonial Medicine', Garry Gottfriedson (2019: 26) describes the shocking stories from survivors of the residential schools: 'and just like that/it all comes out', where it is 'beyond just a story, truth/deep down inside':

> the residential schools
> their stories from survivors
>
> the sun sees all
> surfacing [. . .]
>
> 'reconciliation' so they call it
> is not black and white words
>
> skinning thin layers
> off the tongue

That medicine is a deeply colonial discipline, and that coloniality is a powerful determinant of especially Indigenous (but globally many people's) health, is well-evidenced (Greene et al. 2013; Belcourt 2018). This chapter cannot delve fully into the ways medicine as a discipline, practice, and culture has, since its modern manifestation and standardization under the advent of the 1910 Flexner Report, gone hand-in-glove with colonial expansion and the solidification of colonialism (Rutecki 2020). To understand medicine as colonial unto itself is, in great part, to acknowledge how medicine has pioneered and perpetuated ways of knowing and being that uphold hierarchies and taxonomies of human worth, including devaluing bodies and communities that are 'other' to a fictious norm of being male, white, able-bodied, affluent, and in possession of sociocultural power.

Given the concern of this chapter with criticality, poetry, and poetics in medicine, suffice it to say that a fundamental and governing logic of any colonial ideological framework or system of power is its own sense of uncritical, almost divinely ordained, manifest superiority. Colonial subjugation is so often naturalized for the *benefit* of everything over which the colonial logic presides (Stoler 2002, 2016; Harris 2004). Colonialism works in great part because it perpetuates a sense of its own inherent superiority, which is often cloaked in a quasi-benevolence (Gebhard et al. 2022).

With these broad strokes in mind and given this chapter's moorage in Canadian undergraduate medical education, a few specific points about medicine's coloniality in the country seem important (Allan and Smylie 2015; de Leeuw 2015). Métis Indigenous physician Cassandra Felske-Durksen (2020), a specialist in women's health at the Indigenous Wellness Clinic near Edmonton, recently wrote in the *Journal of the College of Physicians & Surgeons of Alberta* about conflicting Indigenous and Euro-Canadian non-Indigenous worldviews towards medicine. The paper specifically calls out non-Indigenous physicians, requesting that they understand some disquieting realties about the discipline that pays their bills. Felske-Durksen notes that,

> Euro-Canadian non-Indigenous medicine [is] complicit in both historical legacies and present-day colonialism. . . .. Euro-Canadian non-Indigenous medicine supported scientific experimentation on unconsenting patients in Indian Hospitals, including the Edmonton Charles Camsell Hospital. Euro-Canadian non-Indigenous medicine played a key role in the targeted gender violence and violation of body sovereignty through the Alberta Sexual Sterilization Act.

Further, 'Euro-Canadian medicine has acted as an agent of colonial agendas', where 'Euro-Canadian non-Indigenous medicine bestows power and privilege (especially upon settlers and colonial ways of knowing and being)'.

Felske-Durksen is not alone in critiques of historic and contemporary medicine's coloniality as it is widely taught, studied, and practiced across Turtle Island and around the world. Paediatric emergency physician Samir Shaheen-Hussain (2020), writing and practising in Tio'tia:ke (Montreal), documents how colonialism has always been hard-wired into Canada's medical system. Shaheen-Hussain offers expansive present-day examples of Indigenous children being violently removed from families and communities, in ways reminiscent of residential school tactics, in the name of medical care and public health. Medicine, and medical professionals, appear remarkably uninterested about Indigenous children having died in hospitals, hundreds of miles from families and home communities, and under 'state care' purporting to act in the children's best interests. His arguments are nested within a larger assertion: historically, and into the present day, only those who serve colonial agendas are promoted to positions of power. A high-profile example is William Osler, who practised in the early 1900s and is ongoingly lauded as the father of modern medicine and medical education not just in Canada but worldwide. Osler, whose name graces various rooms in some of the country's largest faculties of medicine, appears on the public record insisting that 'Canada should remain a white man's country' (Persaud et al. 2020).

Osler's opinion might not find overt mainstream purchase in medical education, practice, or scholarship in the 21st century. However, for many Indigenous or Black peoples or Peoples of Colour from the World's Majority Populations, the general sentiment of Canada being a white-man's country still undergirds much of the health care system (Dryden and Nnorom 2021; Sexton et al. 2021). Indeed, as a colonial nation, 'Canada' is increasingly grappling with reports about systemic anti-Indigenous racism in the health care system (Turpel-Lafond and Johnson 2021). We (especially Euro-white non-Indigenous settlers) who live in the colonial state of so-called Canada, including physicians and other health care providers, educators, and professionals, are realizing (like UBC's 23/24 makes clear) that coloniality is an organizing and determining force in our all lives. It affords systemic racism.

A state of coloniality results from colonialism's domination, wherein colonialism is best understood as the establishment of sociocultural, legal, political, economic, and discursive grids of power either to buttress colonization or to cohere and validate colonial processes (especially permanent settlement). It is less about direct theft of lands and resources and more about establishing logics and philosophical frameworks that try to make material and grounded theft or settlement invisible. Colonialism is a social construction that (at least to some degree) neutralizes the need for guns and armies (Said 2012), while simultaneously imagining and designing structures like police forces, courts of law, education and medical institutions, and economic structures so that they always and expressly privilege settler rights (LeFevre 2013). This transpires by constructing Indigenous subjects as aberrant and unhealthy, sick, and diseased. Drawing on Maldonado-Torres (2007), colonialism's tenacious extension into the 21st century might best be described as a naturalized state of coloniality.

Here, colonial relations of power leave profound marks on authority, bodies and sexuality, knowledge, and the economy, as well as a general understanding of being, including health and illness. These *marks* are, in essence, coloniality's deep impacts on human health and the ways that health and health care practices are taught, theorized, and enacted. The coloniality of *power* has much to do with interrelations between forms of exploitation and domination. The coloniality of *knowledge* gestures towards the impact of colonization on different areas of knowledge production, including medical education, whereas a coloniality of *being* is anchored in the lived experience of colonization, especially its impact on language, expressions of culture, and encoding of bodies and subjectivities.

Put simply, coloniality manifests in ideological constructs that make White European ways of knowing and being appear, including in disciplines like medicine, to be naturally right and normative. For anyone who is part of the dominant structures of power, the privilege and positionality of dominance can be very difficult to see because they have been naturalized and normalized. How can one see what feels unseeable and invisible? Of course, Indigenous people, and peoples who embody traits of the globe's majority populations, have always resisted, and refused, the power imbalances perpetually visible to them. But a dominance (what can be called a hegemony – see Kulchyski 1995) of White Euro-colonial structures consistently seeks to supress that resistance and refusal, including in medicine. For example, and in part buttressed by medical logics about what was healthy or unhealthy, colonial governments and laws made it illegal for First Nations, Métis, or Inuit people and communities in 'Canada' to have full and unfettered self-determining authority over their own bodies, children, and families. Instead, the colonial state, again deeply buttressed by medical logics (Kelm 1998), decreed that children and youth be placed in residential schools, where amongst many other atrocities, Indigenous children were medically experimented on (Mosby 2013; MacDonald et al. 2014; Mosby and Swidrovich 2021).

When residential schools began to crumble, state coloniality shifted into child welfare programming, also partly buttressed by medical and health care professionals' assertions about Indigenous families and communities being places of aberrance and poor health, that, into the present day, tear them apart. Indigenous peoples have never been well served by colonial structures, a point which extends to health and medical structures. Indeed, in 2023, the Indigenous Physicians Association of Canada (IPAC) released a 'report card' of anti-colonial efforts underway in faculties of medicine across Canada. The 'grades' were not stellar: IPAC noted that nearly 70% of medical students felt their educators were minimally educated or not educated at all on the issues facing Indigenous people in Canada. Fewer than 40% of Indigenous medical students felt satisfied with the amount of cultural support offered by their respective programmes, including mentorship opportunities, cultural activities, Indigenous-specific spaces, and access to Indigenous Elders. In addition, fewer than 30% of Indigenous medical student respondents reported having faculty support and protected time to attend cultural activities, conferences, and events.

Hence, UBC's UGME is unequivocally correct (morally and ethically) both in making space to confront colonial violence in medicine and in teaching future health care professionals, especially physicians, about culturally safe and humble practices. This is not up for debate. What is open for discussion, especially by medical educators working in humanities, is the potential of poetry. This is the case not because poetry is *absent* from anti-colonial cultural safety and humility training but instead precisely because poetry is *present* in the curriculum. Poetry thus deserves to be engaged with critically and with respect, in a context of growing conversations about the roles of arts and humanities in medical education, scholarship, and practice. Digging into some of medical coloniality's organizing logics also provides a means of integrating how medical education's use of poetry might afford yet another colonial move.

In 'A Crook that Signifies Home', Dallas Hunt (2021: 74–76) notes how Indigenous persons carry certain socially ascribed burdens, where he 'read an article/on the CBC today' showing that indigenous people suffer from arthritis 'at a rate/three times higher/than average'. Hunt ponders on what it may be like to not

> have a predetermined
> bundle of
> signifiers rest
> heavily on one's
> shoulders,
> to be able
> to shrug off
> an entire
> discursive field [. . .]

Claims, some of them evidence-based, abound about the potential of creative arts and humanities to transform medical education and medical practices. In early 2021, the American Association of Medical Colleges (AAMC 2021) announced a national commitment to humanities:

> [T]he first two decades of 21st-century medicine have witnessed significant transformation in healthcare delivery, marked health disparities, civil unrest, unprecedented rates of physician burnout and suicide, and unforeseen public health crises . . . .. [The] integration of the arts and humanities into medicine and medical education may be essential to educating a [health care] workforce that can effectively contribute to optimal healthcare outcomes for patients and communities.

Meanwhile, the primacy of biomedical paradigms and a privileging of Euro-colonial epistemologies and ontologies continues within medical culture. This privileging can result in racist othering of Indigenous world views but also a downgrading of any bodies and ways of being that deviate from subjectivities that are settler/white, economically privileged, heterosexual, fit/able-bodied, neurotypical, and/or living in urban geographies.

In response to the dominant discourse, a new force in medical/health humanities has emerged as a potential of humanities to specifically address *these* subjectivities and to mitigate the unique needs of highly marginalized and medically pathologized peoples and communities. These include those who are Indigenous, LGTBQ2S+, experiencing poverty, and/or body-diverse; those with addictions and/or mental illnesses; the elderly and institutionalized; racialized and immigrant peoples; and many other people who live and have for a long time lived with greater burdens of poor health (for exceptions see: Goez et al. 2020; de Leeuw et al. 2021). Tethering humanities in medical education to, for instance, antiracist feminist Indigenous queer neuro/body-diverse and class-conscious social justice activism constitutes a 'second wave', or a *critical*, medical humanities (Whitehead and Woods 2016). Such an approach, however, placed biomedical science in opposition to humanities, the latter acting as saviour of the patient as 'person' within a de-personalizing medicine. A 'third wave' 'translational' medical humanities (Kristeva et al. 2020) has since emerged that places biomedical science in productive conversation with arts and humanities such that the value of innovative science is recognized, where it embraces aesthetic, ethical, political, and transcendental sources (Bleakley 2023).

The health impacts of social inequities and inequalities have increasingly become a focus for the medical/health humanities. For example, a recent project at the Johns Hopkins University School of Medicine Emergency Medicine Residency Program set out to expressly measure the impact of humanities curriculum interventions on anti-Black racism and bias (Balhara et al. 2022). The Health Humanities at Hopkins Emergency Medicine (H3EM) initiative, begun in 2018, demonstrated strong correlation between decreases in anti-Black racism and learners' engagement with humanities traditions such as narrative, literature, and critical self-reflection. In the H3EM project, literary arts (including poetry and fiction) were purposely chosen as agents through which to address systemic prejudice. The literary arts that learners engaged with were studied closely as affording a capacity to transform feelings and thoughts. Indeed, as H3EM project developers note, a conscious effort was made to '[weave] the arts and humanities with an understanding of historical context and critical reconsideration of current practices' (*ibid.*: 292).

In 'Australia', a multidisciplinary team implemented an Indigenist health humanities curriculum that sought to bridge knowledge gaps about Indigenous health by broadening intellectual investment in the topic area. Humanities and social science perspectives and expertise about Indigenous social worlds were called upon to understand the production of health, illness, and inequality (Watego et al. 2021). This project was purposeful in drawing from and integrating Indigenous artists, writers, and philosophers (as practicing and leading experts in their fields) into health and medical education.

In the Australian Indigenist Health Humanities project, humanities and social sciences were expressly and clearly treated as domains unto themselves with histories, conventions, contexts, and principles that could be employed to purposefully target anti-Indigenous racism and bias in health care education. Pedagogically, this is quite different from using one discipline and its practices (for instance poetry) to accessorize another, essentially buttressing a dominant mode of doing 'business as usual' but shifting ever-so-slightly its dominance by adding a few new decorations or trinkets to the mix. Arts and humanities in medicine cannot, in other words, be empty signifiers in a larger curriculum that continues to take for granted its own disciplinary dominance and superiority – or what others have suggested are hollow 'sparks of joy' (Adams and Reisman 2019) that leave learners thinking (and feeling!) that arts and humanities are cute accessories to the principal foci (biosciences and clinical medicine) at hand in medical education.

Critical, detailed, and humble contextualization of arts and humanities (as independent, evolving, powerful modes and practices of thought and being) is a must if medicine is to avoid using arts and humanities disciplines as 'a way of *framing* or *garlanding* a particular discipline [medicine] with another discipline's [humanities] insights or expertise' (Mitchell and Bhabha 1995, my emphasis). In other words, when putting humanities (including poetry) to work in medicine, medical educators might do well to toss aside security blanket or garlanding languages of enrichment or empathy and, instead, prioritize and embrace descriptors like discomfort and disruption (Adams and Reisman 2019). Medical education initiatives like UNBC 23/24 Curriculum appear not to have considered this.

Medicine and medical education are in a cultural and disciplinary crisis (Kuper 2014). Humanities are increasingly being turned to as means of getting medical culture and education out of a bit of a pickle, including – and as UBC's 23/24 curriculum laudably tackles – a propensity in medicine for anti-Indigenous racism and the privileging of white-colonial ways of knowing and being in the world.

What are the implications, however, for uncritical (ahistorical, decontextualized) uptake in medicine of humanities practices like poetry? Can medicine's state of coloniality ever be unsettled if (to return to Homi Bhabha) the use of poetry or other humanities practices remain persistently reduced to garlanding or framing status, a kind of sweetener that makes medicine go down easier while never being afforded the time or space to critically tackle whether the medicine is right in the first place. Is poetry in UBC's 23/24 curriculum being used to decolonize or, instead, to make more palatable conversations about colonial violence, where poetry-writing participants can feel better about the work they are doing towards combating anti-Indigenous racism? If the poetry lacks rigour, will its target of attitude and values transformation ultimately fail?

Poetry's (missed) potential and some concluding poetic musings

Following the lead of Joy Harjo (2015),

> You will have to answer to your children, and their children, and theirs – [. . .]
> By listening we will understand who we are in this holy realm of words.
> Do not parade, pleased with yourself.
> You must speak in the language of justice

Imagine if, in the confines of medical education focused on disrupting bias and assumptions about power and privilege, poetry was called upon for the sake of poetry. Imagine if poetry and poetics appearing in various domains of medical culture were considered not in the *service of* medicine or as things to prop up the interests of medicine but instead as partners in conversations about a healthier and more just world where medicine was destabilized from a place of disciplinary rule. Or medicine and poetics became 'translational'. Imagine if medicine did not open time and space to medical professionals and learners with no previous interest or experience in poetry to comfortably and without question become 'poets'. Does this anointing of disciplinary expertise upon people with no formal training or understanding of the discipline not risk inscribing a sense of mastery and command over things they may know little or nothing about? Is this not, fundamentally, a hallmark of colonial conceit? Not only is the assumed superiority of medicine colonizing poetry as something that doctors can 'do', untutored and unchallenged, but poetry is reduced to a bland medium for 'personal growth' or (temporary at best) cultivation of 'empathy', a space that could just as well be occupied by entry-level guitar playing, glass blowing, or candle making.

Integrating Indigenous poetry, poetics, and poets into curriculum like UBC's 23/24 need not be complicated. For instance, a quick and easy way to ensure poetry, *as poetry*, is felt and experienced in medical education is to invite and remunerate Indigenous poets to read or present during 23/24 classes. Include videos of, and links to, Indigenous spoken word poets in virtual learning platforms. Rather than composing their own work focused purely on themselves, with no sense of what it means to write poetry, medical learners can be asked to reflect on poetry presented by an Indigenous poet. They might be invited to consider the disruption of poetics to traditional medical learning, thereby mulling over what constitutes normative (colonial) medical education. Students might be invited to read aloud, in small group settings, poems penned by First Nations, Métis, or Inuit poets and might extend the reading of poems to larger conversations about voice, clinical engagements, and different ways of knowing and being in the world.

Indigenous-penned poetry might also be specifically paired with the medical teachings that students are being asked to learn. When students learn about the experiences of Indigenous men in emergency wards, they might read Dallas Hunt's words about ways Indigenous peoples are consistently constructed as sickly and abject. Indigenous poetic voice would be directly tethered to clinical learnings. When asked about reconciliation, students might read Garry Gottfriedson on the subject. Medical students could contemplate and reflect on Joy Harjo's lines 'Do not parade, pleased with yourself.//You must speak in the language of justice' and be invited to relate those lines directly to the medical education in which they are being enculturated. In other words, poetry within a context of UBC's 23/24 curriculum would maintain poetic integrity while at the same time deepening the very learnings 23/24 is advancing. Sadly, this is not at all what is transpiring.

It is plain hubris that within the confines of a tiny element of a medicine curriculum, medical students can be anointed poets. Imagine if, like in Joy Harjo's poem 'Conflict Resolution for Holy Beings', medicine instead listened seriously to poetry. Imagine if medicine began, poetically, to consider itself, akin to poetry, a holy realm of words. Imagine if, anchored in instrumental uncritical use of poetry, medical education did not (to again draw from Harjo) parade, pleased with itself. Imagine if, rather than magically turning more than 200 undergraduate medical students into pseudo-poets for an afternoon, UBC's 23/24 curriculum instead introduced medical students to Indigenous poetic traditions, poets, and poetry. If poetry as a practice was explored with depth and rigour, afforded the time, space, and seriousness that all things lauded as bioscientific are allowed, might this not be revolutionary? Might it not combat colonial conceits at the heart of anti-Indigenous racism? A starting point might be to show how reductive biomedical language can so readily colonize patients' experiences, draining traditions of longstanding metaphors.

Medicine is a colonial discipline. Across 'Canada' and beyond, medicine is facing critique as being rife with anti-Indigenous racism and multiple other biases and violences. If poetry were employed in critical anti-colonial ways, it might just play a small, but important, role in unsettling the settler-colonial foundations and norms that undergird medical education and practice. Poetry, as it is currently being taken up in some corners of medical education, may be at risk of normalizing colonial modes of power. Poetry, particularly poetry by contemporary Indigenous poets in Canada and poetry taking aim at White supremacy more broadly, might well be an important means for medical students and professionals, through discomfort and critical self-reflexivity, to reappraise ways medicine has disciplined them into certain modes of knowing and being. Poetry employed to make medical learners simply feel better about themselves might, however, miss that point, acting as another means of colonial oppression.

Notes

1 Throughout this chapter, effort is made at reminding readers that monikers like 'Canada' are a colonial fiction. Hence the iterations of 'so-called' and reference to Turtle Island, thereby erasing colonial borders and state divisions. I extend 'so-called' to apply to other colonial nations.

2 This chapter references a report titled *In Plain Sight: Addressing Indigenous-specific Racism and Discrimination in B.C.* released in British Columbia in 2021. As of 2022, the First Nations identity and achievements of the report's lead author, who for citational purposes is sourced throughout this chapter, have been widely disputed. *In Plain Sight*, however, was authored by many knowledgeable and credible (but unnamed, as often happens in authorship of government reports) Indigenous scholars, writers, and knowledge holders: the findings of the report, that anti-Indigenous racism is prevalent across the health care system, are not disputed.

References

Adams Z, Reisman A. Beyond Sparking Joy: A Call for a Critical Medical Humanities. *Academic Medicine*. 2019; 94: 1404.

Allan B, Smylie J. 2015. *First Peoples, Second Class Treatment: The Role of Racism in the Health and Well-Being of Indigenous Peoples in Canada*. Toronto: Wellesley Institute.

American Association of Medical Colleges (AAMC). 2021. *The Fundamental Role of the Arts and Humanities in Medical Education*. Washington, DC: AAMC.

Axelrod C, Brenna CT, Gershon A, et al. The Companion Curriculum: Medical Students' Perceptions of the Integration of Humanities Within Medical Education. *Canadian Medical Education Journal*. October 31, 2023; 14: 119–24.

Balhara KS, Ehmann MR, Irvin N. Antiracism in Health Professions Education Through the Lens of the Health Humanities. *Anesthesiology Clinics*. 2022; 40: 287–99.

Belcourt BR. Meditations on Reserve Life, Biosociality, and the Taste of Non-Sovereignty. *Settler Colonial Studies*. 2018; 8: 1–15.

Bleakley A. 2023. *Medical Humanities: Ethics, Aesthetics, Politics*. London: Routledge.

Bleakley A, Neilson S. 2021. *Poetry in the Clinic: Towards a Lyrical Medicine*. Abingdon: Routledge.

Brown B. 2015. *Daring Greatly: How the Courage to be Vulnerable Transforms the Way We Live, Love, Parent, and Lead*. London: Penguin.

Browne AJ., Lavoie JG, McCallum MJL, Christa Big Canoe. Addressing Anti-Indigenous Racism in Canadian Health Systems: Multi-Tiered Approaches are Required. *Canadian Journal of Public Health*. 2022; 113: 222–26.

Chrystos. 1988. I am Not Your Princess. In: *Not Vanishing, 101*. Vancouver: Press Gang Publishers.

de Leeuw S. 2015. Introduction to Determinants of Indigenous Peoples' Health. In: M Greenwood, S De Leeuw, NM Lindsay (eds.) *Determinants of Indigenous Peoples' Health: Beyond the Social*. Toronto, ON: Canadian Scholars' Press, 7–18.

de Leeuw S, Larstone R, Fell B, et al. Educating Medical Students' "Hearts and Minds": A Humanities-Informed Cultural Immersion Program in Indigenous Experiential Community Learning. *International Journal of Indigenous Health*. 2021; 88–107.

Dryden O, Nnorom O. Time to Dismantle Systemic Anti-Black Racism in Medicine in Canada. *Canadian Medical Association Journal*. 2021; 193: E55–E57.

Felske-Durksen C. 2020. Physicians' Notes: Decolonizing a Swab: A Commentary From an Indigenous Physician Who Works in Indigenous Health. *CPSA*, August. Available at: https://cpsa.ca/news/decolonizing-a-swab/. Last accessed: 1/12/2022.

Gebhard A, McLean S, St Denis V. (eds.) 2022. *White Benevolence: Racism and Colonial Violence in the Helping Professions*. Halifax, Nova Scotia: Fernwood Publishing.

Goez H, Lai H, Rodger J, et al. 2020. The DISCuSS Model: Creating Connections Between Community and Curriculum – A New Lens for Curricular Development in Support of Social Accountability. *Medical Teacher*. In press.

Gottfriedson G. 2019. *Clinging to Bone*. Vancouver: Ronsdale Press, 26.

Greene J, Basilico MT, Kim H, et al. Colonial Medicine and Its Legacies. *Reimagining Global Health: An Introduction*. 2013; 1: 33–73.

Harjo J. 2015. *Conflict Resolution for Holy Beings: Poems*. New York, NY: WW Norton & Company.

Harris C. How Did Colonialism Dispossess? Comments From an Edge of Empire. *Annals of the Association of American Geographers*. 2004; 94: 165–82.

Hunt D. 2021. A Crooks that Signifies Home. In: *Creeland*. Vancouver: Harbour Publishing, 74–76.

Kelm M-E. 1998. *Colonizing Bodies: Aboriginal Health and Healing in British Columbia, 1900–50*. Vancouver, BC: UBC Press.

Kristeva J, Moro MR, Odemark J, Engebretsen E. 2020. The Cultural Crossings of Care: A call for translational medical humanities. In: A Bleakley (ed.) *Routledge Handbook of the Medical Humanities*. Abingdon: Routledge, 34–40.

Kulchyski P. Aboriginal Peoples and Hegemony in Canada. *Journal of Canadian Studies*. Spring, 1995: unpaginated. Available at: https://caid.ca/AboPeoJCS1995.pdf. Last accessed: 24/12/2023.

Kuper A. When I Say . . . Cultural Knowledge. *Medical Education*. 2014; 48: 1148–49.

MacDonald NE, Stanwick R, Lynk A. Canada's Shameful History of Nutrition Research on Residential School Children: The Need for Strong Medical Ethics in Aboriginal Health Research. *Paediatrics & Child Health*. 2014; 19: 64–80.

Maldonado-Torres N. On the Coloniality of Being: Contributions to the Development of a Concept. *Cultural Studies*. 2007; 21: 240–70.

Mitchell WJ, Bhabha H. Translator Translated. *Artforum*. 1995; 33: 80.

Mosby I. Administering Colonial Science: Nutrition Research and Human Biomedical Experimentation in Aboriginal Communities and Residential Schools, 1942–1952. *Histoire Sociale/Social History*. 2013; 46: 145–72.

Mosby I, Swidrovich J. Medical Experimentation and the Roots of COVID-19 Vaccine Hesitancy Among Indigenous Peoples in Canada. *Canadian Medical Association Journal*. 2021; 193: E381–E383.

Persaud N, Butts H, Berger P. William Osler: Saint in a "White Man's Dominion". *Canadian Medical Association Journal*. 2020; 192: E1414–E1416.

Peterkin A, Beausoleil N, Kidd M, et al. 2020. Medical Humanities in Canadian Medical Schools: Progress, Challenges and Opportunities. In: A Bleakley (ed.) *Routledge Handbook of the Medical Humanities*. Abingdon: Routledge, 364–79.

Raycraft R. 2021. Canadian Medical Association Elects First Indigenous President. *CBC*, February 26. Available at: www.cbc.ca/news/politics/cma-first-indigenous-president-1.5929535. Last accessed: 28/2/2021.

Rutecki GW. Clinical Science After Flexner's 1910 Report on Medical Education: A Research Ethos Inhabited by Racial Prejudice, Colonial Attitudes, and Eugenic Theory. *Ethics & Medicine*. 2020; 36: 51–53.

Said EW. 2012. *Culture and Imperialism*. London: Vintage.

Sexton SM, Richardson CR, Schrager SB, et al. Systemic Racism and Health Disparities: Statement From Editors of Family Medicine Journals. *Canadian Family Physician*. 2021; 67: 13–14.

Shaheen-Hussain S. 2020. *Fighting for a Hand to Hold: Confronting Medical Colonialism Against Indigenous Children in Canada*. Vol. 97. Montreal, Canada: McGill-Queen's Press-MQUP.

Stoler AL. Colonial Archives and the Arts of Governance. *Archival Science*. 2002; 2: 87–109.

Stoler AL. 2016. *Duress: Imperial Durabilities in Our Times*. Durham, NC: Duke University Press.

Turpel-Lafond ME, Johnson H. In Plain Sight: Addressing Indigenous-Specific Racism and Discrimination in BC Health Care. *BC Studies: The British Columbian Quarterly*. 2021; 209: 7–17.

Watego C, Whop LJ, Singh D, et al. Black to the Future: Making the Case for Indigenist Health Humanities. *International Journal of Environmental Research and Public Health*. 2021; 18: 8704.

Whitehead A, Woods A. (eds.) 2016. *The Edinburgh Companion to the Critical Medical Humanities*. Edinburgh: Edinburgh University Press.

27

WHEN CAGED BIRDS SING

Black critical feminist poetry as a tool for political resistance, empowerment, and healing

Thirusha Naidu and Lynne Richards

When caged birds sing

Maya Angelou's (1983: Stanza 3) 'Caged Bird' chronicles her life story and that of many women of colour, in which she states

> The caged bird sings
> with a fearful trill
> of things unknown
> but longed for still
> and his tune is heard
> on the distant hill
> for the caged bird
> sings of freedom

In this chapter, we introduce the rich histories of Black, critical feminist poets who were also political activists, educators, and liberators. Through their writing, we show how they amplify issues of health inequities and inequalities. They are the caged birds who, through voice, art, and written word, envisioned and created new possibilities futures for themselves and women of colour who followed them. These poets were selected as illustrators of poetry as a tool for political activism and empowerment, highlighting structural and social determinants that mould the lived experiences of women of colour. At a foundational level, we centre poetry as a modality of healing both the psyche and the physical body. We present the works of Black, influential female poets who deploy poetry as a mechanism of change in their socio-political contexts in North America. Maya Angelou, Audre Lorde, and the more contemporary Nikki Giovanni offer perspectives on the experiences of women of colour, spanning the civil rights and black consciousness movements to current social and structural challenges.

On the Indian subcontinent, the poetry of Sarojini Naidu, known as 'the Nightingale of India', provides a depiction of the lives of Indian women in the 1800s during a period characterized by colonialism and the oppression of women's rights. Olive Senior's work offers the blurred perspective of living between the marginalized and the affluent as she navigates her childhood and later

DOI: 10.4324/9781003341796-35

adulthood as a Jamaican poet in Canada. South African poet Makhosazana Xaba's writings bridge the chasm between colonial and Apartheid South Africa and a democratic South Africa in which the rights of women were denied. Finally, we present one of the author's (TN) works depicting the use of art in academia. Her work laces the chapter together with threads of critical feminism, health, empowerment, and self-acceptance.

The desire for freedom that Angelou refers to in the poem 'Caged Bird' reflects the universal struggle for the empowerment of women. While the poem echoes her life story of racism, sexism, and child sexual abuse described in her first autobiographical book, *I Know Why the Caged Bird Sings*, Angelou uses the imagery of a cage to depict the circumstances of women universally. Angelou experienced a tumultuous upbringing with her parents separating at an early age where she subsequently moved between various family members. At age seven, she was abused by her mother's then boyfriend, who was later killed by her maternal uncles (Neubauer 1987). Blaming herself for voicing the abuse and then for his death, Angelou became selectively mute (Harisunker and du Plesis 2021). She later found solace in writing about these experiences.

Her early adulthood was marked by significant changes, including the birth of her son and financial difficulties. She was challenged by motherhood and struggled to find meaning in her romantic relationships (Neubauer 1987). It was not until the early 1950s, in her late twenties, that she discovered a love for dance and a career in writing. She used this platform to challenge political ills and became a prominent figure in the New York Civil Rights Movement, the Pan-African Movement, the Black Power Movement, and the Black Arts Movement (Harisunker and du Plesis 2021). Angelou believed that her work was immortalized in word and provided a guide for future generations to understand the past and challenge unjust practices (Ramsey 1984):

But a caged bird stands on the grave of dreams
his shadow shouts on a nightmare scream
his wings are clipped and his feet are tied
so he opens his throat to sing.
(Angelou 1983: Stanza 5)

Throughout history, women of colour have experienced unjustified discrimination and oppression as a result of the intersectionality of race, class, and gender, to name a few of the social determinants of health (Perry et al. 2013). Oppressive regimes, including colonialism, imperialism, and country-specific political instability, have been driven and shaped by ideologies of patriarchy, white global supremacy, and cultural hegemony as staged histories of oppression in which women suffered most. Despite the illusion that the oppression of women was secondary to these regimes, the 'othering' of women and women of colour served as a mechanism to maintain the existing rule.

Colonial policies sought the possession of indigenous land and the exploitation of labour and material resources, maintaining this through the imposition of a new form of education and devaluing of cultural practices and language (Spencer-Wood 2016). Ideologies of ideal womanhood and motherhood, often differing from matriarchal traditions, confined women to the domestic sphere. This denigrated women to a lowly status of unskilled and unpaid labour, denying women's rights in the public sphere and imposing strict laws and social mores on sexuality and so-called immorality (*ibid.*). White women were responsible for the preservation of a 'pure' race, setting them against women of colour, who were imbued with the value of attaining pureness or 'whiteness' (Frankenberg 1993; Spencer-Wood 2016; Besson 2021). Ultimately, this created a divide among women of different races which would lead to a division in feminisms.

One of the author's (TN) poems (*Affirmative Activism*), written in contemporary South Africa, battles with the concept of ethnic and racial belonging for the person of colour. Indigenous individuals must learn that they are 'other' and will never be White:

> . . . If you find yourself in places
> Where your ancestors walked
> You'll want to add "native" to your name.
> Who needs to know you belong?
> And why?
> Your grandmother was Negro, Indian or Coloured.
> Sometimes all three. Always nothing.
> Your mother was Black, Asian or Native.
> Free to choose
> Anything but White.
> You might want to calculate your percentage
> Of the now popular "Indigenous"
> With a capital I
> Whatever gets you ahead
> in the Race
> Stop to ask and you'll lose your place.
> Who needs to know where you came from?
> And why?
>
> (Thirusha Naidu)

This poem captures how contemporary generations of women continue to grapple with their sense of belonging and ascription to Western white practices. Detachment from Indigenous knowledge systems and ways of being provide for the internalization of ideologies of femininity and womanhood. These ensured that the oppressed were self-regulated and, in turn, child rearing was compliant with the dominant culture (Hamilton et al. 2019). The women who deviated from these social norms were deemed immoral, uncivilized, witches, and social outcasts. This is captured in Lorde's (1997: Stanza 3) poem 'A Women Speaks'. Lorde says that she has 'been woman'

> for a long time
> beware my smile
> I am treacherous with old magic
> and the noon's new fury
> with all your wide futures
> promised
> I am
> woman
> and not white.

Lorde (1981) describes how Black women have been written out of history. Black women have experienced a history of slavery and emerged resilience. Lorde's work speaks about the 'treacherous old magic' and 'divinities' of women referring to feminine intuition, ancient indigenous knowledge, and sexuality. She further notes 'her sister witches' in reference to the White woman's suspicion and paranoia, and the White man's intrigue of the Black woman as a sexual conquest.

Lorde was born in New York to parents from Barbados and Grenada (Rowell and Lorde 2000). She had trouble expressing herself as a child and turned to poetry as a means of expression (Sala-hub 2017). Through poetry she found her voice as a Black African American mother, lesbian, and activist. Like Angelou, Lorde became actively involved in the Black Power Movement, the Black Arts Movement, and later the Gay-Lesbian Movement (*ibid.*). Her essays and poetry tackled poignant social topics. Furthermore, her literary works became a personal coping mechanism to transcend physical pain and suffering from living with cancer (Rowell and Lorde 2000). In her revolutionary essays 'The Master's Tools Will Never Dismantle the Master's House' and 'Poetry is not a Luxury', Lorde calls on Black women to not concern themselves with writing to educate the White man or woman that keeps us occupied with the 'master's concerns' (Lorde 1984: 3; Bowleg 2021). Instead, she calls on women to use poetry to create action, as more than words.

Of the weapons in the 'Master's' arsenal, none is as powerful as language used in the oppression of marginalized groups. Language shapes the construction of our social worlds and influences consciousness (Jeewa and Bhima 2021). According to Fanon (1963), to speak is to exist. The imposition of English and the re-storying of histories to depict a dominant White saviour rescuing the illiterate, savage 'other' has fractured the sense of belonginess among cultural minorities. The aim for the colonizer is cultural hegemony and acculturation ensuring obedience. Eventually, it creates a universal culture and legitimates imperialism (Shakib 2011). This allows no room for alternate realities and experiences thought to be inferior, affecting social structures including academia.

Nikki Giovanni, in her 1968 sharp-witted poem 'Nikki Rosa', explains that her experience as a Black woman can never be understood for its value by a White individual. She asserts,

> and I really hope no white person ever has cause
> to write about me
> because they never understand
> Black love is Black wealth and they'll
> probably talk about my hard childhood
> and never understand that
> all the while I was quite happy

Giovanni's poetry emerged from the Civil Rights Movement of the later 1960s (Jago 1999). Interestingly, Giovanni denies being a feminist or even a Black feminist, asserting that feminism places the problems of all women before the problems of racism in America. Furthermore, she expresses dismay at the failure of the women's movement to ignore other struggles. Her beliefs seem to resonate with the thoughts of intersectional and critical feminist writers. In her poem 'Nikki-Rosa' she fondly reminisces about her early childhood, underprivileged by Western standards. However, she vehemently rejects the notion of 'underprivilege', indicating that the love she experienced was sufficient privilege. Her experience transcended the physical. Giovanni, and the female poets presented here, found the means to claim and express their voices through vernacular lyrical poetry with strong roots in storytelling, folktales, lullabies, and protest or activism (George 2017).

Sarojini Naidu, dubbed 'the Nightingale of India', or 'Bharat Koklia', takes a political stance in her poem 'To India' in which she pleads with the country to fight against the oppressive British regime. India, 'Mother', is urged to 'rise', to 'regenerate' and 'beget new glories':

> The nations that in fettered darkness weep
> Crave thee to lead them where great mornings break . . .

Mother, O Mother, wherefore dost thou sleep?
Arise and answer for thy children's sake!

Thy Future calls thee with a manifold sound
To crescent honours, splendours, victories vast;
Waken, O slumbering Mother and be crowned,
Who once wert empress of the sovereign Past.

Naidu was born to a family of a high social caste (Indian National Congress 2021; Sarojini Naidu College for Women n.d.), but despite her caste, Naidu understood that as a woman there were certain freedoms that she would not be afforded. At an early age, she had good command of various languages and began to write plays and poetry. She earned a scholarship to study at Kings College and Cambridge, where she would later be introduced to the suffrage movement (Indian National Congress 2021). She married a man who was of a lower caste. On her return to India, she continued her fight for women's empowerment and joined the Indian National Congress that fought the British rule. She was integral to the Civil Disobedience Movement, under the leadership of Mahatma Gandhi, and endured numerous imprisonments for her beliefs. Her literary works were imbued with themes of womanhood, sexuality, marriage, and the richness of life in India.

The subjugation of ethnic minority culture through the imposition of a dominant language and the imposition of Christianity separated long-established social bonds and fractured the psyches of these collectives (Oliver and Oliver 2017; Gouws and Coetzee 2019). Razack (2016) describes the vulnerability of women of colour and indigenous peoples to poor health outcomes and high rates of violence as 'gender disposability', or expendability.

Olive Senior, a Jamaican poet, described herself as a child of a mixed social and racial world, characterized by different cultures, norms, and mores (Rowell 1988). As a child, she struggled to find an identity between these worlds. Her early childhood in an underprivileged community without entertainment led her to creative expression, where she attributes her first contact with expressive art to oral traditions including storytelling and praying (*ibid.*). This connected her to the traditions of those before her. When Senior entered high school, she discovered a passion for English literature, asserting that writing had been the 'strongest single force in [her] life', allowing her to affirm an identity (Rowell 1988: 484). Despite emigrating to Canada, Senior uses her poetry to discuss experiences from the Caribbean diaspora, colonial existence in Jamaica, and, more broadly motherhood, caregiving, and health (Westall 2019). Senior's (2021) *Pandemic Poems*, is an anthology she wrote during the first wave of the COVID-19 pandemic. 'V for Vaccine' says,

How quickly COVID-19 has been upstaged
By a more insidious injection of hate
Into the black body that has gone viral
Boots on the ground
And no social etiquette required
Unless there is rigorous commitment
to eradicating poisonous infection
no vaccine to counteract this one
will ever be found

In this poem, Senior describes the perpetuance of Black violence masked by law and fuelled by an ideology of inferiority.

Where the personal is political and poetry is political

In the above accounts of the poets who are also women of colour, we offer perspectives on their lives and histories that intersect with their social contexts, forming their poetic voices. These women were selected as representative of their ages because of their engagement with revolutionary Black critical feminist and civil rights movements. While their work is undoubtedly essential in conveying the use of poetry as a liberatory mechanism, it is also of course open to critique. However, such critique can merely reinforce oppression where literary quality is defined by White northern hemisphere traditions.

Maya Angelou's work continues to be popular with emerging generations of women of colour. However, this may be due more to her activism and autobiographies, considered to be more important than her poetry. Some critics consider her poetry to be lacklustre and without depth (DeGout 2005; Tetteh and Derx-Takyi 2015). But again, this may be mis-directed critique where Angelou's poetry speaks not to northern hemisphere notions of poetic diction but to a politics of identity and what it means to be an African American. Her work reflects the African traditions of praising, singing, and the beat of a drum, along with African American music genres including be-bop jazz (Traylor 2005). Her poetry reflects African American vernacular, while her tendency to use laughter and ridicule to alleviate suffering may be representative of how the women she speaks of respond to multiple intersecting oppressions over generations (Tetteh and Derx-Takyi 2015)

Sarojini Naidu was undoubtedly a committed activist in the struggle against British colonial influence, establishing and re-establishing Indian culture (Reddy 2010). She was encouraged by her compatriots in the Indian independence movement to write poetry to inspire Indians to the cause. However, her poetry reflects the coloniality hidden in her voice and is reflective of her position of privilege. Her poems, in structure and language, reflect the British or English poetic style (*ibid.*). Perhaps unintentionally, and by means of her British education, Naidu's work reflects the deep infiltration of a colonial mindset. It sets the reader wondering that if a privileged and educated activist was so influenced by colonial thought, how much more ordinary women's lives and health must have been affected by colonial oppression. A contradictory view is posited by Reddy (*ibid.*), who suggests that this image, parallel to Naidu's nationalism, may have asserted her position as a mechanism of change. Naidu's grasp of the English language and eloquent poetry was unthreatening to the colonialists. While Naidu is respected for her role in history, her poetry is no longer as popular in India, probably because the country has long moved on from independence. Naidu's poetry did not speak to Indian women to rise for themselves but to rise to a cause, despite internal oppressions such as ritual Sati and the widespread discrimination against widows (Staggs 2021).

Giovanni's work offers a counterpoint to Naidu's where she deliberately positions herself first as a poet with the task of documenting activism through her words. A chronological look at her poetry shows how she positions herself as an observer while experiencing the effects of oppression and activism in her own life (Standford 1994; Walters 2000). In some ways this is reminiscent of women – even today – who must be activists in addition to, and despite, their gender-based social demands. Giovanni's work has received both popular and academic acclaim, and she has been described as the primary voice for Black activism in the United States (Standford 1994; Harris 2012).

Giovanni is an academic poet of standing (Jago 1999) having lectured in literature. Her deeply reflective and complex body of work that mirrors social contexts is considered of high literary quality, yet Angelou's poetry remains popular without literary pretensions. This raises the question: 'what makes good poetry?', especially in the context of a consciousness-raising politics. Does poetry have to meet a literary standard to endure? And, again, whose 'standards' are we drawing on? We might think of Linton Kwesi Johnson's protest dub poetry that draws on Anglicized

Jamaican vernacular and recited against dub music, creating a new genre. This once experimental verse is now part of the canon. Poetry can no longer be thought of exclusively as 'art for art's sake' where it has an essential role in liberation of the oppressed within the political sphere.

Lorde's work is perhaps the most deeply personal of all the poets we discuss in this chapter. However, her work reminds the reader that the personal is political. While she discusses and inspires activism, she positions herself firmly as a poet. She is unapologetically self-indulgent in her poetry as reflected in her autobiographical works (Rowell and Lorde 2000). The reader gets the sense that she uses personal experience as material to consider wider social ills that women of colour experience. She is indeed held together by her poetry. When her love life, family relationships, and health fail, her poetry remains (Salahub 2017). Lorde's death from cancer further elevated her voice as poet, where she has been canonized.

Olive Senior was named poet laureate of Jamaica from 2021 to 2024 (Montout 2006). Her work has been described as intertextual, inflected with power relations even within a highly canonical British literary context. Senior's work echoes that of Sarojini Naidu in style though not in content (Phillips 2003). Senior's work speaks more openly and critically about the power relations of oppression in the Caribbean (*ibid.*, Bucknor 2009). She does not need to subtly motivate Caribbean people to activism but does so through clear, even drastic, descriptions of colonial oppression long after colonialism was apparently over (Westall 2019). Her later pandemic poems (titled poems from A to Z) reflect neglected or hidden aspects of the experiences of, and responses to, the pandemic. Future critics will likely find many of these poems wanting in relation to Senior's usual quality of work. However, the fact that Senior chose to publish these poems almost daily on Twitter during the pandemic may reflect an intention to connect contemporary audiences to the intersection of how poetry, health and activism can draw attention to the experiences of marginalised people. Senior shows how poetry could respond to communal issues, uncertainty, fear, hopelessness, and isolation

Health inequalities and racism

So what does this poetry disclose in relation to medicine and health? Society remains riddled with inequality and racism. The social and structural determinants of health created by histories of inequality have affected every aspect of social life and, in turn, the physical and mental health of the oppressed in particular. In populations of colour, these determinants have created significant health crises, including the spread of infectious disease, lack of access to quality services, and increased maternal mortality rates (Howell 2018). Studies have also found that women of colour are disproportionately affected by anaemia, cardiovascular disease, and obesity, due to poor nutrition (Chinn et al. 2021). Additionally, women of colour are more likely to die from breast cancer due to inequality in access to care and to poor nutrition and education while receiving insufficient pain management (Gehlert et al. 2021).

Racism and ensuing hostility, discrimination, and marginalization may understandably precipitate and perpetuate mental illness, but studies on the prevalence of mental illness among different populations have yielded an unclear picture (McLaughlin et al. 2019; Williams 2019). While the prevalence of mental illness is similar to or lower in black populations than in others, mental illness within this population tends to have a chronic course and poorer prognosis (Louie and Wheaton 2018; Williams 2019). In addition, the literature reports a historic overdiagnosis of severe psychopathology and psychosis amongst African American and Latino American and Hispanic communities (Faber et al. 2013; Schwartz and Blankenship 2014). However, the relevance of the application of diagnostic categories to cultural minorities has been questioned.

In a South African context, one of us (TN) has written about isiZulu patient encounters with Western mental health systems in the poem 'Mental Status Extrication'. A patient's nuanced experience of being misunderstood is reduced to no more than a multiaxial diagnosis:

I, poised on the edge
of reason, sway.
While you, weighing differentials,
strike a diagnostic match
igniting fiery thoughts and
cogitating a multi-axial symptom overload.
I, wording my life, flounder.
Gasp, a fish on the table.
You and I fray over
shattered mirrors reflecting only
I in mine and you in yours.
You ask about my mother.
She was there, but not where
I, could find a history
In the splayed shards that
You, compose into me
With an assertive air.
Pill purveyor, dream voyeur.
I have seen izangoma, priests, witchdoctors.
Did they see me? I cannot know.
You a doctor of Which? When? What?
Questions to throw my bones.
To read where they lie.
To determine my status of mind.
I rise unpatient-like and cross a canyon in bare feet,
encountering you midway, adrift.
You trying to put yourself in my shoes
You still in your own feet.

Unsurprisingly, discrimination towards individuals of minority racial and ethnic identities impacts self-esteem and belonging (Harris-Britt et al. 2007). Studies have shown that self-concept is linked to racial identity (Perry et al. 2016). Watson and colleagues (2016) found that racism resulted in lower self-esteem, and increased trauma.

Reclaiming the voices of marginalized women through poetry

Women must re-write themselves into history from the margins (Rasool and Harms-Smith 2022). The reassertion of voice among the marginalized gives testimony to their lived realities and serves as a political act of self-determination. However, women continue to face exclusion from mainstream publication and academia (Attfield 2006). Western knowledge published in dominant academic journals continues to be considered the gold standard in Western academia (Mazzocchi 2006). The reliance on language conventions, rigid methods, and colonized and male-dominated publishing panels has served as a gatekeeping mechanism perpetuating the marginalisation of minority voices, particularly women of colour (WOC).

This act of coloniality devalues the 'knowledge production and knowledge dissemination' of marginalized communities and creates a knowledge hierarchy (Hungwe and Ndofirepi 2022: 55). Epistemic violence results when the marginalized community 'is silenced by both the colonial and indigenous patriarchal power' (Moletsane 2015: 40). Epistemic dominance establishes a sense of legitimacy while claiming neutrality and objectivity (Akena 2012; Moletsane 2015). This legitimacy of knowledge is interconnected with the socio-economic status and ethnic identity of the producer.

Furthermore, the established hegemony has resulted in marginalized communities being the object of studies that perpetuate discrimination (Vaditya 2018). These individuals have rarely been the researcher or authors of their own experiences and the experiences of engaging with the dominant class (*ibid.*). In this way, knowledge-creating organizations commit epistemic violence towards marginalized populations. As a result, WOC and Global South scholars have resorted to Northern ventriloquism, maintaining local knowledge within local spaces or enacting epistemic disobedience (Naidu 2021). New forms of poetry and prose that serve the needs of WOC have been developed. This form of poetry, with its unique structure, form, and register, provides an opportunity to voice the experiences of the marginalized. In this way, poetry is an act of epistemic disobedience. It provides access to historical information for those without epistemic access and voices sensitive topics (Godsell 2019). Further, this poetry implicates medicine and health issues as it challenges systemic inequities and inequalities.

This evolution has been described in Xaba's (2019) anthology of poems *Our Words, Our Worlds*. The South African Black Women's Poetry movement, described by Baderoon (2021), has evolved over the past century in response to women being excluded from mainstream poetry and related publishing. This marginalization has resulted from a history of colonialism, imperialism, and apartheid, as well as contemporary struggles against post-apartheid patriarchal ideologies. The literary movement arose from the need to describe South African women's experiences of surviving trauma, violence, and injustice to celebrate joy, sexuality, and resistance through identity. It represented the idea of the personal as political. Intuitively, the movement imbued prominent South African Black women's poetry with collectivist and feminist notions, serving as both gate openers and publishers (*ibid.*). The movement has created new forms and themes in poetry. This draws on new registers challenging the established control of language that continues to marginalize black women. Such a challenge to the established hegemony includes stylistic experiments. Further, this form of poetry embraces the use of different vernaculars, including those representing a mixed language of individuals from lower socioeconomic groups.

Makhosazana Xaba's work is grounded in her experiences as a psychiatric nurse, midwife, journalist, and activist. She was active in the African National Congress Women's League and Umkhonto we Sizwe. She went into exile, returning in 1990 with the League (*ibid.*), writing poetry in 2000 and subsequently authoring four collections of poetry. An extract from her poem 'The alkalinity of bottled water' (2019) presents a call to activism. Xaba tells the reader that while working on the poem, she receives a call from a literary scholar who tells her that a poetry session has been cancelled at the University of Pretoria. This is during a period of 'flaring fires' both literally and metaphorically (as 'rising students' discussing decolonizing, and now ten years on we look back, to find that,

> This poem has settled with the analysis of the alkalinity of the water we are drowning in
> As our arms flail in desperation, we hope to start seeing a hard rock below

Now 'Waiting for us at the unfathomable bottom. Fezekile, the four sisters ensured/That we never forget: Kufezekile! And for that, the pH rises and we with it'. So,

> As the rock becomes visible, we strengthen our arms & legs, some pray, others start a song
> We dive with smiles on our faces because we realize that the turning point is close
> We would be singing out loud if we were not under water, so we focus on not drowning
> So that we can rise again, resurface and realize the dreams of the democracy we want

Xaba's poem addresses contemporary challenges in post-apartheid South Africa, including student unrest, a failure to decolonize education, violence against female political activists, and sexual abuse by members of the ruling class. She notes that the work is not complete, while to write is to ensure that future generations have a road map. Further, one of the author's (TN) poems, 'Give Girl', calls women to overcome the oppressive realities of their existence to pursue fulfilment and self-affirmation:

> Girl you got to give
> Give up, give in,
> give over, give off
> Who say you can't?
> He don't know what you got
> She don't think your head's worry
> You your mother's child
> Who say you can't?
> He don't know your shoe pinch
> She don't want your word sorry
> You your gran'ma's gold
> Girl you got to give
> Give up, give in,
> give over, give off
> Give it
> All you got
> Who say you can't?
> He don't want your skinny body
> She don't feel your baby hungry
> You your people's story
> You go
> You go on over, go on under
> You go on top
> Who say you can't?
> He don't stomach your troubles

She don't know your blood
You your own queen lady
You go
You go on over, go on under
You go on top
Who say you can't
              Thirusha Naidu

Through these ground-breaking shifts in acquiring voice, Black women's poetry – in the tradition of protest literature – acts as a modality for healing both the individual and the collective. The voice of protest acts as a health intervention. It marks the new ways in which the caged bird sings of freedom.

References

Akena FA. Critical Analysis of the Production of Western Knowledge and Its Implications for Indigenous Knowledge and Decolonization. *Journal of Black Studies*. 2012; 43: 599–619.

Angelou M. 1983. *Shaker, Why Don't You Sing?* New York, NY: Random House.

Attfield S. Worth Our Salt: Australian Working Class Women's Poetry. *Hecate*. 2006; 32 (1): unpaginated. Available at: https://go.gale.com/ps/i.do?p=AONE&u=googlescholar&id=GALE|A150966352&v=2.1&it=r&sid=googleScholar&asid=bbdeeba7. Last accessed: 29/4/2023.

Baderoon G. 2021. Forward. In: M Xaba (ed.) *Our Words, Our World*. Scotsville, SA: UKZN Press.

Besson EK. Confronting Whiteness and Decolonising Global Health Institutions. *The Lancet*. 2021; 397: 2328–29.

Bowleg L. "The Master's Tools Will Never Dismantle the Master's House": Ten Critical Lessons for Black and Other Health Equity Researcher of Colour. *Health Education & Behaviour*. 2021; 48: 237–49.

Bucknor MA. Sounding Off: Performing Ritual Revolt in Olive Senior's "Medication on Yellow". *Mosaic: An Interdisciplinary Critical Journal*. 2009; 42: 55–71.

Chinn JJ, Martin IK, Redmond N. Health Equity Among Black Women in the United States. *Journal of Women's Health*. 2021; 30: 212–19.

DeGout Y. The Poetry of Maya Angelou: Liberation Ideology and Technique. *The Langston Hughes Review*. 2005; 19: 36–47.

Faber S, Roy A, Michaels T, Williams M. The Weaponization of Medicine: Early Psychosis in the Black Community and the Need for Racially Informed Mental Healthcare. *Frontiers in Psychology*. 2013; 14: 1098292.

Fanon F. 1963. *The Wretched of the Earth*. New York, NY: Grove Press.

Frankenberg R. 1993. *White Women, Race Matters: The Social Construction of Whiteness*. Minneapolis, MN: University of Minnesota Press.

Gehlert S, Hudson D, Sacks T. A Critical Theoretical Approach to Cancer Disparities: Breast Cancer and the Social Determinants of Health. *Frontiers in Public Health*. 2021; 9: 674736.

George A. Slam Poetry – A Link Between Black Feminism and Oral Poetry Traditions. Canterbury. *International Journal for Intersectionist Feminist Studies*. 2017; 3 (2). Available at: https://ir.canterbury.ac.nz/bitstream/handle/10092/14522/George.pdf?sequence=1. Last accessed: 29/4/2023.

Godsell S. Poetry as Method in the History Classroom: Decolonising Possibilities. *Yesterday and Today*. 2019; 21: 1–28.

Gouws A, Coetzee A. Women's Movements and Feminist Activism. *Empowering Women for Gender Equity*. 2019; 33: 1–8.

Hamilton L, Armstrong E, Seeley J, Armstrong E. Hegemonic Femininities and Intersectional Domination. *Sociological Theory*. 2019; 37: 315–41.

Harisunker N, du Plesis C. A Journey Towards Meaning: An Existential Psychobiography of Maya Angelou. *Europe's Journal of Psychology*. 2021; 17: 210–20.

Harris T. Nikki Giovanni: Literary Survivor Across Centuries. *Appalachian Heritage*. 2012; 40: 34–47.

Harris-Britt A, Valrie C, Kurtz-Costes B, Rowley S. Perceived Racial Discrimination and Self-Esteem in African-American Youth: Racial Socialization as a Protective Factor. *Journal of Research on Adolescence*. 2007; 17: 669–82.

Howell E. Reducing Disparities in Severe Maternal Morbidity and Mortality. *Clinical Obstetrics and Gynaecology*. 2018; 61: 387–99.

Hungwe J, Ndofirepi A. A Critical Interrogation of Paradigms in Discourse on the Decolonisation of Higher Education in Africa. *SUN Journals*. 2022. Available at: www.scielo.org.za/pdf/sajhe/v36n3/04.pdf

Indian National Congress. 2021, March 5. *Congress Sangesh*. Sarojini Naidu (13 February, 1879–2 March, 1949). Available at: https://inc.in/congress-sandesh/tribute/sarojini-naidu-13-february-1879–2-march-1949. Last accessed: 29/4/2023.

Jago C. 1999. *Nikki Giovanni in the Classroom: The Same Ol' Danger But a Brand New Pleasure*. Ann Arbor, MI: University of Michigan. National Council of Teachers of English.

Jeewa T, Bhima J. Discriminatory Language: A Remnant of Colonial Oppression. *Constitutional Court Review*. 2021; 11: 1–17.

Lorde A. 1984. The Master's Tools Will Never Dismantle the Master's House. In: A Lorde (ed.) *Sister Outsider: Essays and Speeches*. Berkeley, CA: Crossing Press, 110–14. Available at: https://collectiveliberation.org/wp-content/uploads/2013/01/Lorde_The_Masters_Tools.pdf. Last accessed: 29/4/2023.

Lorde A. The Uses of Anger. *Women's Studies Quarterly*. 1997 (originally pub. 1981); 25: 278–85.

Louie P, Wheaton B. Prevalence and Patterning of Mental Disorders Through Adolescence in 3 Cohorts of Black and White American. *American Journal of Epidemiology*. 2018; 187: 2332–38.

Mazzocchi F. Western Science and Traditional Knowledge: Despite Their Variations, Different Forms of Knowledge Can Learn from Each Other. *EMBO Reports*. 2006; 7: 463–66.

McLaughlin KA, Alvarez K, Fillbrunn M, et al. Racial/Ethnic Variation in Trauma-Related Psychopathology in the United States: A Population-Based Study. *Psychological Medicine*. 2019; 49: 2215–26.

Moletsane R. Whose Knowledge is It? Towards Reordering Knowledge Production and Dissemination in the Global South. *Educational Research for Social Change*. 2015; 4: 35–47.

Montout M. The Intrinsic Written Quality of the Spoken Word in Olive Senior's Short Fiction. *Journal of the Short Story in English*. 2006; 47: unpaginated. Available at: http://journals.openedition.org/jsse/805. Last accessed: 3/5/2023.

Naidu T. Says Who? Northern Ventriloquism, or Epistemic Disobedience in Global Health Scholarship. *The Lancet Global Health*. 2021; 9: e1332–e35.

Neubauer C. An Interview with Maya Angelou. *The Massachusetts Review*. 1987; 28: 286–92.

Oliver E, Oliver W. The Colonisation of South Africa: A Unique Case. *HTS Theological Studies*. 2017; 73: a4498.

Perry B, Harp K, Oser C. Racial and Gender Discrimination in the Stress Process: Implication for African American Women's Health and Well-being. *Sociological Perspectives*. 2013; 56: 25–48.

Perry S, Hardeman R, Burke S, et al. The Impact of Everyday Discrmination and Racial Identity Centrality on African American Medical Student Well-being: A Report from the Medical Student CHANGE Study. *Journal of Racial and Ethnic Health Disparities*. 2016; 3: 519–26.

Phillips G. Personal and Textual Geographies in Olive Senior's Literary Relationship With Jean Rhys. *Journal of Caribbean Literatures*. 2003; 3: 199–206.

Ramsey P. Transcendence: The Poetry of Maya Angelou. *A Current Bibliography on African Affairs*. 1984; 17: 139–53.

Rasool S, Harms-Smith L. Retrieving the Voices of Black African Womanists and Feminists for Work Toward Decoloniality in Social Work. *Southern African Journal of Social Work and Social Development*. 2022; 34: 1–30.

Razack S. Gendering Disposability. *Canadian Journal of Woman and the Law*. 2016; 28: 285–307.

Reddy S. Cosmopolitan Nationalism of Sarojini Naidu, Nightingale of India. *Victorian Literature and Culture*. 2010; 38: 571–89.

Rowell C, Lorde A. Above the Wind: An Interview With Audre Lorde. *Callaloo*. 2000; 23: 52–63. Available at: www.jstor.org/stable/3299518. Last accessed: 28/4/2023.

Rowell CH. An Interview with Olive Senior. *Callaloo*. 1988; 36: 480–90.

Salahub J. (2017, February 20). *Black History Month: Audre Lorde*. Fort Collins, CO: Colorado State University. Available at: https://english.colostate.edu/news/black-history-month-audre-lorde/. Last accessed: 29/4/2023.

Sarojini Naidu College for Women. n.d. *Sarojini Naidu*. Sarojini Naidu College for Women. Available at: www.sncwgs.ac.in/profile/about-sarojini-naidu/. Last accessed: 29/4/2023.

Schwartz R, Blankenship D. Racial Disparities in Psychotic Disorder Diagnosis: A Review of Empirical Literature. *World Journal of Psychiatry*. 2014; 4: 133–40.

Senior O. 2021. *Pandemic Poems: First Wave*. La Vergne, TN: Olive Senior, Distributed by Ingram Book Co.

Shakib M. The Position of Language in Development of Colonization. *Journal of Languages and Culture*. 2011; 2: 117–23.

Spencer-Wood S. Feminist Theorizing of Patriarchal Colonialism, Power Dynamics, and Social Agency Materialized in Colonial Institution. *International Journal of Historical Archaeology*. 2016; 20: 477–91.

Staggs M. From Poet to Activist: Sarojini Naidu and Her Battles against Colonial Oppression and Misogyny in 20th Century India. *Armstrong Undergraduate Journal of History*. 2021; (1): Article 5. Available at: https://digitalcommons.georgiasouthern.edu/aujh/vol11/iss1/5/. Last accessed: 3/5/2023.

Standford A. The Complications of Being Nikki Giovanni. *African American Review*. 1994; 28: 481–84.

Tetteh U, Derx-Takyi C. The Literary Merits of Maya Angelou's Choice of Narrative Style in Her Autobiographies. *International Journal of English Language, Literature and Humanities*. 2015; III: 26–49.

Traylor E. Maya Angelou Writing Life, Inventing Literary Genre. *The Langston Hughes Review*. 2005; 19: 8–21.

Vaditya V. Social Domination and Epistemic Marginalisation: Towards a Methodology of the Oppressed. *Social Epistemology*. 2018; 32: 272–85.

Walters J. Nikki Giovanni and Rita Dove: Poets Redefining. *The Journal of Negro History*. 2000; 85: 210. Available at: www.journals.uchicago.edu/doi/abs/10.2307/2649078. Last accessed: 3/5/2023.

Watson LB, DeBlaere C, Langrehr KJ, et al. The Influence of Multiple Oppressions on Women of Color's Experiences With Insidious Trauma. *Journal of Counseling Psychology*. 2016; 63: 656–67.

Westall C. An Interview with Olive Senior. *The Journal of Commonwealth Literature*. 2019; 54: 475–88.

Williams D. Stress and the Mental Health of Populations of Colour: Advancing Our Understanding of Race-Related Stressors. *Journal of Health and Social Behaviour*. 2019; 59: 466–85.

Xaba M. 2019. *The Alkalinity of Bottled Water*. South Africa: Botsotso Publishing.

CREATIVE WRITING IN MEDICAL EDUCATION

Michael Hanne

Introduction

'Creativity and being a good doctor are one and the same thing', Art Nahill (24 March 2022) declared to the medical humanities class I co-teach with Elisabeth Kumar to student doctors at the University of Auckland, New Zealand. Nahill is one of the extraordinary number of doctors in many countries who are also outstanding writers. As we read the work of doctor–writers, we also explore the value for the students themselves of writing creatively during their training and in their future careers. We invite several outstanding local doctor–writers to the course to read their work, to talk about why (and how) they combine the two professions, and to mentor the students in their own creative writing.

Resisting the specificity of the title of this volume, the course we teach draws attention to the fact that while some of the best doctor–writers are indeed poets, many have excelled in writing short stories (Anton Chekhov), novels (Abraham Verghese), essays (Richard Selzer), autobiography (Gabriel Weston), and case studies (Oliver Sacks) or have mixed writing in poetic and in narrative form (William Carlos Williams) directly relating to their medical experience.

Why many doctors feel the need to write

'Medicine engages life's essential mysteries: the miraculous moment of birth, the jarring exit at death, the struggle to find meaning in suffering . . . [I]t is literature that most vividly grapples with such mysteries, and with the character of physician and poet'. These are the powerful words of Jerome Groopman (2007), a researcher in cancer and HIV-AIDS and a regular contributor to the *New Yorker* and the *New York Times*. He is referring as much to reading as to writing and as much to the work of patients as to that of medical professionals. As many doctor–writers testify, these mysteries are the fundamental subject of their writing, and the doctor–patient consultation is the spark that so often ignites their creativity.

The consultation relating to a serious medical condition requires complex intellectual and intuitive activity on the part of the physician for diagnosis in the context of a privileged intimacy between doctor and patient and, hopefully, of empathy and subtlety in communication between the two. In the words of doctor–poet Rafael Campo (2014), Director of Literature and Writing

 DOI: 10.4324/9781003341796-36

Programs of the Arts and Humanities Initiative at Harvard Medical School: 'It is those moments when I am in physical proximity to my patients where I am often most drawn to an imaginative experience of writing, when I want to be writing'.

Many doctors feel the need to compose creative works that distil the intensity and cognitive and emotional complexity inherent in the consultation. Indeed, writing – and reading – creative works may imaginatively develop and hone the imaginative skills that doctors depend on not only in communicating with their patients but also in the deeply intuitive business of diagnosis (Hanne 2015). Art Nahill (2022) continues,

> Both poetry and good doctoring are centred around observation, close observation, and pay-ing particular attention to the things that are not said rather than the things that are said. Letting a poem and a patient relationship and even a diagnosis develop before your eyes, rather than trying to force them into a particular construct.

Campo is one of several doctor-writers who refer to themselves as 'bearing witness' to their patients' experiences. Art Nahill (*ibid.*) insists on the symbiotic relationship between writing and medical practice thus:

> Poetry has both informed my clinical life and also been informed by it . . .. The skills that I have learned by sheer determination around writing poetry, I think have made me a better doctor and my experiences as a doctor have also helped me become a better poet'.

He particularly highlights the relevance of the ambiguities that are characteristic of poetry to his clinical work: '[Poetry] has helped me to sit much more comfortably with uncertainty . . . once you get into clinical medicine the vast majority of what you deal with is uncertainty'. More broadly, much writing by doctors stems from the fundamental paradox identified by Jennifer Okwerekwu, an American psychiatrist and writer, in the film *Why Doctors Write: Finding Humanity in Medi-cine*, that medicine is 'maddeningly beautiful' (Browne 2020). A specific instance of this paradox is captured by New Zealand oncologist/poet Rae Varcoe (2007) in the first lines of her poem 'The Cancer Cells Sum Up'. The poem begins: 'I am startled by the blue beauty/of the cancer cell'.

The descriptions our visiting doctor–poets give of the relationship between their two profes-sions are richly varied. Probably most vivid is that of Glenn Colquhoun (2016: 23), who recalls that he used to joke that

> poetry was the first girl I ever loved, the one I always wanted but never felt confident enough to ask out, and . . . medicine was the girl I got pregnant behind the bike shed and thought I had to make an honest woman of'.[1]

This is a (no-doubt conscious) variation on Chekhov's famous, but now distasteful, 'Medicine is my lawful wife, and literature my mistress. When I get fed up with one, I spend the night with the other'.[2]

My view is that most good doctors experience some kind of 'excess' that is left over from many of their consultations: of emotion, of curiosity, of diagnostic uncertainty, of things unsaid, and of doubts about their own effectiveness. I say 'good doctors' because it is clear that the medical professionals who engage most fully with their patients are those who listen best to them and are therefore likely to gain and retain the strongest sense of the patient as an individual.

Rafael Campo (2014) asserts that, 'poems really enact empathy'. Indeed, he suggests that there is an extent to which his writing serves as a medium through which patient experience may be communicated: 'my patients are in some sense writing through me'. Some doctor–writers productively imagine those large parts of the life stories of their patients that they cannot see. Greg Judkins (2020), another wonderful New Zealand doctor–writer, has written several short stories in a collection titled *Biopsies* in which he imagines the thoughts and home lives of patients he sees only briefly in his consulting room (see for instance the short story 'Makalofi'). Glenn Colquhoun (2002) wrote a pair of poems contrasting his emotions on different days: 'Today I do not want to be a doctor' and 'Today I want to be a doctor'. The first ends: 'Disease will not listen to me/Even when I shake my fist', and the second, 'Disease has gone weak at the knees./I expect him to make an appointment'.

Not just metaphor, not just poetry

An unfortunate tendency has grown up in medical humanities to view metaphor and narrative as rival approaches to medicine and to place poetry in opposition to narrative writing. Members of the narrative medicine movement assert the crucial role of story in communication between medical professionals and patients. While some of them record their patients' use of striking metaphors, and many employ vivid metaphors themselves about medical issues – Arthur Frank (2013), for instance, writes that 'Serious illness is a *loss* of the destination and *map* that had previously guided the ill person's life' – when they come to discuss metaphor in a medical context, they mostly treat it as a mere servant of story. So, Rita Charon's (2008) classic book *Narrative Medicine: Honoring the Stories of Illness* has just four lines in its index devoted to metaphor as against 36 devoted to narrative.

This shabby treatment of metaphor by narrative medicine has been valiantly called out in recent years by a number of commentators, most notably and effectively by the editors of this volume, Alan Bleakley (2017; Bleakley and Neilson 2021) and Shane Neilson (2022). They seek to 'challenge the dominance of narrative frames' and cite approvingly Cecile Alduy's (in Bleakley and Neilson 2021: 189) call 'to find ways to "release the grip" of the narrative impulse which permeates the way we think about ourselves and the world'. In defending metaphor and poetry against what they see as the domineering stance of narrative medicine and narrative writing, they mistakenly, I believe, privilege metaphor and poetry.

I don't think that is helpful. I subscribe to the grand claim made by philosopher of history Louis Mink (1978: 31) more than 30 years ago that narrative and metaphor are both 'primary cognitive instruments . . . irreducible ways of making the flux of experience comprehensible', and I insist that metaphor and narrative are complementary and most productively explored in combination. In the field of medicine, one of the few to have emphasized our reliance on narrative and metaphor in combination is Phil Barker (a professor of psychiatric nursing) (2000): 'life is a story best understood as an evolving narrative', to which he adds 'it is impossible to relate any aspect of my life experience directly. I need to use a foreign word or phrase to evoke its near inexpressibility. Life is so real I can meaningfully represent it only in metaphor'.

'Unexamined metaphors, uncharted stories'

The course I co-teach with Elisabeth Kumar, titled 'Unexamined metaphors, uncharted stories', takes the narrative medicine exponents to task for undervaluing metaphor but equally pushes back against those who seek to privilege metaphor at the expense of narrative. It utilizes insights from both the well-established narrative medicine movement and more recent work in metaphor studies around health, sickness, and offering and receiving treatment. We assert the need to view health, sickness, and medicine through the lens of metaphor and the lens of narrative *in combination*, thereby achieving a stereoscopic, three-dimensional image of the scene. This course and the conference I had the privilege of convening at UC Berkeley in 2010, titled Binocular Vision: Narrative and Metaphor in Medicine, both derive from that assertion (Hanne 2011).

We focus not only on explicitly literary work by doctors and medical students but on the many creative ways in which human beings employ narrative and metaphor to help us make meaning around health, sickness, and medical treatment. In addition to the abundant scholarly work that exists (most often on *either* narrative *or* metaphor, rarely both), we make use not only of creative writing by doctors, patients, and loved ones but also films and videos to illustrate each strand. (In their seminars, students occasionally bring our reference list up to date by presenting powerful works by musicians, especially rap artists such as Kendrick Lamar, on depression, grief, and the experience of cancer.

We accept the basic claims of narrative medicine that our individual identity is largely defined in terms of the 'library of stories' (Bruner 2002: 3–9) we tell ourselves and others and that serious illness disrupts the patient's self-narrative. We note, however, that in the consultation, patients not only tell a story of the symptoms they are experiencing but also use metaphors to convey physical sensations, emotional reactions, and their understandings of what is happening to them. Doctors need to attend closely to those stories and metaphors and invite the patient to elaborate on them, not only for strictly diagnostic purposes but also to gain a clear sense of the person as an individual, and what their condition means to them. Glenn Colquhoun (2002) writes,

> You probably think
> when I listen
> to your chest
> with my stethoscope
> I am listening
> to your heart.
> But I'm not.
> I am listening
> to your stories.
> I am throwing a line
> from one old ship
> To another.
> And swinging aboard.

The doctor who aspires to patient-centred, holistic care will attend closely to patients' own phrasing and assist them to elaborate on, or sometimes modify, that phrasing. We argue that respect for each patient, and the empathy doctors aspire to in best practice, are manifested very largely in the form of engagement with the narratives and metaphors of patients. 'Stories', write Rita Charon and Laurie Zoloth (2002: 21–36), 'call for response'. 'Metaphors', writes philosopher Ted Cohen (1978: 3), are 'an invitation . . . to intimacy'. Moreover, it is only possible for patients to make informed choices if such engagement has occurred. To the requirement referred to by Charon (2008) and others that doctors demonstrate 'narrative competence' should be added an insistence on 'metaphor competence'.

New Zealand poet Tracey Slaughter (2022) illustrates a failure of such competence as she writes of telling a doctor that, as each new drug was administered for the appalling pain she had been suffering for months,

> my body seems to turn the pain dial with each new dosage, forcing the nerve signals up, red hot and shrill over the block. The first time I stammer this out to a doctor he pats my hand patronisingly, saying 'My, you have a lively imagination'.

Many people who have experienced severe pain echo Emily Dickinson's description of the difficulty of communicating its severity to anyone else: 'Pain – has an element of blank'. Yet pain specialists have long used the McGill Pain Questionnaire, which offers a comprehensive array of metaphors from 'quivering' to 'pinching' to 'burning', among which the patient selects those terms that correspond most closely to their experience of pain (Melzack 1975). And wonderful poems, stories, and whole books have been written which seek to convey some sliver of the experience of pain. A fine example we refer to is Stephanie de Montalk's (2014/2018) book of creative nonfiction, *How Does it Hurt?*

The point has been well made by Saul Frederiksen (2002) and others that the introduction of X-ray and other imaging technology has resulted in diseases being increasingly 'concealed' from the patient's own sensory perception, with the result that metaphor is often the only way the patient can experience their own condition, let alone communicate it. As Susan M. DiGiacomo (1992) says, 'No-one ever experiences cancer as the uncontrolled proliferation of abnormal cells'. Regarding this and many other points, we draw attention to the inadequacy of Susan Sontag's (1978) assertion that we should liberate ourselves from the use of metaphor in medicine.

As doctors come to lay out diagnosis, prognosis, and treatment options to their patients, so it is incumbent on them to fashion stories and metaphors to fit the specific person, not just to get patients to grasp instructions but also to engage with their world. And when it comes to selecting among treatment options, narrative medicine proponent Howard Brody (1994) proposes the term 'co-authoring' for the process by which patient and doctor may jointly construct a story of management of the patient's condition. Narrative refers to agency to an extent that metaphor cannot. It is crucial, however, that metaphors within that narrative be jointly constructed, too.

Several doctors have created a repertoire of language devices for communicating with patients in relation to their specialism. A well-known example is G. Lorimer Mosely's (2007) *Painful Yarns: Metaphors and Stories to Help Understand the Biology of Pain*. Discussion of around the metaphors and narratives used by oncologists to discuss cancer and its treatment options with their patients has flowered, in the hands of Elena Semino and others, as a 'metaphor menu for people living with cancer' (see: https://wp.lancs.ac.uk/melc/the-metaphor-menu/). This goes beyond the contrasting 'battle' and 'journey' metaphors to other metaphors by which patients may acknowledge that their cancer is not something that has come from outside or see themselves as in some kind of personal relationship with cancer. In an interview shortly before he died, New Zealand industrialist and philanthropist Rob Fenwick (2020) explained,

> For five years, I have danced with cancer. I refuse to call it a struggle or a battle – I am dancing with the disease. We swing, we twist, sometimes we lift, and too often we step on each other's feet. But my determined dance partner will end our dance before I'm ready.

Narrative therapy has been developed as a means by which psychologists and counsellors work with people to explore the self-narratives by which they define themselves, focusing especially on dysfunctional stories ('I can be relied on to mess up any relationship I get into' and so forth) that can be amended in a therapeutic context. While they often term themselves 'narrative therapists' (Polkinghorne 2004), they clearly work as often on the dysfunctional metaphors that patients use as on their stories. So, another visitor to our course, narrative therapist Sarah Penwarden (2006), who works with school students, explains the strategies she uses to assist them. When someone talks of being 'sucked down a well of depression', the therapist elaborates stories by which the patient might escape the well or avoid approaching it, so that the patient can play with them and develop alternative stories and metaphors.[3] Doctors can readily borrow these strategies and use them with their patients – if their appointment schedules permit, of course! As for psychiatrists and psychologists, it is worth noting that the former, relying as they primarily do on chemical medication, make much less use of narrative and metaphor than the latter. More broadly, it may also be said that the two vocations operate in terms of very different explanatory and treatment narratives.

One of the most pervasive emotions witnessed (and experienced) by medical professionals is grief. We draw attention to the variety of health contexts in which grief is experienced: you receive a life-limiting diagnosis, either for yourself or, worst of all, for your child; you witness the suffering of a loved one; you discover that you have inherited a predisposition to a serious health condition; you face your own death or that of a family member. (Many doctors would echo the lament of Atul Gawande (2014: 1) that 'I learned a lot of things in medical school, but mortality wasn't one of them'.) While the work of Elizabeth Kűbler-Ross on death and dying in the 1960s and 70s was extraordinarily valuable in bringing both medical professionals and the general public to focus on a topic they had preferred to ignore, her suggestion that we may experience 'stages of grief' has been adopted by many health professionals as an over-rigid narrative formula, with 'denial' being inevitably followed by 'anger', then 'bargaining', then 'depression', then 'acceptance'. Sasha McAllum Pilkington, a therapist at a local hospice, visits the course and acquaints us with the most recent research, which shows that people experience and express grief in much more individual and less orderly ways. To illustrate this point, we read Anatole Broyard's (1989) wonderful essay 'About Men: Intoxicated by my illness', in which he comments,

> When my friends heard I had cancer, they found me surprisingly cheerful and talked about my courage. But it has nothing to do with courage, at least not for me. As far as I can tell, it's a question of desire – to live, to write, to do everything. Desire itself is a kind of immortality. While I've always had difficulty concentrating, I now feel as concentrated as a diamond, or a microchip.

Pilkington describes how she engages with terminally ill patients to assist them to unpack and review their life stories in ways that encourage them to see the value of their story and to decide how they will live out the final chapter. By also presenting her research articles in narrative form, rather than the traditional scholarly analytical form, she leads the reader through the process she employs (see: www.researchgate.net/profile/Sasha-Pilkington).

Students consider some of the many poems, essays, and stories that reflect on the nature of death and how to face it, from John Donne's 'Death be not proud' to Dylan Thomas's 'Do not go gentle into that good night', concluding with the folk wisdom of the cemetery sexton in a story by funeral director and writer Thomas Lynch (2000: 31–37): 'Copulation, population, inspiration, expiration. It's all arithmetic'. A local poet, Johanna Emeney (2017), reads poems to the class about witnessing her mother's experience with terminal breast cancer. In a poem titled 'And then it spreads', she writes,

Of course, I'd read up –
Bought every heavy oncology tome
on the tendency of this cancer
to spread metastases to bone,
like the ugly towels of tourists
all over the beach in summer.

But she then records that her mother's life ended in a quite different way:

My mother wasn't
supposed to die

in a car crash caused by a boy racer
who took a chance at the crossroads:
she was destined for cancer – staged.

Key insights are gained from articles by palliative care workers, who seek to ensure that the metaphors which pass backwards and forwards between them and terminally ill patients and their families are as constructive and comforting as possible. They find poetry in the words of a family member who says. 'Losing your parents is like losing the tent poles out of your tent' (Spall et al. 2001).

The students are invited to recognize, as many medical practitioners do not, that modern bio-medicine – while it is rigorously scientific in that it is based on experimental evidence – is actually structured around three major metaphors: mechanical, military, and informationist. Using an essay by Scott Montgomery (1996) as our guide, we briefly trace the history of the adoption of these metaphors: first, the mechanical, which developed alongside the evolution of hydraulics, the combustion engine, and telegraphy; then the military, which developed out of Pasteur's theories around bacterial infection as he applied them in the context of the Franco-German War; and, most recently, the informationist metaphors, with their prime source in computing.

We highlight the extent to which each set of metaphors has generated valuable research and possibilities for intervention while also acknowledging that they are inadequate for achieving psycho-social goals in that they do not focus attention on the overall wellbeing of the patient. For this reason, medical professionals need to build more human metaphors into their repertoire. It is the lack of these that enables proponents of much alternative or complementary medicine to gain the trust of so many people with the use of metaphors such as 'energy system', 'equilibrium', 'cleanse', 'purify', and 'wholeness' – that are almost empty of scientific meaning (for a more positive view see Stibbe 1998). A number of researchers (including practising homeopaths) have found that claims for the validity of homeopathy are best understood as expressing belief in the therapeutic power of metaphor (Konitzer et al. 2002).

There is a strong focus in the course on issues around cross-cultural medical practice. The understanding that patients bring to the medical consultation reflects their education and personal views but, above all, their cultural backgrounds. Ethnographers identify the distinctive conceptual metaphors employed by different cultures to convey their understanding of health and disease (e.g. Traditional Chinese medicine's (TCM) 'flow' and 'balance' versus Western 'attack' and 'defence' – see for example Pritzker 2003). While biomedicine is increasingly the dominant approach worldwide to health and sickness, and evidence-based discoveries from non-Western countries are feeding into biomedicine, we highlight the fact that patients may bring with them very different frames of reference and understanding. Doctors should not, however, assume that an ethnic Chinese patient will necessarily have a deep knowledge of TCM or that an indigenous Māori patient will have a detailed knowledge of Rongoā Māori (see: www.healthnavigator.org.nz/ health-a-z/r/rongo%C4%81-m%C4%81ori/). Like most Western patients, they are likely to have a rudimentary acquaintance with some of the main metaphors of their traditional medical systems. So, the Chinese patient may see their condition as determined by the balance between hot and cold in the food they consume, or the Māori patient may believe that their illness has been caused by the breaking of *tapu*, or even by *makutu* (sorcery). In either case, doctors ignore that understanding at their – and the patient's – peril. Indeed, in a loose sense, they should recognize the poetry embodied in indigenous understandings of health and medicine.

While it is unrealistic to expect doctors to study closely the traditional medical thinking of all the cultures they encounter, it is crucial that they engage in some way with the explanatory metaphors and narratives patients bring with them. The question 'How do you understand what is happening to you?' (whether referring to symptoms or to treatment) seems the best way to engage with the patient's thinking. By and large, it will not be helpful simply to deny the validity of what the patient says. Many doctors have a good relationship with some traditional healers and, where there is mutual respect, it may be possible for them to collaborate in treating the individual patient. A doctor may attend respectfully to the traditional metaphors that patients bring with them, while explaining 'the way we look at your condition is . . .'. Overall, 'success' from a holistic (psychosocial) approach will involve contributing to the patient's personal and cultural wellbeing as well as to their clinical health. We view a fine video, made in 2003 by Maren Grainger-Monsen for the Stanford Program in Bioethics and Film, titled *Worlds Apart* in which a pious Muslim patient has refused a chemotherapeutic implant because he believed he would not be able to fulfil the purity requirements for daily prayer with it inside him. The message that chemotherapy could have been administered by means other than the implant had not been adequately communicated to him.

Many of the issues which arise under the broad heading of 'medical ethics' are usefully approached with insights from narrative studies. Philosopher Alasdair MacIntyre (1984), a major proponent of narrative ethics, asks, 'How can I know what I should do if I don't know what story I am part of?' We explore some of the many medical contexts in which this question is relevant, including abortion and euthanasia. Sharon Olds' (2004) poem 'The Promise', in which the speaker and her partner affirm once again their commitment to kill the other out of love if either is suffering incurable distress, dramatizes the latter issue. The poet illustrates beautifully the claim by philosophers such as Mark Johnson that ethics depends as much on metaphor as it does on narrative, with her use of images of 'binding' and 'tying'. She recalls the grandmother so afflicted by dementia that she was *tied* to a chair; she reflects on the way in which they are *bound* to each other in sex but concludes, 'if the ropes/*binding* your soul are your own wrists, I will *cut* them'. We also draw students' attention to the ethical implications of the many competing narratives at work in medical schools and hospitals. We view extracts from Mike Nichols's film *Wit*, starring Emma Thompson, which exemplifies the clash that may occur when the research narrative is given priority over the care narrative as a gruelling chemotherapy treatment is employed on a patient with an incurable cancer long after it might have been useful.

Big ethical questions arise in the fields of epidemiology and public health. We follow Nancy Krieger (1994) in evaluating different metaphorical models for causation and for inequities in the incidence of illness. The cover of a report developed by the MacArthur Foundation – *Reaching for a healthier life: Facts on socioeconomic status and health* – offers a vivid image of fundamental health inequities: a set of shelves, with five apples arrayed on the top shelf, four on the next shelf, descending to half an apple on the sixth, a quarter apple on the seventh and no apple at all on the eighth (see: https://scholar.harvard.edu/davidrwilliams/reports/reaching-healthier-life). We read the story told by sociologist Irving Zola of the doctor who says that he has no time as he repeatedly dives into the river to save drowning patients to ask the crucial question 'who the hell is throwing them in?' (Tones and Tilford 2003). One of our students with a background in public health gave a seminar on the inadequacies of the image of the 'fence at the top of the cliff and the ambulance at the bottom' for prevention and treatment of illness. Increasingly, as Janine Talley (2011) explains, '[s]tories and metaphors are seen as tools for empowerment, valuable social and cultural assets containing knowledge and resources for building community, solving problems, creating resilience, and galvanizing action'. In a specifically New Zealand context, we examine the causal connection between colonization, with the disastrous dispossession of land, language, and culture suffered by Māori and their current shocking health status. (Māori die at twice the rate of non-Māori from cardiovascular disease. Māori children have a mortality rate 1.5 times the rate for non-Māori children. Māori are more likely to be diagnosed late and die from cancer. Māori die on average seven years earlier than non-Māori; see: www.healthnavigator.org.nz/clinicians/m/m%C4%81ori-health-overview/). We read poems and creative pieces which record personal experience of these issues, such as doctor Greg Judkins' (2022) poem 'Wheel of Fortune':

> When you go with a list of four problems
> but the doctor has time for just two,
> when you've scraped up his fee since last pay day
> and there's scarcely enough left for food,
>
> how does it feel to be bound to a wheel
> in a life as surreal as a circus?

And we assess recommendations for public policies which might gradually tackle the health inequities experienced by Māori (and by Pasifika migrants and their families), including, at this moment, the setting up of a state-funded separate Māori Health Authority (Te Aka Whai Ora), to reset health policy in ways that respond to Māori values, needs, and demands. We draw attention to the metaphors of *te whare tapa whā* (the house of wellbeing), *te pae mahutonga* (the Southern Cross), and *te wheke* (the octopus of health), devised by Māori public health professionals to represent the kind of health care system they want to see, which would value family, ancestral, spiritual, environmental, and other perspectives on wellbeing alongside mere physical health (see: www.health.govt.nz/our-work/populations/maori-health/maori-health-models). The metaphor-narrative connection in public policy is something that philosopher Donald Schön (1993) has illuminated, pointing out that when we adopt a specific metaphor to characterize a situation, we will tend to assume the validity of narratives generated by that metaphor to solve it.

During the COVID-19 pandemic, policy makers, and the media have employed an abundance of metaphors and associated narratives to refer to the process by which the infection spreads and mutates and the interventions which might be used to control its spread and reduce its health, economic, and other impacts (see Special issue on COVID-19 of *Metaphor and Symbol* 2022; 37: 2). If, as so many national leaders (including Donald Trump, Boris Johnson, and Emmanuel Macron) did, you assert the metaphor of 'a war' on the pandemic, then you become 'commander-in-chief', and a limited array of policy narratives is presented to the public. Hanne (2022) argues that countries which seized on the 'war' metaphor were, by and large, the least successful in dealing with the pandemic. Earlier researchers (Hanne and Hawken 2007) examined the fact that metaphors employed by the media to represent different health conditions (from cancer to HIV-AIDS and avian flu) shape public perception of the condition and those who suffer from it in important ways.

Students' writing

As for how creative writing may feel relevant and useful to medical students and junior doctors, our students, both in their writing and in discussion, offer many insights. Unsurprisingly, much of their writing relates to the stresses associated with acquiring so much medical knowledge and mentally filing it away in the hope that it will be accessible for exams and future practice. They hear from both Art Nahill (who grew up and trained in Massachusetts) and Glenn Colquhoun (who grew up and trained in NZ) that, at times when they felt like quitting, it was their focus on writing poetry that kept them in their medical training.

Students take our course just before they begin the clinical component in their education, which means they have actually met very few patients. The one 'patient' they have got to know well is the cadaver from which they have gained much of their knowledge of anatomy, and their writing about cadaver dissection is always fascinating. The questions our students put to the visiting medical professionals most commonly begin with the phrase 'What's it like when . . . ?' They read with great attention the documentary, as well as the poetic and fictional, accounts by doctors of their work lives, especially those working in the New Zealand health system. They read not only *Things that Matter: Stories of Life and Death* by experienced intensive care specialist David Galler (2016) but also the wonderful *Vital Signs*, by Izzie Lomax-Sawyers (2022), which tells 'heartbreaking, sometimes hilarious stories of a junior doctor's first year working in a hospital'. They read the writings of a graduate from our programme, Maria Yeonhee Ji, including her poem 'Thirteen Ways of Looking at a Patient'[4] and her critical essay 'The Truths We Bury about Childbirth in Aotearoa'.[5]

Each student builds up a portfolio of work, and a selection from these portfolios is circulated as an anthology at the end of the year. We draw students' attention to the many national and international competitions for creative work by medical professionals and students[6] and the prestigious medical journals which accept creative submissions.[7] In the poems and short prose pieces they write, they convey both their eagerness to enter practice and their anxiety about whether they will be ready to do so. They are acutely aware that they will be applying their book-learning and technical skills to real human beings and, with our encouragement, reflect on the emotional, moral, and communication issues they will be facing when they do so. They use their own experiences of ill health in their family, of medical treatment, and for example of grief at the death of a grandparent as touchstones for imagining aspects of future practice.

One of the many challenges we put to them is the question of whether, before they start practice, they need to confront the fact of their own mortality. The title of the film *Why Doctors Write: Finding Humanity in Medicine* captures the essence of what they and we are seeking to do. One of the student contributors to that film comments that 'As a medical student you can go an entire day without talking' and that writing courses serve 'to help students develop a voice'. Another student in the film observes, 'I had no idea when I started medical school that it was going to be connected to so many large questions in life and society, and so I think being able to write gives you a repository for all those experiences'. Writing will often assist students – and, of course, practitioners at any stage in their career – to work through problems they encounter. In the words of Jennifer Okwerekwu, writing is especially productive when you are 'stuck' in any context.[8]

However widely our students range in their reading and reflections, much of their writing returns to the mixture of delight and terror that they experience as we meet them, halfway through their basic medical education. Here is a piece by Eileen O'Reilly, who studied with us in 2009, that captures that ambivalence, in a delightfully simple form somewhere between poetry and prose:

Medicine is the backyard I played in with my sister when I was young./It is a sprawling overgrown garden with hiding places, wildflowers and ladybugs, and so many exciting possibilities./The patients are the broken sparrows we cared for after the wind blew them into the thick green bristling hedge line./And the sick hedgehog who died, vulnerable, bringing a sense of sadness and compassion./My knowledge is the tree house we built in the giant pine in the corner. There is pride in achievement, and anticipation of further building./Medicine is also the swamp in the back paddock. Fear rises at the thought of the unknown and a feeling of doom at being caught in the dark weed strewn mud.

Notes

1 Colquhoun acknowledges that in recent years, the faces of the two lovers have merged: 'On my best days there is no separation at all between both disciplines'.
2 In a letter to his friend Alexei Suvorin, 11 September 1888. See www.gutenberg.org/files/6408/6408-h/6408-h.htm#link2H_4_0041
3 Stephen S. Pearce (1996) is one of the few who explicitly employ the binocular vision we recommend in treating mental distress.
4 This poem was awarded third prize in the prestigious international Hippocrates Prize for Poetry and Medicine. Hear her read it at www.youtube.com/watch?v=fxqlglkgNgE. The title and structure of the poem are modelled on Wallace Stevens' poem 'Thirteen Ways of Looking at a Blackbird', which can be found at www.poetryfoundation.org/poems/45236/thirteen-ways-of-looking-at-a-blackbird
5 *The Pantograph Punch*, May 2019.[0]
6 http://hippocrates-poetry.org/ For other competitions for medical students, see www.alphaomegaalpha.org/programs/the-pharos-poetry-award/; www.neomed.edu/wcw-poetry-competition/; www.bcm.edu/departments/surgery/education/debakey-poetry-contest; https://nzmsj.scholasticahq.com/section/1782-creative-arts; https://medicine.uiowa.edu/md/student-support/opportunities-growth/writing-and-humanities-program/creative-writing-contest; www.ucl.ac.uk/news/2021/feb/yale-ucl-poetry-competition-winners-announced
7 See https://yasminealimd.com/5-medical-and-healthcare-publications-that-accept-non-research-submissions/
8 Those perspectives are developed in a panel discussion chaired by a central figure in that film, Danielle Ofri: www.youtube.com/watch?v=ncGnmI8IKSU.

References

Barker P. Working with the Metaphor of Life and Death. *Journal of Medical Ethics*. 2000; 26: 97–102.
Bleakley A. 2017. *Thinking With Metaphors in Medicine: The State of the Art*. Abingdon: Routledge.
Bleakley A, Neilson S. 2021. *Poetry in the Clinic: Towards a Lyrical Medicine*. Abingdon: Routledge.
Brody H. My Story is Broken; Can You Help Me Fix It? Medical Ethics and the Joint Construction of Narrative. *Literature and Medicine*. 1994; 13: 79–92.
Browne K. (Director.) 2020. *Why Doctors Write: Finding Humanity in Medicine*. Newton, MA: Center for Independent Documentary. Trailer available at: www.whydoctorswrite.org/about. Last accessed: 22/12/2023.
Broyard A. 1989. About Men: Intoxicated by My Illness. *New York Times Magazine*, November 12.
Bruner J. 2002. Narratives of Human Plight: A Conversation with Jerome Bruner. In: R Charon, M Montello (eds.) *Stories Matter: The Role of Narrative in Medical Ethics*. New York, NY: Routledge, 3–9.
Campo R. 2014. *The Arts of Healing, Paul Holdengraber in Conversation With M.D and Poet Rafael Campo*. Available at: www.youtube.com/watch?v=-LksXrCQN5Y. Last accessed: 4/1/2023.
Charon R. 2008. *Narrative Medicine: Honoring the Stories of Illness*. Oxford: Oxford University Press.
Charon R, Zoloth L. 2002. Like an Open Book: Reliability, Intersubjectivity, and Textuality in Bioethics. In: R Charon, M Montello (eds.) *Stories Matter: The Role of Narrative in Medical Ethics*. New York, NY: Routledge, 21–36.

Cohen T. Metaphor and the Cultivation of Intimacy. *Critical Inquiry*. 1978; 5: 3–12.

Colquhoun G. 2002. *Playing God*. Wellington: Steele Roberts.

Colquhoun G. 2016. *Late Love: Sometimes Doctors Need Saving as Much as Their Patients*. Wellington: Bridget Williams.

de Montalk S. 2014. *How Does it Hurt?* Wellington: Victoria University Press. Republished as: *Communicating Pain: Exploring Suffering Through Language, Literature, and Creative Writing*. London/New York: Routledge, 2018.

DiGiacomo SM. Metaphor as Illness: Postmodern Dilemmas in the Representation of Body, Mind, and Disorder. *Medical Anthropology*. 1992; 14: 109–37.

Emeney J. 2017. *Family History*. Wellington: Mākaro Press.

Fenwick R. 2020. Shelter From the Storm. *New Zealand Listener*, March 7–13.

Frank A. 2013. *The Wounded Storyteller: Body, Illness & Ethics* (2nd ed.). Chicago, IL: University of Chicago Press.

Frederiksen S. Diseases are Invisible. *Medical Humanities*. 2002; 28: 71–73.

Galler G. 2016. *Things That Matter: Stories of Life and Death*. Auckland: Allen and Unwin.

Gawande A. 2014. *Being Mortal: Illness, Medicine, and What Matters in the End*. London: Profile Books.

Groopman J. 2007. Prescribed Reading. *New York Times Book Review*, May 13.

Hanne M. The Binocular Vision Project: An introduction. *Genre: Forms of Discourse and Culture*. 2011; 44: 223–37.

Hanne M. Diagnosis and Metaphor. *Perspectives in Biology and Medicine*. 2015; 58: 35–52.

Hanne M. How We Escape Capture by the "War" Metaphor for Covid-19. *Metaphor and Symbol*. 2022; 37: 88–100.

Hanne M, Hawken SJ. Metaphors for Illness in Contemporary Media. *Medical Humanities*. 2007; 33: 93–99.

Judkins G. 2020. *Biopsies: Stories of Struggle and Hope in South Auckland*. Auckland: Greg Judkins.

Judkins G. 2022. *Shrapnel: Fragments We Carry for Life*. Auckland: Greg Judkins.

Konitzer M, Wiebke S, Freudenberg N, Fischer GC. Therapeutic Interaction Through Metaphor: A Textual Approach to Homeopathy. *Semiotica*. 2002; 141: 1–27.

Krieger N. Epidemiology and the Web of Causation: Has Anyone Seen the Spider? *Social Science and Medicine*. 1994; 39: 887–903.

Lomax-Sawyers I. 2022. *Vital Signs*. Auckland: Allen and Unwin.

Lynch T. 2000. *Bodies in Motion and at Rest: On Metaphor and Mortality*. New York, NY: W.W. Norton.

MacIntyre A. 1984. *After Virtue: A Study in Moral Theory* (2nd ed.). Notre Dame, Indiana: University of Notre Dame Press.

Melzack R. The McGill Pain Questionnaire: Major Properties and Scoring Methods. *Pain*. 1975; 1: 277–99.

Mink L. 1978. Narrative Form as a Cognitive Instrument. In: RH Canary, H Kosicki (eds.) *The Writing of History: Literary Form and Historical Understanding*. Madison, WI: University of Wisconsin Press, 31.

Montgomery SL. 1996. Illness and Image: An Essay on the Contents of Biomedical Discourse. In: *The Scientific Voice*. New York, NY: Guilford Press, 134–95.

Mosely GL. 2007. *Painful Yarns: Metaphors and Stories to Help Understand the Biology of Pain*. Canberra: Dancing Giraffe Press.

Nahill A. 2022. Personal Correspondence.

Neilson S. A Logical Development: Biomedicine's Fingerprints are on the Instrument of Close Reading in Charonian Narrative Medicine. *Medical Humanities*. 2022; 48: e9.

Olds S. 2004. *Strike Sparks: Selected Poems 1980–2002*. New York, NY: Alfred A Knopf.

Pearce SS. 1996. *Flash of Insight: Metaphor and Narrative in Therapy*. Needham Heights, MA: Allyn and Bacon.

Penwarden S. Turning Depression on Its Head: Employing Creativity to Map Out and Externalise Depression in Conversations With Young Women. *The International Journal of Narrative Therapy and Community Work*. 2006; 1: 65–70.

Polkinghorne DE. 2004. Narrative Therapy and Postmodernism. In: LE Angus, J McLeod (eds.) *The Handbook of Narrative and Psychotherapy: Practice, Theory and Research*. Thousand Oaks, CA: Sage, 53–58.

Pritzker S. The Role of Metaphor in Culture: Consciousness, and Medicine: A Preliminary Inquiry into the Metaphors of Depression in Chinese and Western Medical and Common Languages. *Clinical Acupuncture and Oriental Medicine*. 2003; 4: 11–28.

Schön D. 1993. Generative Metaphor: A Perspective on Problem-Setting in Social Policy. In: A Ortony (ed.) *Metaphor and Thought*. Cambridge: Cambridge University Press, 254–58.

Slaughter T. 2022. Notes on a Scale of Silence. *The Spinoff*, December 17.

Sontag S. 1978. *Illness as Metaphor*. New York, NY: Farrar Strauss Giroux.

Spall B, Read S, Chantry D. Metaphor: Exploring its Origins and Therapeutic Use in Death, Dying and Bereavement. *International Journal of Palliative Nursing*. 2001; 7: 345–53.

Stibbe A. The Role of Image Systems in Complementary Medicine. *Complementary Therapies in Medicine*. 1998; 6: 190–94.

Talley J. Metaphor, Narrative and the Promotion of Public Health. *Genre*. 2011; 44: 405–23.

Tones K, Tilford S. 2003. *Health Promotion: Effectiveness, Efficiency, and Equity* (3rd ed.). London: Chapman and Hall.

Varcoe R. 2007. *Tributary*. Wellington: Victoria University Press.

29

ON THE READING LIST FOR ALL TRAINEE MEDICS

Autobiography of a Marguerite by Zarah Butcher-McGunnigle

Johanna Emeney

Published when the poet was 24, the poems in *Autobiography of a Marguerite* tell the story of a young writer, Marguerite, navigating the health care system as she seeks treatment for an unnamed autoimmune condition. At her side is her mother, also named Marguerite. The enmeshed nature of the pair's relationship and the young woman's struggle for autonomy and identity are central to the collection. Another of the book's key preoccupations is the tension inherent in doctor–patient communication. Zarah Butcher-McGunnigle forces readers to experience the frustration and powerlessness of the patient-speaker's position by means of strategic linguistic choices. She presents readers with the depersonalizing effects of the health care system by demonstrating its clinical and excluding language in poems about medical encounters. In these poems, she also illustrates the ways in which playful, repetitive diction, and an insistence on the ambiguous and subjective, can become a mode of resistance.

It is of significance that the poet's own emotionally damaging experiences in the New Zealand health care system led her to eschew medical care for 10 years, during which her autoimmune disease worsened considerably. This collection is a clarion call for a medicine that is more holistic, compassionate, and personal. I would recommend *Autobiography of a Marguerite* to any medical student and to any medical humanities course coordinator. It has the capacity to enrich understanding and empathy in medical students and medical practitioners with regard to the experience of chronic pain and to encourage different communication behaviours that allow for the psychosocial life of the patient to be more actively attended to during consultations and during the formulation of treatment plans. For, as we have known for several decades, giving attention to psychosocial issues improves health outcomes.

Since the 1980s, sociolinguists have found that doctors and patients approach the chronicling of illness differently, particularly in the doctor–patient interview. Doctors, seeking foremost to find diagnostic clues and 'to accomplish their clinical tasks as systematically and efficiently as they can' (Hydén and Mishler 1999: 178), focus on timelines involving dates and the appearance and exacerbation of various symptoms. Patients, however, find biomedical data inextricable from diurnal realities – illness occurs alongside family troubles or key life events; it affects job performance; it may be worsened by stress, grief, or anxiety; it might respond well to alternative

DOI: 10.4324/9781003341796-37

therapies. These conflicting communicative approaches have been studied extensively by sociologists and psychologists:

> In typical interviews, physicians either ignore or interrupt patients' storied accounts. The traditional medical "story" of illness is in the form of a chronicle in which signs and symptoms are ordered sequentially but removed from the larger context of patients' lives. In their stories, patients try to restore this context, locating the trajectory of symptoms within their daily experiences, specifying their impact on how they can function personally and socially, reporting their own remedial and reparative efforts.
>
> (Hydén and Mishler 1999: 178)

For Butcher-McGunnigle, the patient's placement of the biomedical within the framework of the personal and the social is of great importance. She is at pains to convey that no part of experience can be excised and appraised in a purely clinical chronology. To this end, the poet chooses to give overt focus to the subjective in *Autobiography of a Marguerite*. She seeks out ambiguity and exploits it in a way that is both humorous and pointed. Her writing employs figurative language counter to the concreteness of medical language's precision. The poet demonstrates a fine understanding of medical terminology throughout the collection, but she also balances medicalese against deliberate opacity and homonymous repetition. Take for example this extract from her poem in which the speaker, attempting to make bread, is beset by medical anxieties as well as the smothering presence of her mother:

> . . . I cannot stand in
> one place for very long, because of my knees. The cookbook
> on the bench is called I Hate to Cook. My mother comes
> into the kitchen and says, I need the oven soon, so hurry
> up.
>
> . . .
>
> I look at my knees and
> they are like dough.
>
> . . .
>
> I'm not
> articulate. What am I trying to prove. My mother comes into
> the kitchen and says, I need you.
>
> (Butcher-McGunnigle 2014: 16)

Of note in this poem is the way in which Butcher-McGunnigle consciously eschews the word 'knead', instead choosing to employ its definition (see original full poem lines 1–2), its near-homonyms 'knees' (3,10) and 'knee' (line 11) and its full homonym (lines 8, 15). It is in the same vein that, throughout the book, she will not name her chronic autoimmune condition. This deliberate withholding is a sort of powerplay which she presents here for the first time. She, of course, knows the word 'knead'; she can give us words which are very similar; she will even give us the synonym 'prove' (15), but she will not give the readers the one word for which they are searching. The thing that she is 'trying to prove' (15) despite her claims otherwise is how 'articulate' (14) she is despite the problems with her joints' articulations. She is also making the reader sit with ambiguity, however frustrating and testing it may feel. For this is what a patient does very often: awaiting a diagnosis; not knowing how an illness will progress; wondering if tests will yield poor or good results.

In Danielle Ofri's (2017: 1657) article regarding the value of the humanities to medical training, she makes the point that

> the humanities can offer doctors a paradigm for living with ambiguity and even for relishing it. Great works of literature, art, theater, and music specialize in ambiguity, confusion, and frailty. Unlike medicine, the humanities do not shy away from uncertainty. They revel in the depth and breadth that ambiguity affords.

In many ways, this 'living with ambiguity' (*ibid.*) is what *Autobiography of a Marguerite* enacts. Not only does the reader have to accept ambiguity, but also the reader comes to understand the constant state of flux experienced by the patient as she seeks diagnosis and treatment. There is little *revelling* (*ibid.*) as in Ofri's description, but an expansive empathetic leap is definitely required of the reader. For example, one of the early poems enables the reader to feel something of Marguerite's frustration with endless appointments and appraisals by means of repetition and ambiguity:

> It is not even a story. Every day I have to cross a bridge.
> The patient back and forth motion. The patient
> back and forth. The patient's back. The patience.
>   (Butcher-McGunnigle 2014: 7, lines 1–3)

Auckland Hospital is accessed via Grafton Bridge. Crossing a bridge is a commonly used metaphor for travelling between two states of being: in this case, from Sontag's kingdom of the well into the kingdom of the sick, and back. 'The patient/back and forth' (2–3) not only suggests the regular visits to and returns from the hospital but also perhaps the way in which she might be asked to walk up and down for doctors as they assess her proprioception, stability, and movement (2), as well as the alignment of her spine (3). All of these possible readings suggest that what the patient is going through takes a good deal of 'patience' (3). The repetitions are somewhat tedious for the reader and must be so for the 'I' who is constantly in movement and never finished with the task of being a 'patient' (2). 'It is not even a story' (1) because it lacks a beginning and ending. There is only this bridge (1).

In this first section of the book, the speaker describes her daily experiences, peppering them with the ways in which her chronic illness impinges on everyone, from making bread to breaking it at the dinner table with her increasingly estranged parents. Butcher-McGunnigle uses these diurnal snapshots to invite the reader into the larger dysfunction of her life. What she presents in these poems is essentially social psychologist Elliot Mishler's (1984: 190) 'voice of the lifeworld', communicating the ways in which her condition affects the everyday, and the ways in which the everyday affects her condition.

In his ground-breaking monograph *The Discourse of Medicine: Dialectics of Medical Interviews*, Mishler (*ibid.*) studied doctor–patient appointments, finding that 'lifeworld' talk (*ibid.*: 190) – about the patient's family, life, job, social and economic status – often went unheard or unencouraged by doctors who chose to focus on the biomedical realities of the patient's situation, drowning out the 'voice of the lifeworld' with the more dominating 'voice of medicine' (*ibid.*). To make doctor–patient talk more interactional and less biomedically controlled, Mishler posited, would be to acknowledge the core relationship between the psychosocial and the biophysical and therefore to make diagnosis and treatment more accurate, personalized, and successful.

Poems in *Autobiography of a Marguerite* 30 years on from Mishler's studies seem to match his findings,[1] summarized here:

> physicians controlled the flow of the clinical interview: (1) through their ways of asking questions; (2) by interrupting patients' efforts to say more than was asked for, often in the form of stories; (3) and by ignoring, that is, refusing to acknowledge or respond to patients' accounts of the effects on their daily lives of symptoms of their illness.
>
> (Mishler 2005: 437)

One poem, describing a pain clinic appointment, presents a scenario in which communication between doctor and patient is hindered by medicalized language – both written and oral – and questions which seek to elicit precision despite their fundamental vagueness. The poem opens with the ubiquitous pain scale:

> . . . On a scale
> of one to ten, I can never just pick a number. On a scale
> of one to then. The doctor is looking at my form. I nod and
> smile when she says something I don't hear. On the desk is a
> packet of "non-sterile" latex gloves. She leans closer to me,
> pointing to the form. So, when rating your progress, from
> the choices of: quicker than expected, as expected, and
> slower than expected, you circled *my progress is slower than*
> *expected*. Why did you circle that?

Butcher-McGunnigle says that she doesn't know: 'Because I'm still in pain, because I noticed/ improvement before and now I don't?' She looks at her watch and then realises that she is not wearing a watch. The doctor interrupts with a conundrum: 'is progress slower than you expected or slower than you hoped?' (Butcher-McGunnigle 2014: 22).

The poem presents biomedicine as characterized by a desire to narrow down, to close in on – to rate pain on a 1–10 scale. The patient, however, is clearly frustrated and constrained by form-filling; she seems to express a desire to explore more complex concepts, such as the difficulty of dealing with the difference between her life before the illness and since the illness ('On a scale/of one to then' (3–4)).[2] The patient's thoughts are far more multifaceted and equivocal than a scale might reflect: retrograde steps after seeming improvement (12–13) cannot be described as 'progress' (15), and we are led to believe that being able to talk about the disappointment and confusion associated with this unexpected trajectory instead of choosing between two variations of numbered explicatory statements would be better suited to this patient – indeed to many patients. Throughout the collection, Marguerite's highly personalized story works in this way; her individual situation, anonymized condition, and utterly singular voice transcend uniqueness, becoming universal.

As noted by doctor and writer Iona Heath (2016), there is a temptation in medicine to choose the numerical over the lexical despite the fact that words are the things that convey the trust and empathy patients need from their doctors when dealing with and adjusting to complex and frightening health issues:

> At its starkest, the rift is between numbers and words. Numbers have seductive beauty and purity that suggest solidity and certainty. Words are infinitely malleable and adaptable but can communicate much more. We try to define disease using numbers, but this has separated the map from the territory even further. Words are essential to help patients to understand what is happening to them and what might help. Only with words can we forge trust, relieve fear, and find meaning.

Numerically based forms and questionnaires with absurdly utilitarian medical metaphors and similes feature frequently in the collection. Butcher-McGunnigle uses them as lines of found poetry to articulate how useless such documents are to the speaker, and, by ironic implication, how useful some form of empathetic human interaction might be:

> . . . Question: How would you
> describe the pain? For example, is it like being stabbed with
> a piece of glass. My mother takes the paper from me, Would
> it be helpful if I did the writing. But I don't know, I say, I've
> never been stabbed with a piece of glass.
> (Butcher-McGunnigle 2014: 12, lines 6–10)

Part of this acquisitive play with the language of the forms is, of course, dark humour. However, the main point is Butcher-McGunnigle's critique of pain scales such as the McGill Pain Questionnaire – tools designed to measure treatment outcomes and patient progress. The intent of such documents is to combine sliding scales and distilled language to assess the patient's physical and affective state and the efficacy of treatment modalities. However, what has been found in recent research regarding the expression of pain in a clinical setting is that living with pain is 'a phenomenon that cannot be categorized straightforwardly as a sensation or feeling, since it involves the totality of the human self' (Miglio and Stanier 2022: unpaginated). As such, 'imaginative expression – through means such as "words, rhythm, and ritual" – can be meaningfully employed to transform painful experiences beyond pain scales in medical settings' (*ibid.*). This is what we see at work in *Autobiography of a Marguerite*. Butcher-McGunnigle appropriates the impractical material and transforms it meaningfully.

Contrapuntal to the narrative prose poems in which Marguerite describes her daily experiences in the first section of the collection, Butcher-McGunnigle positions associative, cryptic poems from the genre of language poetry. These place the reader directly in the position of meaning-maker. Here, the poet knows her full intent, while the readers may only intuit meaning in a limited way, as in the following example:

> Ached, pillaging, dampen. Lollygag. (But mother.
> You bought her an ice cream the last time she went
> to the doctor.) Nothing rhymes with orange, but I
> like orange-flavoured confectionery. Confect, infect.
> Regarding pain, regarding value. (Yes but she was
> really sick, her headache was very bad.)
> (Butcher-McGunnigle 2014: 13, 1–6)

The strands of meaning onto which the reader holds suggest some of the tenuousness of the I-patient's position as she sits in front of a new pain-related document or attends an interview with her doctor. Without context or prior knowledge, unfamiliar vocabulary is pure guesswork. To 'lollygag' is to laze about. It is an unfamiliar word to most readers in the Antipodes. In the context of the poem, and to readers without a dictionary at hand, it may seem like a sweet treat (lolly) to make someone quiet (gag), bought for them as a bribe or reward: 'You bought her an ice cream last time she went/to the doctor' (1–2). Sweets and illness go together again ('Confect, infect') in line 4, and it appears as if the ice cream is being justified because 'she was/really sick, her headache was very bad' (5–6). We might imagine that the person to whom the treat is being explained is a jealous sibling, tired of seeing her sister rewarded by their mother just for malingering and paying another visit to the doctor. The poem can therefore be intuited to be about the way in which 'pain' (5) has its 'value' (5), and how it causes internal rifts and alliances within families.

There is a lot of room for (mis)interpretation in this poem, but it is also very cleverly assembled in order that we are led towards particular modes of (mis)interpretation. It offers a person who is unfamiliar with 'language poetry' a unique experience of meaning-making as well as the experience of feeling removed from the way in which an otherwise familiar language is being used. The effect is disorienting and uncomfortable.

To construct these poems, Butcher-McGunnigle used words and sentences from the text quoted in the collection's epigraph: *Love Your Disease: It's keeping you healthy* by Dr John Harrison. These include 'Describe the worst event/in your childhood' (2014: 15, lines 5–6); 'Who chose your name, Did your parents want a boy/or a girl' (2014: 27, lines 5–6). She also made the central tenet of Harrison's book – that psychology, past trauma, familial roles and tensions, key beliefs, and behaviour patterns can shape and perpetuate chronic conditions – a focal preoccupation of these poems. To have knowledge of this intertext's importance to the poems' nascence is to better understand them. However, not to know this information is to be in a similar position to a patient reading biomedically dense documents or being dominated by the 'voice of medicine' (Mishler 1984: 190).

The language poems which feature on the alternate pages of the first section are certainly destabilizing. They make the story and the meaning slightly out of focus, but we know, at least, who the central character is. However, when we come to the next part of the book, Butcher-McGunnigle begins to disassemble the speaker's identity. In this second part of the collection, the lines are incomplete. They end on random words or pieces of punctuation. They are from two different points of view: 'I' (Marguerite the daughter) or 'she' (Marguerite the mother). There are also footnotes on every page from the works of Marguerite Duras and Marguerite Yourcenar which add to, refute, or comment on individual words, phrases or lines.

The polyphony has a rather maddening effect. The reader feels overwhelmed with vying voices, none of whom seems able to finish what she is saying or to complete a full account of herself. The style of this section reflects the difficulty of locating the self within the family and the self within the ill body, which is key to Butcher-McGunnigle's presentation of chronic illness and its psycho-social impact. It is also in keeping with the work of Katharine Galloway Young (1997) on the self-body separation which occurs in a clinical setting. Furthermore, in the collection as a whole, Marguerite struggles to find who she is without the mother of the same name who insists that she sleep in the same bed 'because [she] need[s] looking after' (Butcher-McGunnigle 2014: 38, line 16) and because her father is currently inhabiting her bedroom, having been disgraced after an affair.

How can she individuate when her therapist is 'the same woman[her]/mother had seen fifteen years earlier, and . . ./also friends with [her] grandmother' (*ibid.*: 72, lines 5–7). What sort of weight is it to bear that the mother tells Marguerite, 'I will never be happy until you/are well' (*ibid.*: 78, 6–7). Butcher-McGunnigle has commented that an autoimmune illness itself can be seen to symbolize 'the struggle for a sense of self' (O'Neill 2014):

> The immune system is a boundary between you and the outside world, and the first task of the immune system is distinguishing self from non-self. Autoimmunity occurs when the immune system cannot recognise what is self and non-self, and begins to attack its own tissues. In the book, it is sometimes difficult to distinguish the mother and the daughter, particularly in the second section with the footnotes.

It is clear that the concept of this this section of the book is a close examination of identity in the midst of illness, and it is noteworthy that the poet has stated that one of her aims for *Autobiography of a Marguerite* was 'to give visibility to chronic illnesses because they are often "invisible" . . . in that there may be no physical signs apparent to friends or people on the street' (O'Neill 2014). It follows that the book as whole is replete with incidents where the speaker's suffering goes unseen by those around her. Take for example this exchange with a neighbour:

> . . . She asks me where I am going. I am going
> to the hospital, I say. It is the third time I've broken my arm
> this year. She bends down to cut the head off a dandelion.
> Is that so, she says. Well, did you know, once I went to three
> weddings in a month.
> (Butcher-McGunnigle 2014: 20, lines 12–16)

More poignant is this interaction with her father:

> My father said that we didn't do anything together
> anymore, and suggested we go kayaking – when I told
> him I couldn't go kayaking, he seemed bewildered
> (*ibid.*: 76, lines 8–10)

There is a thread of loneliness which runs through *Autobiography of a Marguerite* which is deeper and more poignant than mere isolation. The way in which the poet conveys the abject aloneness of the speaker is possibly most affecting because of the use of humour alongside the devastating admissions of being misunderstood or unseen in her physical and mental suffering.

Autobiography of a Marguerite has a lot to teach its readers about the alienation, depersonalization, frustration, and anxiety associated with chronic illness. The language and form of this collection deliberately enact the experience of being a patient in a manner that is more experiential than that of prose pathography. Readers are forced to encounter the equivocal being shaped into the numerical; they suffer tedious repetition and a confusing lack of context which makes a foreign tongue of a first language. What is more, they are privy to a lifeworld that is both claustrophobic and lonely – a lifeworld that goes unheard at the many clinical appointments Marguerite attends and one which clearly impacts her illness and quality of life. This is a book with the potential to communicate the need for physicians to address the existential needs of patients with chronic illnesses, giving time to conversations about the unpredictability of treatment, disease progression, and the management of associated anxiety. *Autobiography of a Marguerite* tells its readers more than any textbook or memoir possibly could about how important it is that doctors help patients towards managing the impacts of chronic illness on identity and social/familial relationships in order that unavoidable new uncertainties are made more tolerable.

Notes

1 Mishler's findings were replicated in the UK in 2001 by Christine A. Barry et al. (2001), who found that 'poorest outcomes occurred where patients used the voice of the lifeworld but were ignored (Lifeworld Ignored) or blocked (Lifeworld Blocked) by doctors' use of voice of medicine (chronic physical complaints)'. The analysis supports the premise that increased use of the lifeworld makes for better outcomes and more humane treatment of patients as unique human beings.

2 Butcher-McGunnigle describes this eloquently in her interview with Rachel O'Neill (2014):

> illness is a way of measuring time . . . ('Oh, I used to swim every week back then, before I got sick'; 'We moved here a year after I got so sick, so that must be seven years ago, now'; 'That was the summer your father got so ill he almost died'). I'm talking about chronic illness in particular. And in my experience, you can feel both as if you've lost time and as though you're stuck in time. You remain [the age you were when you were diagnosed] . . . you didn't have the chance to live in a way like other people did [at that age] to have the experiences other people did, because of your illness. If you have to spend months at home resting, you can feel as if you are wasting time or losing time. And the trauma that illness may bring can also lead to not being able to remember a period of time very well, as a defence mechanism . . . so you look back [on your life] and you say, ok, I remember going to the hospital and I remember sitting in the lounge for a while, but I don't know what else happened during those five months. Illness also means you locate yourself in time differently because the way you use your time and the way you view the future will most likely change. Maybe the future seems much more uncertain and frightening now that you are ill. The symptoms you have are not just concerning because they are happening right now, but because of what they mean for how your life will be from this point on. Time passes, and you are still sick, so you have to get used to it, or you have to get used to not getting used to it.

References

Barry CA, Stevenson FA, Britten N, et al. Giving Voice to the Lifeworld. More Humane, More Effective Medical Care? A Qualitative Study of Doctor – Patient Communication in General Practice. *Social Science & Medicine*. 2001; 53: 487–505.

Butcher-McGunnigle Z. 2014. *Autobiography of a Marguerite*. Auckland, New Zealand: Hue & Cry Press.

Heath I. How Medicine Has Exploited Rationality at the Expense of Humanity: An Essay by Iona Heath. *British Medical Journal*. 2016; i5705.

Hydén, L-C, Mishler EG. Language and Medicine. *Annual Review of Applied Linguistics*. 1999; 19: 174–92.

Miglio N, Stanier J. Beyond Pain Scales: A Critical Phenomenology of the Expression of Pain. *Frontiers in Pain Research*. 2022; 3. Available at: www.frontiersin.org/articles/10.3389/fpain.2022.895443/full. Last accessed: 20/4/2023.

Mishler EG. 1984. *The Discourse of Medicine: Dialectics of Medical Interviews*. Norwood, NJ: Ablex.

Mishler EG. Patient Stories, Narratives of Resistance and the Ethics of Humane Care: A La Recherche Du Temps Perdu. *Health: An Interdisciplinary Journal for the Social Study of Health, Illness and Medicine*. 2005; 4: 431–51.

Ofri D. Medical Humanities: The Rx for Uncertainty? *Academic Medicine*. 2017; 92: 1657–58.

O'Neill R. 2014. The Marguerites: Rachel O'Neill Interviews Poet Zarah Butcher-McGunnigle for Poetry Shelf. Other. *Poetry Shelf*. Paula Green, June 12. Available at: https://nzpoetryshelf.com/2014/06/10/the-marguerites-rachel-oneill-interviews-poet-zarah-butcher-mcgunnigle-for-poetry-shelf/. Last accessed: 27/12/2022.

Young KG. 1997. *Presence in the Flesh: The Body in Medicine*. Cambridge, MA: Harvard University Press.

30

HAS THE POETRY OF MEDICINE BURNT OUT?

Sophie Ratcliffe and Andrew Schuman

Introduction

The idea that engagement with the arts, particularly literature, is good for one's health goes back thousands of years (Hurwitz 2015; Bate and Schuman 2016; Ratcliffe 2016b; Billington et al. 2019). It's no surprise, then, to find that physicians have been drawn to heal themselves through literary means. The relationship between poetry and doctoring has a strong pedigree, and for a reason. Medical student John Keats may have left his apprenticeship early, but he carried on practising, after his own fashion. A poet, for Keats (1978) in *The Fall of Hyperion*, was a 'physician to all men'. And when not busy writing about plums in iceboxes, paediatrician and imagist poet William Carlos Williams was making house calls and treating the children of New Jersey.

Doctors, both then and now, have been known to prescribe pages and not pills – the vogue for 'bibliotherapy' is nothing new (Dovey 2015). But physicians have, historically, also felt the need to heal themselves. Sir William Osler, whose work on what we now call the 'bedside manner' broke new ground at the turn of the twentiety century, insisted that medical students should 'start a bed-side library' (Osler 1904: 385), read widely, and nod off with the works of Shakespeare. Nowadays, 'Poems in the Waiting Room'– packs of cards printed with poems – provide a welcome alternative to the usual battered copies of *Take a Break* (www.poemsinthewaitingroom.org/). The Hippocrates Prize celebrates poetry written by those in the National Health Service, and a new initiative in Scotland means that all graduating medics receive a poetry anthology along with their degree (https://bjgp.org/content/65/636/341.2).

Over the last 30 years, medical and health humanities scholars have attempted more rigorous explorations of the ways in which reading narrative and poetry may make a difference to clinicians (Charon 1995; Epstein and Hundert 2002). Much emphasis in these accounts is placed on the idea that reading literature can improve clinical competence, particularly the development of empathy (Shapiro et al. 2004). Accounts also make the case for literary texts as useful material by which clinicians may practice thinking around ethical issues and making clinical judgements (Jones 1999).

Scholarship – on occasion but to a lesser degree – points to the analogy between reading a text and reading a patient (Leder 1990; Kottow and Kottow 2002) and the idea that the ambiguities of literary texts may allow doctors to practice their medical reading skills ('the perusal of literary pieces helps teach graduate students the humane and ethical aspects of medicine') (*ibid.*: 41).

DOI: 10.4324/9781003341796-38

Some argue that reading about medical encounters may offer a 'rarely explored path towards obtaining a comparative and critical picture of diverse forms of medical practice' (*ibid.*). Further accounts argue that the reading of literary texts may counter burnout (Mangione et al. 2018). This connection is potentially important, as burnout is a key concern for general practitioners and in the profession at large. For example, George and Gerada (2019: 116) note that GPs report experiencing 'specific work pressures compared with other doctors, such as: working beyond rostered hours; a significant proportion of high pressure days; feeling unable to cope with workload'. Further,

> as a specialty, GPs do more face-to-face patient contact as core to their expected work than any other specialty, adding to the risk of burnout and exhaustion; poor satisfaction with work-life balance; and an increase in the number of referrals to manage workload pressures.
>
> (*ibid.*)

Work in the field

In reflecting on current continuing professional development (CPD) provision for GPs, it is useful to explore the history of how such work has come about and which disciplines and demographics have been involved. Over the last 50 years, there has been a considerable body of theoretical and philosophical work concerning the relationships between illness and the humanities. Scholars in humanities departments, such as Sontag (1978) and Scarry (1987), have explored the ideas of illness and the limits of language more generally, as well as exploring the power plays implicit in metaphorical framings of specific health conditions and the ways in which narrative and empathy relate to each other (Hanne 2010; Conway 2013; Wohlmann 2017). There is also a wide body of research by scholars in the field of linguistics, drawing on patient experience narratives as raw material, that reflects on the density and variety of metaphors and similes employed in everyday speech. Work in the health humanities might be seen as the natural springboard for knowledge exchange.

Recent work by Anita Wohlmann (2022) offers useful 'sample exercises' by which individuals may sharpen and practice thinking about metaphor usage. Other important work in this area is by Patterson and Kitchington (2019) and Louise Younie (2019). It is clear that some of this work feeds back into medical training for both medical students and GP registrars (trainees) with recommended reading including Greenhalgh and Hurwitz (1998), Launer (2019, 2023 this collection),[1] and Roger Neighbour (2005, 2018).[2] As Angela Andrews writes in her discussion about 'ways of seeing', '[m]ost often, poetry is put forward as having the potential to humanize medicine: by promoting, for example, empathy, ethical sensitivity, and an appreciation for diverging interpretations (Ahlzén and Stolt 2001; Wolters and Wijnen-Meijer 2012)'.

Scholarship from philosophy, literary criticism, linguistics, and the medical/health humanities also finds its way into the hands of clinicians, and a proportion of this reaches those in primary care. Excellent independent ventures, including the *Medicine Unboxed* festival curated by Sam Guglani, conferences, Facebook groups, and day workshops have doubtless reached some GPs. Resources about medical education and the humanities are, at times, shared amongst GP trainers in informal and ad hoc ways.[3] A particular standout for CPD in terms of visibility and efficacy is John Launer's *Conversations Inviting Change* project, as well as the MindReading Project at the University of Birmingham.[4]

Nevertheless, the dispersed nature of CPD resources, the cost of workshops, and the absence of any central forum means that once a GP has qualified, she is unlikely to find herself engaging with work in the medical/health humanities unless she actively seeks it. At the time of writing, there are no materials on the Royal College of General Practitioners website offering any courses on 'poetry', 'humanities', or 'literature'. As Desmond O'Neill (2012) argues, while there is much provision in the medical and health humanities for medical students, medical humanities rarely feature as an aspect of CPD (Shapiro et al. 2004). If our medical students do not see the medical humanities figuring in postgraduate educational programmes for the trainees, CPD events for specialists, or the clinical lives of their teachers, then it is likely that this cognitive and professional dissonance will weaken the case for the value of medical humanities, an area already suffering from lack of definition.

O'Neill (*ibid*.: unpaginated) notes that while 'major generalist medical journals' give the medical humanities generous coverage, 'this is much less often the case in specialty journals'. He also comments on the rarity of arts and health provision in hospitals. We need, he notes, 'a better understanding of what the medical humanities mean, both in definition and content, to the full spectrum of our colleagues'; otherwise, 'the subject is in danger of preaching to the converted, of those with a natural affinity for a particular palette of artistic activities'. Further, the medical/health humanities in general, and specifically the literary medical/health humanities, have very little stake in policy conversations. A case in point is a 2018 Royal College of Physicians document, 'Talking About Dying: How to Begin Honest Conversations about what lies ahead'. The document includes 'signposts to tools and educational resources to support physicians and other health care professionals', listing numerous stakeholders. But there are no named figures or institutions from the field of poetry or literature. Even a medical project with an explicitly medical/health humanities bent – Semino and colleagues' (2017) 'Metaphor in End of Life Care' (http://ucrel.lancs.ac.uk/melc/non_aca_dissemination.php) – draws on the expertise of team members with (primarily) linguistic, rather than literary, expertise.

True interdisciplinarity?

All language users are, by nature, experts in metaphor, simile, and storytelling. However, the absence of those who have training in the reading of literature in the provision of medical/health humanities material (for both medical students and at CPD level) may be of import, and the question of field expertise in relation to the use of the arts and humanities in medical/health humanities has rarely been addressed. Medical conversation, as Paul Komesaroff (2005) argues, proceeds 'at the level of metaphor, similes and other devices that are used to capture and tame elusive meanings . . . [s]omewhat like talking in poetry' (see also Vyieyanghi and Periyakoil 2008; Bleakley 2017). Launer (2019), commenting on Komesaroff's work, says that 'all effective communication . . . involves the careful, tentative use of "the same devices, rhetorical forms, figures and tropes generally eschewed by philosophers and scientists, but embraced by poets and creative writers"'.

If this is true, then the best medical training, policy making and ongoing CPD will be alert to the need to practice such reading skills. While any engagement with the medical/health humanities at a CPD level may be of benefit (although, as will be discussed later, such benefit is difficult to measure), there is, arguably, dilution of benefit if those with literary expertise are not included in the interdisciplinary conversation. The value of including literary experts in health humanities conversations includes:

1) Technical Expertise

A literary expert may be able to offer those engaged in the medical humanities a wider range of literary texts and an increased knowledge of technical insights surrounding those texts, relating to questions of genre, style, metaphor, tone, and narrative form.

2) *Expertise in the ethics of reading*

There is little evidence about concrete benefits of reading for doctors, but the most common suggested benefit of engaging with literature is that it might offer an improvement in clinician 'empathy' (Winkel et al. 2016). Literary experts with knowledge of theories of reading and the philosophy of mind bring new knowledge to these claims (and may indeed cast doubt, in a useful way, on the equation between literature and empathy).

3) *Inclusive interdisciplinarity may bring a more complex understanding of the relationship between reading and empathy*

In the literary/philosophical field, the imagining of other minds is an unquantifiable and unmeasurable (and for some philosophers), impossible task (Ratcliffe 2016a). Nevertheless, many medical articles about patient communication often lionize 'empathy' while leaving its complexities unexamined (Halpern 2003).[5] While one could argue that a pragmatic understanding of 'empathy' is useful, such a pragmatic understanding maps uneasily onto literature, which often involves a much more complex understanding of reading practices.

4) *Inclusive interdisciplinarity may prevent complacency*

An easy embrace of the concept of 'empathy' (and the co-opting of the reading of literature into this) has ethical risks. Doctors engaged in literary CPD may be enlisted in what the critic Andrew Scull (2018) refers to as a kind of simplified 'march-of-progress narrative', in which reading doctors are seen as 'better doctors'. 'There is the view', as the poet John Ashbery (in Blume 1989) wryly remarked, 'poetry should improve your life. I think people confuse it with the Salvation Army'.

5) *Inclusive interdisciplinarity may bring new benefits, and improve clinician wellbeing*

Literary expertise may allow for a more complex, and arguably more accurate, discussion about the realities of imagining the minds of others and about what happens when we read. The inclusion of literary expertise guards against literature being co-opted or instrumentalized and allows for a broader exploration about the process of reading (arguably involving us in failures of sympathy, fascination, horror, boredom, arousal, disgust, amusement, interest, and so forth). There is evidence that repeated pressure on improving physician empathy may have negative effects on doctors, or at least that 'empathy does not come without a cost'(Gleichgerrcht and Decety 2012; Samra 2018). The inclusion of literary expertise may prevent the occlusion of the different benefits that literature brings to doctors themselves that are not primarily patient centred (but which may indeed bring additional benefits to patients). Uncoupling literature and empathy, through the lens of the literary expert, may be beneficial.

Measurement

A key issue relating to the presence of literary reflection in CPD for those in primary care – or more generally – is the distinct lack of empirical evidence that such activity is of value. Schoonover and colleagues' (2020: 127) systematic review of studies of the impact of poetry on both empathy and burnout in health care workers noted 'a relatively small number of studies', where 'the studies themselves were limited interventions with small sample sizes, and the study groups were heterogeneous'. More fundamentally, perhaps, literary engagement presents itself as a test case for the difficulties of measuring activities in two distinctly separate spheres. Measuring the value and efficacy of a literary workshop is not possible in the same way as one might measure the outcomes of a new drug. Literary engagement provokes questions about what kinds of 'evidence' might be gathered, or measured, and what is meant by value or measurement.

Work on measurement in the medical/health humanities can be roughly categorized. Some, echoing Schoonover's study, try to record measurable, accurate evidence-based results. This kind of scholarship can be seen in Josie Billington and colleagues' (2019: 264) chapter that 'rises to the challenge posed by health commissioners and public health providers when they require evidence of the benefits of reading according to standard and widely used measures of health and well-being'. Such scholarship is challenging. As the authors note, some of the 'standard self-report measures of mental health and well-being' (*ibid.*: 266) are distinctly different from 'measures' we might adopt from a readerly perspective. Put more simply, reading might provoke negative emotions and therefore register badly on a conventional measure of mental health, but such an experience of negative emotions might, in the long term, be positive, in a way that clinical measurement might not comprehend.

This mismatch of ways of measuring is, fundamentally, difficult to overcome. It may suggest a kind of blindness, metaphorically speaking, on the part of the clinical framework to happenings both within and outside its framework. As Angela Andrews (2016) writes, 'the clinical training of doctors cultivates a "way of seeing" that both highlights and obscures aspects of medicine'. Reading can be seen as both a metaphor and a literal action, and, as Alan Bleakley (2017) argues, there is a certain figurative 'illiteracy' in medical culture, when it comes to contemplating the benefits of the arts: 'The vacuum created by slack philosophical thinking in medicine is filled by simplistic managerialist approaches and by the instrumental ethics approach of principlism, which ignore messy, context-based human judgement'. This illiteracy, as Glenn Regehr (2010: 31) notes, can only be rectified when we begin to think about a different kind of reading: 'Reorienting education research from its alignment with the imperative of proof to one with an imperative of understanding, and from the imperative of simplicity to an imperative of representing complexity well'. Such an approach may deflect researchers' interests away from 'search for proofs of simple generalizable solutions' towards 'the generation of rich understandings of the complex environments in which our collective problems are uniquely embedded'.

These arguments are compelling. However, those in the medical/health humanities are themselves potentially blinded or conflicted or at risk of 'slack' thinking. The imperative to justify the value of the humanities, driven both by personal investments and a climate in which the humanities are under threat, may lead to the kinds of conflicts of interest that are difficult to overcome – a fetishizing of reading, where, as Adam Phillips and Philip Davis (2020: 366–67) suggest, for some people 'it is reading that helps. But it does not have to be'. As Phillips and Davis discuss, one might equally think about the consolations of birdwatching, or horse-racing, or 'whatever it is that matters' to a person – it is, at heart, 'what the philosopher Gilles Deleuze calls "the capacity to be affected"'. This is not to deny the interest of the work in the field or the potential benefits of continuing to create structures that encourage work of a true interdisciplinary nature. It is more to suggest that searching for measurable proofs of evidence may not be the best use of the limited resources available in either medicine or the humanities.

Case study

In 2018, a workshop was held for 14 general practitioners.[6] The workshop leaders had held 20 similar workshops in the past and believed that the value of literary encounters cannot be measured conventionally, however nuanced. The aim of the workshop was threefold:

1) to provide a forum in which literary texts could afford a lens through which GPs could discuss their working lives

2) to record GPs' reflections to provide a qualitative, shared account of this conversation
3) to attempt to apply conventional measuring techniques to the workshop to find out more, through practice, about the specific challenges and opportunities of measuring literary experiences

Metaphor and communication in general practice

The first part of the workshop focused on metaphor, using a poem which was densely metaphorical as a prompt for the discussion: 'Balloons' by Sylvia Plath. Written from the perspective of a caregiver, the poem describes a domestic scene of some children and some deflating balloons. The balloons are seen variously as 'Oval soul-animals', or 'free/Peacocks'. At the end of the poem, a balloon bursts and a child is left holding a 'red/Shred' of rubber 'in his little fist' (Plath 1999: 75–76). At a more general level, the burst balloon could be read as a metaphor for the depleted caregiver, the female postpartum body, or even the fate of poetry itself. After probing the meanings and interpretations of the poem, and thinking about its language, the workshop moved on to discuss metaphor in medical practice. One participant noted that she found

> it difficult when patients are trying to explain how they feel metaphorically and I don't quite understand what they mean – for example, "I feel foggy-headed" and I'm trying to pick out what they mean by that medically, and they find it hard to explain, so I have to sort of try to guess based on asking more questions.

Another doctor noted the 'danger of metaphors', by which 'you assume you know what they mean . . . so I wonder whether it's sometimes worth picking them up, you know, unpicking that again'.

Echoing both Launer's and Komesaroff's observations about the push for 'clarity' in medical communication, the group reflected on the inherently metaphorical nature of language. One doctor reflected that,

> the idea of lack of metaphor is quite interesting. I think I probably do use a lot of metaphor. We see a lot of patients for whom English is not their first language, and actually it's a real struggle sometimes . . . there are so many ways to describe and express things that it's actually sometimes very difficult – I sometimes wonder if I use metaphor and it's just completely misunderstood because sometimes it doesn't translate.

Another added that, 'the other group that this idea also works for is patients with Asperger's and autism who don't have that recognition . . . just very flippantly saying, "how do you feel in yourself?", and them saying, "oh I don't know what that means"'.

Many participants commented on the potential for misunderstanding and the sense that both patients and doctors may use different kinds of metaphorical language:

> we want patients to speak our language . . . we have a menu of words that we like, and what you're saying makes me wonder whether they're any more meaningful than the ones that they offer in the first place – so I feel happy when they use one of my words, but maybe we're not talking about the same thing at all.

The doctors considered the way in which metaphor, as Shklovsky (1917) argues, makes ordinary things seem 'strange', like that a post-natal woman might think of herself as a deflated balloon (in a manner both witty and tragic) or that a balloon might be like a poem (playful and potentially pointless but also joyful, or signalling). The way in which poetry might illuminate the complex and symbolic nature of everyday things was seen as a fascinating element of joint reading.

This discussion then took a provocative turn away from the drive towards clarity of language in relation to terminal illness. Participants reflected on the way in which thinking through poetry made them look upon issues in different, metaphorical ways. One doctor reflected on her experience of discussing terminal illness and watching others do so:

> there's something quite comforting about metaphor – and saying something without actually saying it sort of provides you with a little cushion, but again it only works if the other person understands where you're coming from and understands the metaphor in that sense.

The discussion of metaphor concluded with the sense that the idea of 'clear and honest' language, so important in instructions concerning medical communication, was less transparent than it seemed.

Dealing with uncertainty

Tolerating uncertainty is frequently cited as one of the most challenging and difficult aspects of being a doctor, and arguably this is nowhere more apparent than in primary care, where the seriousness or not of the vast array of unsorted problems that a GP deals with is, so often, uncertain and unclear. In their manual for GPs, Penny Moore and Simon Curtis (2008: 7–8) offer the following analogy, drawing on the work of Marshall Marinker:

> You know the old joke about hearing horses' hooves in the distance, and the hospital physician saying "Aha! I hear a unicorn!". Marshall Marinker famously differentiated hospital doctors from GPs like this:
>
> Hospital doctors have to reduce uncertainty, explore possibility and marginalize error. ("Could be a unicorn, better organise a serum hoof count and a PET scan, just in case it is a unicorn and it scratches us with its nasty sharp pointy horn").
>
> Whilst GPs must tolerate uncertainty, explore probability and marginalize danger. ('It's most likely a horse, there are lots of horses around at the moment and I recognise that hoof beat. Most horses go away by themselves. If it's a unicorn, we'll find out soon enough and then deal with it . . . those expensive tests would use valuable resources and aren't needed yet.')[7]

As a springboard for talking about uncertainty, the room was divided into groups of four, with each group discussing their experiences of living with uncertainty. We dwelt on whether there were better or worse ways of dealing with the experience of slowly coming to the right diagnosis, waiting for the outcome of a patient complaint, or dealing with feelings of anxiety after a difficult consultation. We asked how (and whether) they had learned to cope with uncertainty and fear of unicorns, and whether it might be seen, in some ways, as analogous to John Keats' 1817 letter describing the idea of 'Negative Capability' – the state 'of being in uncertainties, Mysteries, doubts, without any irritable reaching after fact & reason' (Keats 1958: 193).

In the discussion that followed, much was made of the positive aspects of uncertainty. One participant noted that they liked 'those bits when you don't know, because [. . .] if you then go back and look at it, that's when you kind of learn [. . .] you develop an understanding'. The lasting and ongoing value of dealing with uncertainty was prized by many:

> I think that uncertainty is the bit that makes the job really interesting. I love the fact that I come to work . . . and I still don't know what I'm going to encounter, and I love that . . . there aren't many people who are middle-aged who actually really enjoy bits of their jobs still, because they've been doing the same job, which is really predictable.

A kind of Keatsian pragmatism came out in discussion, too:

> That's so much of our job though, isn't it, I suppose. We deal with so much uncertainty and ambiguity, and a lot of stuff is quite messy . . . of course there is that irritation where you're sitting there and just really want to understand what this patient is trying to say to you, but we're probably fairly comfortable . . . I think you develop a sense of comfort with not really knowing.

Uncertainty in medicine was seen, by the participants, as something that they had often been able to manage positively, and how they might enable trainee doctors and medical students not to be overwhelmed by it. Here, peer support was seen to be central. As one participant noted, 'that's one of the things I found quite comforting from experienced GPs, saying, "yeah, we don't know" – and when you see them doing it, you think, "oh it's okay that I don't know either"'.

The group reflected on whether there might be an analogy between reading difficult or ambiguous poems and encountering complex and uncertain medical scenarios and whether literature and the arts might be of help. The participants generally supported this idea, noting the absence of the arts in medical training:

> But that's the strange thing . . . medical students are traditionally selected from those who've done sciences, and it's about empiricism, and certainly round here, you know, the better you are at 'science' and 'knowing answers' the better you are, and if you say you're interested in primary care and uncertainty then it's all a bit soft.

A clear consensus emerged about the lack of training in relation to medical uncertainty:

> Looking back, when I was at medical school a lot of the talks we would get and the focus we might have was from specialists . . . so you would have the renal specialist talk to you, who often is dealing with comparative certainty. From primary care we would often have communications skills, which is obviously very important in primary care, but it was often focusing on the consultation, not so much on the uncertainty, which I think has only become more apparent to me the further into training I've got . . . it's only when something maybe doesn't go quite according to plan when you think 'gosh, I thought I really knew what was going on there', and subsequently I found out I didn't. And then go into primary care and that's magnified even more, and it's that juxtaposition between, 'okay I'm thinking in terms of science, blood tests, findings', but not necessarily focusing on the fact that – and it's something that I'm doing a lot more now – is saying that, actually, we may never understand what's causing these symptoms.

It was perhaps appropriate that no certain answer was generated in the discussion about uncertainty, but one further clear theme emerged near the end:

> I think – taking it a step back – that some of the problem is, why is uncertainty a problem in the first place? [. . .] in fact, what we deal with is uncertainty, but I think that's shorthand for 'fear' most of the time: it's patients' 'fear' and they bring it to us to manage, or it's our fear that there's something awful going on and that we might just have missed it – and we never have that conversation in training, really, at all.

The idea of 'fear' as 'a kind of [unspoken] narrative' in the doctor's brain struck a chord with many of the participants, with some highlighting the loneliness of the GP role in relation to this fear:

> there is fear there, and I think consultants probably also have the fear because all of the responsibility comes back to them, I think just sometimes perhaps its shared a little bit more because you've got registrars and things, rather than when you're the GP you are the only person that sees them . . . maybe it's the lone working that enhances the fear.

Dealing with space

A further section of texts and images focussed on the idea of medical space and whether the concept of the 'poetics of space' could be a helpful lens by which to consider the space in which the clinician and patient meet. We reflected together on a series of paintings and photographs of both the doctor's room and the waiting room in time, commenting on the ways in which doctors might use furniture, and arrangements of objects, to consciously or unconsciously signal power, learning, expertise, and intimacy. We also looked at photographs of the doctors' own rooms, which the participants had shared in advance.

Some doctors had not thought consciously about the way in which their workspace was relatively impersonal (two doctors agreed that 'actually looking at that picture we can't even work out whose room it is'). One doctor participant spoke of the importance of her room reflecting her personality:

> one of the things about lots of these rooms is that they're very anonymous . . . actually mine's quite messy, but it's messy with *my* stuff, it's got *my* photos of *my* children, *my* children's drawings, and it's a kind of way to, you know, say something about me in a space that has so many other people in it . . .

A participant recalled that, historically, the GP would be practicing out of his home. In this sense, the patient would, essentially, be hosted by the doctor and, often, the doctor's spouse (historically, his wife). Another doctor, citing the work of Nancy Klein and the idea of a 'thinking environment', commented that the space of the consultation room 'needs to make both the doctor and the patient feel important'.

Practicality played into the ways doctors arranged their rooms: 'I have a little toy table and chairs in my room . . . because I decided I would have more time and space in the consultation if children were occupied', but many participants also thought clearly about the power dynamics of their room, either in the basic set up ('[W]hen I first came the doctor's table was in front of me and then it was the patient, and on the first morning, I just moved it all round, because I couldn't work like that') or in the individual adjustments they made for consultations ('sometimes during a consultation I'll flip that switch and make my chair go lower because I don't want to feel like I'm towering over a patient.')

The group found the idea of the 'palimpsest' useful as a literary metaphor to describe the way in which patients and doctors experience the clinical environment differently. For the doctor, the clinical space is layered with numerous encounters. As one participant put it: 'it's when they walk in and they think you remember them, and you don't . . . because that last conversation we had was the last conversation you had in this room, but I've had hundreds since then'.

Images of contemporary and nineteenth-century waiting rooms, prompted a conversation about patient privacy. In the nineteenth century, consultations were sometimes carried out in communal spaces, as demonstrated in a painting by Vladimir Makovsky (figure 30.1).

The image reminded one doctor of her elective in Sri Lanka, where 'the patients would be queuing outside the medical rooms to be seen, and they would be there for days, waiting their turn, and they would sleep there'. The participants reflected on the value of waiting, both personally and in their role as doctors. One admitted to enjoying her time, 'waiting at the GP' and noted that there is 'the odd patient who comes early because it's a social thing, that they'll see people that they know'. Another agreed that 'I've had patients moan at me because I've called them in

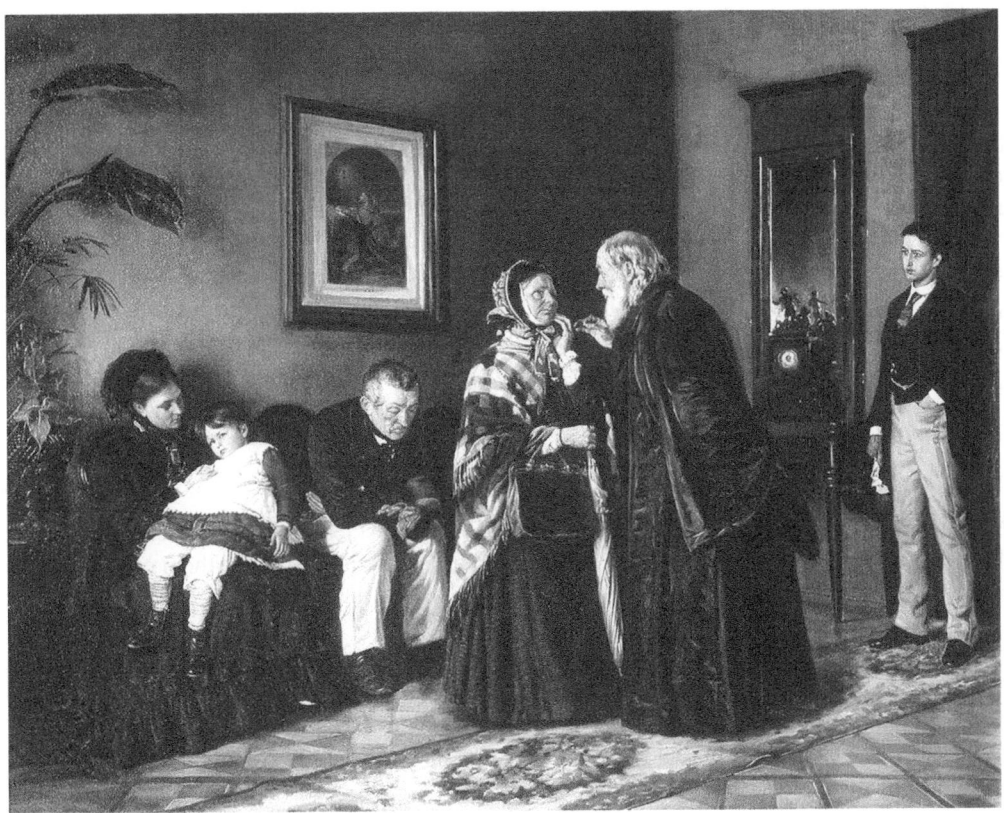

Figure 30.1 Vladimir Makovsky 'The Doctor's Waiting Room' (1870).

too early . . . because they wanted that time'. The conversation unfolded to consider the value of virtual forums for discussing illness and wellbeing, as kinds of 'waiting rooms' and communal consultation rooms, where it 'changes the dynamic totally, though, doesn't it, because the doctor's no longer the healer, it's the patients who are trying to heal themselves'.

Kafka's 'A Country Doctor'

While there has been considerable work on the value of narrative in developing empathy, less attention has been paid to discussions of the emotions and wellbeing of doctors themselves. For this reason, the workshop leaders involved a discussion of Franz Kafka's short story 'A Country Doctor'. The tale offers an account of a doctor's urgent night-time visit to an unwell patient at home. Kafka's doctor ends up misreading and misunderstanding his patient and is eventually humiliated and hounded out of the house by the patient's relatives. All the participants seem to agree that the surreal qualities of the story captured something central to general practice; for some, it recalled 'those weird work dreams' but was also strangely resonant with the act of consultation:

> We felt like he did have amazing insight into a visiting doctor's life, so even though it has this crazy dreamlike, kind of, aspect to it – and the dream is the kind of explanation for why this is crazy – that's what everyone kind of jumped on to, there are huge events that are completely reminiscent to all of us . . . situations we've been in with families, anxieties, and the work life . . . so there's a strange fluctuation between very recognisable and then very sort of abstract and odd . . . and the dream is our way of explaining that.

The main character in the story suffers great pressure from the fact that he doesn't have the horses to make his night visit and speculates on whether he might have to ride a pig. The idea of being under-resourced struck a chord with the participants:

> We talked a bit about them being resources in a way – you know, the doctor in this circumstance couldn't do the visit without the horses, but then the horses also bearing over into the consultation itself, so, you know, the system in which we work, we rely upon, we need the computer systems, we need the way funding works, but then it's also perhaps something we're battling against. . . . We were also saying that, in terms of resources that we have where we now just work with whatever we have got available, because at some point he says, 'I would make do with pigs I suppose'.

Another trauma in the story is the way in which the doctor must leave his home life, which is under threat, and go to work. Again, many doctors in the session felt this reminded them of the pressures of preserving boundaries and the way work and home life collide:

> I think what struck me is that he's got all this stuff going on at home that he'd quite like to be dealing with . . . often patients come in and say to me . . . 'well where's your child today?', and I say, 'oh, she's at nursery', and they say 'oh, that's sad', and I'm like, 'if I'm not here, you're moaning at me because I'm not here' . . . now I'm thinking about my child at nursery being without me!'

In a dramatic scene, Kafka's doctor finds himself stripped naked, an image which resonated with at least two members of the discussion group:

> I thought the vulnerability and the nakedness was very much how you are as a doctor when you do a home visit, and that, looking through my career, when we used to do home visits, we'd take our doctor's bag and whatever, and it'd be a symbol of pride in a way, and we'd have our bit, and we'd arrive and we'd get a cup of tea and it would all be fine . . . and then the bag became something that was a threat because it had prescriptions, drugs, we used to take morphine on home visits, and all that, and then actually you were vulnerable because of who you were, and then how vulnerable you are as a doctor going into someone's home, that it's not always a safe thing, so you are dressed down and you are on your own, you don't have your colleagues around you, so I very much got the vulnerability of the naked-ness, because that is how it often can be . . . We also talked a little bit about exposure, and I suppose it all kind of relates to what is expected of the doctor to start with, because actu-ally what happens is that he gets it wrong, potentially, you know, he misses the wound, but what the boy said or somebody says into his ear is that 'you haven't helped me'. But what does he mean by 'help', what's he expecting the doctor to do? Because if he'd got it right he wouldn't necessarily have been able to help anyway, but he's not helped because he's got it wrong . . . so perhaps being exposed . . . it exposes someone who doesn't *know* everything, someone who *isn't* a god . . .

The doctors discussed the question of self-doubt in the narrative and how that related to their own doubts: 'it's sort of a theme running through it isn't it, about his own self-doubt', noting that 'his failure to do the things that he's asked to do' and the issue of 'whether he wants to do them' was central to the story:

> we also talked about the fact that it's often our fear isn't it, that you go in and you make a decision and actually you miss the other bit completely. So that may be why . . . it's part of his vulnerability isn't it? We all might miss the wound if we don't look for it.

One of the doctors praised Kafka's writing:

> I reckon he's a genius for being able to do what he's done, because I started off saying this isn't anything about a home visit, it's just so bizarre, but actually by the end I was saying it's all about a home visit – but it's all about a home visit, and it's all about all the stuff that isn't at the front of your mind, but is actually going on, the darker parts, or the bits that you can't necessarily be conscious of . . . being overstretched, being pulled in all the different directions, that confusion, and that's kind of all there in the story . . .

One of the workshop leaders raised the idea of 'patient-centred care' and asked the question 'where is the doctor placed in patient-centred care?', adding 'it's quite interesting that it's very, very simi-lar to our experience . . . nothing has really changed has it? . . . It's very much like the life of a doctor today, and our health system is entirely different in a way, but it isn't.' Another added, 'he's really quite bitter about it all I think . . . the family seems to be wanting more of him than he can give, they don't understand him . . . he's certainly not enjoying his job, is he?'

Points for change, qualitative vs quantitative data

At the end of the session, the workshop leaders asked the participants to share anything they might be more aware of or do differently, in the light of the day's discussion. Some doctors spoke about the ways in which the day had highlighted issues of language:

> I suppose with metaphors it's noticing them . . . to start with – that it's okay, but we don't always think about them . . . It's awareness of using it and thinking what you mean by it . . . And I suppose when you're reading, you think about the ways that other people use metaphors, and see if that can enhance your own use.

Others discussed the idea of the poetics and resonance of physical space: 'I think sometimes by changing you can change . . . even just a change of furniture can change a situation – even just standing up'. One final remark related to question of practitioner burnout. Reflecting on Kafka's 'A Country Doctor', a participant noted "Well sometimes you get that sense from a patient . . . they forget that you're human'.

Modes of measurement

A sheet was distributed to each doctor before and after the session. The question sheet offered two questions and the chance to offer a numerical answer and free text. The questions were:

a) *How useful are books and reading in relation to your wellbeing as a doctor?*
b) *How useful are books and reading in relation to your clinical practice?*

Some participants gave answers to both questions and free text comments. Some chose to only give numbers or to only answer one of the two questions (see Table 30.1).

The numerical responses give the impression that this session increased practitioners interest in reading by an average of about 25%. The qualitative responses bear this out, with a shift in emphasis on the value of reading to prevent practitioner burnout and the fact that GPs generally have read less and less for pleasure since qualification. Nevertheless, the complexities of measuring this sort of work are enough to render this 'evidence' as signifying very little. This is a very small sample size. Even if the workshops were replicated on a large scale, the question of leadership must be considered. It would always be very difficult to determine if the 'benefits' of such a discussion were created by the group discussion, the texts chosen, the combination of participants, or the individuals leading the group.

Conclusion

Convincing evidence for the value of literary interventions in medical education and continuing professional development is necessarily elusive, and the benefits of activities such as literary discussion groups are difficult, if not impossible, to quantify and measure. However, this does not mean that activities which engage with the intersections between literature and medicine are not meaningful or valuable. It is always important to note that any benefits may also be due (to varying degrees) to the way in which a literary workshop fosters a nurturing and facilitative group dynamic and a feeling of group solidarity, a change of pace (at the end of a busy working week) – as well as interests, insights, or even 'lightbulb moments' that exploration and discussion of literary texts might provide.

Table 30.1 Participants' responses to the workshop.

Number	Score out of 10 and comment before the Session	Score out of 10 and comment after the session
1	a) *How useful are books and reading in relation to your wellbeing as a doctor?* 10/10 Essential relaxation and helps with looking at other perspectives b) *How useful are books and reading in relation to your clinical practice?* 8/10 I have used text in consultation with the right patient	a) *How useful are books and reading in relation to your wellbeing as a doctor?* 10/10 Essential for preventing burnout b) *How useful are books and reading in relation to your clinical practice?* 10/10 Especially for mental health problems
2	a) *How useful are books and reading in relation to your wellbeing as a doctor?* 7/10 I try to read to unwind/distract myself from work related worries b) *How useful are books and reading in relation to your clinical practice?* 9/10 essential to keep up to date	a) *How useful are books and reading in relation to your wellbeing as a doctor?* 9/10 I feel inspired to look at poetry and novels in a different way, to try to understand both my feelings and to look at patients' feelings in a different way b) *How useful are books and reading in relation to your clinical practice?* 9/10 To keep up to date but also to keep my empathy and understanding 'topped up'
3	a) *How useful are books and reading in relation to your wellbeing as a doctor?* 8/10 Important for giving perspective	a) *How useful are books and reading in relation to your wellbeing as a doctor?* 8/10
4	a) *How useful are books and reading in relation to your wellbeing as a doctor?* 9/10 Finding time to read is difficult, I've been 'reading' audiobooks and this has changed my reading habits very much b) *How useful are books and reading in relation to your clinical practice?* 8/10 For thinking about, and finding ways to articulate feelings	a) *How useful are books and reading in relation to your wellbeing as a doctor?* 9/10 More consciously so after coming today b) *How useful are books and reading in relation to your clinical practice?* 9/10 For different reasons to those I gave earlier, thinking and articulating un-thinkable things
5	a) *How useful are books and reading in relation to your wellbeing as a doctor?* 3/10 I don't make any time for reading for pleasure or relaxation b) *How useful are books and reading in relation to your clinical practice?* 6/10 Most information for clinical practice is via website and electronic devices but I still have some books to refer to!	a) *How useful are books and reading in relation to your wellbeing as a doctor?* 7/10 I struggle to read anything not directly clinical but I have a long list b) *How useful are books and reading in relation to your clinical practice?* 7/10 I only read technical medical books but I have plenty of books by doctors and others regarding the practice of medicine

(Continued)

Table 30.1 (Continued)

Number	Score out of 10 and comment before the Session	Score out of 10 and comment after the session
6	a) *How useful are books and reading in relation to your wellbeing as a doctor?* 10/10 My number 1 way of taking my mind away, the honesty and the insight into the inside of people's minds in books, especially fiction, and poetry, are a great tonic to the fear endemic to practising medicine b) *How useful are books and reading in relation to your clinical practice?* 8/10 For the above reason and for giving me insight into the lives of different people	a) *How useful are books and reading in relation to your wellbeing as a doctor?* 10/10 b) *How useful are books and reading in relation to your clinical practice?* 10/10
7	a) *How useful are books and reading in relation to your wellbeing as a doctor?* 8/10 b) *How useful are books and reading in relation to your clinical practice?* 7/10	a) *How useful are books and reading in relation to your wellbeing as a doctor?* 8/10 b) *How useful are books and reading in relation to your clinical practice?* 8/10
8	a) *How useful are books and reading in relation to your wellbeing as a doctor?* 5/10 I don't read as much as I would like but definitely find much benefit when I do b) *How useful are books and reading in relation to your clinical practice?* 10/10 essential to keeping up to date	a) *How useful are books and reading in relation to your wellbeing as a doctor?* 8/10 b) *How useful are books and reading in relation to your clinical practice?* 8/10
9	a) *How useful are books and reading in relation to your wellbeing as a doctor?* 9/10 b) *How useful are books and reading in relation to your clinical practice?* 5/10	a) *How useful are books and reading in relation to your wellbeing as a doctor?* 9/10 I need to escape into another world at the end of the day b) *How useful are books and reading in relation to your clinical practice?* 8/10

10.
a) *How useful are books and reading in relation to your wellbeing as a doctor?*
6/10
b) *How useful are books and reading in relation to your clinical practice?*
8/10

11.
a) *How useful are books and reading in relation to your wellbeing as a doctor?*
6/10 Don't always have/make time – though I find it v useful
b) *How useful are books and reading in relation to your clinical practice?*
7/10 Textbooks/professional literature

12.
a) *How useful are books and reading in relation to your wellbeing as a doctor?*
7/10 Reading is relaxing and enjoyable, helps sleep, distraction
b) *How useful are books and reading in relation to your clinical practice?*
5/10 Textbooks add to knowledge. I read less about medicine, health care, patients since I became a doctor

13.
a) *How useful are books and reading in relation to your wellbeing as a doctor?*
8/10
b) *How useful are books and reading in relation to your clinical practice?*
8/10

14.
a) *How useful are books and reading in relation to your wellbeing as a doctor?*
5/10 I have reading as one of my appraisal tasks this year – it is always a good barometer of how much space I have in my life. I enjoy podcasts/audiobooks when I am tired
b) *How useful are books and reading in relation to your clinical practice?*
5/10 Less so than the used to be as online. I have read about patients' stories and enjoy books and poetry but often forget to remind patients to use specific books

10.
a) *How useful are books and reading in relation to your wellbeing as a doctor?*
8/10
b) *How useful are books and reading in relation to your clinical practice?*
8/10

11.
a) *How useful are books and reading in relation to your wellbeing as a doctor?*
7/10 may become more important
b) *How useful are books and reading in relation to your clinical practice?*
7/10

12.
a) *How useful are books and reading in relation to your wellbeing as a doctor?*
8/10 Maybe I should read more, make more time for me and perhaps consider poetry
b) *How useful are books and reading in relation to your clinical practice?*
8/10 Reading books from patients' perspectives may be helpful

13.
a) *How useful are books and reading in relation to your wellbeing as a doctor?*
8/10
b) *How useful are books and reading in relation to your clinical practice?*
8/10

14.
a) *How useful are books and reading in relation to your wellbeing as a doctor?*
10/10 this has reminded me of how useful they are
b) *How useful are books and reading in relation to your clinical practice?*
10/10 I plan to prescribe more books

It is our belief – based on more than a decade of qualitative comments and feedback – that such provision is of considerable value, particularly if it can be continued long term, throughout a person's career. Here are a few excerpts from feedback from the Poetry of Medicine sessions, collated over a decade and stored on the Poetry of Medicine website (https://poetryofmedicine. web.ox.ac.uk/feedback):

> So much of my education is factual or evidence-based about 'what to do', 'how to manage'; yet so much of my experience of coalface general practice fails to fit those models. To attend a course which seeks to explore, through literature, the experiences of doctors and patients as people within a consultation was so refreshing and so relevant to me. No right or wrong answers. No tick-boxes or protocols . . . an excellent forum to hear the perspectives of other doctors.
>
> A very enjoyable and stimulating course – liberating not to have to feel that you have to try and remember a lot of stuff which one generally feels at a 'conventional' medical course.'
>
> The perfect antidote to the rest of my PDP . . . it feels like there's a real need for this sort of space.
>
> I found the seminar enjoyable, thought-provoking, but perhaps most of all cathartic. How wonderful to meet like-minded colleagues from a variety of backgrounds (and of different ages!)
>
> Another stimulating thought-provoking day – have taken the thoughts about space and am aware I have integrated it into my consultations – looking forward to next year.
>
> I particularly enjoyed being introduced to new literary terminology and definitions . . . a wonderful antidote to the more mechanistic aspects of our day job.

Ultimately, the richness of this qualitative feedback counts for little as far as 'hard evidence' goes. Further, the current state of the National Health Service is dire: plummeting morale amongst record numbers of doctors, many newly qualified and junior doctors leaving, senior doctors retiring at a greater rate than ever, and paramedics, nurses, and doctors willing to strike for better working conditions. As Tim Adams (2022) notes, in conversation with a GP, 'it will soon reach a threshold where there is a collapse'. '[A]ccording to the latest figures from the BMA, there are 1808 fewer full-time GPs than there were in England in 2015, while each practice has on average 2,131 more patients' (Anonymous 2023). For practising medics, professional survival over the past ten or more years has felt desperately fraught, leaving little to no time or mental space for activities such as literary discussion groups. Perhaps the poetry of medicine, much like the doctors who once engaged with it, is all but burnt out.

Notes

1 These first two works are cited in the 'Narrative Based Medicine' section of the GP Training.Net website www.gp-training.net/communication-skills/communication-skills-theory/narrative-based-medicine/
2 www.gp-training.net/educational-theory/adult-learning/inner_apprentice/
3 See, for example, the active Facebook group Humanities in Medical Education, run by Tara George.
4 See also 'Expressions of Medical Creativity Employee Wellbeing in Healthcare', *Kent*, January 10, 2020. Available at: https://creativethought.co.uk/ and www.conversationsinvitingchange.com/
5 See, for example, Jeremy Howick's account of the importance of empathy, described variously as 'doctor-patient communication' and 'bedside manner': https://podcasts.apple.com/gb/podcast/empathy-jeremy-howick/id1325020720?i=1000397219043. The blurriness around the philosophical concept of empathy is sometimes clarified by the creation of a seemingly new hybrid concept.

6 This study, 'The Poetry of Medicine Workshop', was CUREC approved by the University of Oxford's Medical Interdivisional Research Ethics Committee [R60193/RE001]. The authors assert that the ethical approval included permission given for the publication of the quotations from participants included in this manuscript. The authors disclose a conflict of interest as the founders of the Poetry of Medicine educational initiative. The workshop cited was partially funded by a grant from *ReLit: The Bibliotherapy Foundation*, and research relating to interview transcription was partially funded by a grant from the University of Oxford's centre for interdisciplinary research in the humanities, TORCH.

7 Curtis and Moore are drawing here on some phrases from Marinker (2000), but the reframing of the horse/unicorn analogy is their own.

References

Adams T. 2022. Stress, Exhaustion, and 1000 Patients a Day: The Life of an English GP. *The Guardian*, November 27. Available at: www.theguardian.com/society/2022/nov/27/stress-exhaustion-1000-patients-a-day-english-gp-nhs-collapse. Last accessed: 6/4/2023.

Ahlzén, R, Stolt C. Poetry, Interpretation and Unpredictability: A Reply to Neil Pickering. *Medical Humanities*. 2001; 27: 47–49.

Andrews A. 2016. The Ground Itself: Concealment and Revealment in Poetry and Medicine (PhD Thesis). Victoria University of Wellington, Wellington.

Anonymous. 2023. GPs aren't Just Exhausted: We are Broken. *The Guardian*, April 3. Available at: www.theguardian.com/commentisfree/2023/apr/03/broken-gp-nhs. Last accessed: 6/4/2023.

Bate J, Schuman A. Books Do Furnish a Mind: The Art and Science of Bibliotherapy. *Lancet*. 2016; 387: 742–43.

Billington J, Corcoran R, Watkins M, et al. 2019. Quantitative Methods. In: J Billington (ed.) *Reading and Mental Health*. London: Palgrave Macmillan, 265–92.

Bleakley A. 2017. *Thinking With Metaphors in Medicine: The State of the Art*. Abingdon: Routledge.

Blume M. 1989. John Ashbery, Making Nothing Happen. *International Herald Tribune*, October 2, 14.

Charon R. Literature and Medicine: Contributions to Clinical Practice. *Annals of Internal Medicine*. 1995; 122: 599–606.

Conway K. 2013. *Beyond Words: Illness and the Limits of Expression*. Ann Arbor, MI: University of Michigan Press.

Dovey C. 2015. Can Reading Make You Happier? *The New Yorker*, June 9. Available at: www.newyorker.com/culture/cultural-comment/can-reading-make-you-happier. Last accessed: 6/4/2023.

Epstein RM, Hundert EM. Defining and Assessing Professional Competence. *Journal of the American Medical Association*. 2002; 287: 236–85.

George S, Gerada C. Stressed GPs: A Call to Action. *British Journal of General Practice*. 2019; 69: 116–17.

Gleichgerrcht E, Decety J. 2012. The Costs of Empathy Among Health Professionals. In: J Decety (ed.) *Empathy: From Bench to Bedside*. Cambridge, MA: MIT Press. 245–61.

Greenhalgh T, Hurwitz B. (eds.) 1988. *Narrative Based Medicine: Dialogue and discourse in clinical practice*. London: BMJ Books.

Halpern J. What is Clinical Empathy?' *Journal of General and Internal Medicine*. 2003; 18: 670–74.

Hanne M. The Binocular Vision Project: An Introduction. *Genre: Forms of Discourse and Culture*. 2010; 44: 223–37.

Hurwitz B. Medical Humanities: Origins, Orientations and Contributions. *Anglo-Saxonica*. 2015; 10: 13–29.

Jones AH. Narrative in Medical Ethics. *British Medical Journal*. 1999; 318: 253–56.

Keats J. 1958. *The Letters of John Keats, 1814–1821* (HE Rollins, ed.). Cambridge: Cambridge University Press.

Keats J. 1978. The Fall of Hyperion. In: J Stillinger (ed.) *The Poems of John Keats*. London: Heinemann.

Komesaroff P. Uses and Misuses of Ambiguity: Uses of Ambiguity. *Internal Medicine Journal*. 2005; 35: 632–33.

Kottow M, Kottow A. Literary Narrative in Medical Practice. *Medical Humanities*. 2002; 28: 41–44.

Launer J. 2019. Metaphors and Ambiguity in Healthcare. *Chronicle of Healthcare and Narrative Medicine*, February 11. Available at: www.medicinanarrativa.eu/metaphors-and-ambiguity-in-health-care. Last accessed: 30/4/2023/.

Launer J. 2023. Medicine as Poetry. In: A Bleakley, S Neilson (eds.) *Routledge Handbook of Medicine and Poetry*. Abingdon: Routledge.

Leder D. Clinical Interpretation: The Hermeneutics of Medicine. *Theoretical Medicine*. 1990; 11: 9–24.

Mangione S, Chakraborti C, Staltari G, et al. Medical Students' Exposure to the Humanities Correlates With Positive Personal Qualities and Reduced Burnout: A Multi-Institutional U.S. Survey. *Journal of General and Internal Medicine*. 2018; 33: 628–34.

Marinker M. The Medium and the Message. *Patient Education and Counselling*. 2000; 41: 117–25.

Moore P, Curtis S. 2008. *My First nMRCGP Book*. London: Remedica.

Neighbour R. 2005. *The Inner Consultation: How to Develop an Effective and Intuitive Consulting Style*. London: Radcliffe Publishing.

Neighbour R. 2018. *The Inner Physician: Why and How to Practise 'Big Picture' Medicine*. Abingdon: Routledge.

O'Neill D. 2012. Bicycle Helmets and the Medical Humanities. *BMJ*, August 3. Available at https://blogs.bmj.com/bmj/2012/08/03/desmond-oneill-bicycle-helmets-and-the-medical-humanities/. Last accessed: 30/4/2023.

Osler W. 1904. *The Master Word in Medicine. Aequanimitas. With Other Addresses to Medical Students, Nurses and Students of Medicine*. Philadelphia, PA: P. Blaikiston's, 363–88.

Patterson J, Kitchington F. (eds.) 2019. *Body Talk in the Medical Humanities: Whose Language?* Newcastle: Cambridge Scholars Press.

Phillips A, Davis P. 2020. Reading and Psychoanalysis. In: J Billington (ed.) *Reading and Mental Health*. London: Palgrave Macmillan, 366–67.

Plath S. 1999. Balloons. In: *Ariel*. London: Faber, 75–76.

Ratcliffe S. 2016a. *On Sympathy*. Oxford: Oxford University Press.

Ratcliffe S. The Poetry of Medicine. *London Journal of Primary Care*. 2016b; 8: 39–41.

Regehr G. It's NOT Rocket Science: Rethinking Our Metaphors for Research in Health Professions Education. *Medical Education*. 2010; 44: 31–39.

Samra R. Empathy and Burnout in Medicine – Acknowledging Risks and Opportunities. *Journal of General and Internal Medicine*. 2018; 33: 991–93.

Scarry E. 1987. *The Body in Pain: The Making and Unmaking of the World*. Oxford: Oxford University Press.

Schoonover KL, Hall-Flavin D, Whitford K, et al. Impact of Poetry on Empathy and Professional Burnout of Health-Care Workers: A Systematic Review. *Journal of Palliative Care*. 2020; 35: 127–32.

Scull A. 2018. What is Empathy? *Times Literary Supplement*, April 13.

Semino E, Demjén Z, Demmen J, et al. The Online Use of Violence and Journey Metaphors by Patients With Cancer, as Compared With Health Professionals: A Mixed Methods Study. *BMJ Supportive and Palliative Care*. 2017; 7: 60–66.

Shapiro J, Morrison E, Boker J. Teaching Empathy to First Year Medical Students: Evaluation of an Elective Literature and Medicine Course. *Education for Health*. 2004; 17: 73–84.

Shklovsky V. 1917. Art as Technique. In: LT Lemon, MJ Reis (eds.) *Russian Formalist Criticism: Four Essays*. Lincoln, NE: University of Nebraska Press.

Sontag S. 1978. *Illness as Metaphor*. New York, NY: Farrar, Strauss & Giroux.

Vyieyanghi S, Periyakoil V. Using Metaphors in Medicine. *Journal of Palliative Medicine*. 2008; 11: 842–44.

Winkel AF, Feldman N, Moss H, et al. Narrative Medicine Workshops for Obstetrics and Gynecology Residents and Association with Burnout Measures. *Obstetrics & Gynecology*. 2016; 128 (1): 27S–33S.

Wohlmann A. Of Termites and Ovaries on Strike: Rethinking Medical Metaphors of the Female Body. *Signs: Journal of Women in Culture and Society*. 2017; 43: 127–50.

Wohlmann A. 2022. *Metaphor in Illness Writing: Fight and Battle Reused*. Edinburgh: University of Edinburgh Press.

Wolters F, Wijnen-Meijer M. The Role of Poetry and Prose in Medical Education: The Pen as Mighty as the Scalpel? *Perspectives on Medical Education*. 2012; 1: 43–50.

Younie L. 2019. *Flourishing through Creative Enquiry*. Queen Mary University of London. Available at: www.creativeenquiry.qmul.ac.uk/?page_id=213. Last accessed 22/12/2022.

31

CONCLUSIONS

Conclusion as lyric essay: imagined unity

Shane Neilson

After a long and – we trust – productive read that's been full of theoretical concerns occasionally interleaved with poetic reflections as well as actual poems, we suspect that you, the reader, would like to land on a more personal narrative that, perhaps, describes our peregrinations in medical poetryland. We certainly want to loosen our ties and share our experience, but our desire to escape the tyranny of narrative is strong. Balancing this desire is recognition that the ambiguity of poetry might obscure our message, and any attempt to mitigate the beautiful obscurity we treasure would result in a didactic, dead, completely clear – and perfect rhyming – poem. Thus, we resist narrative by insisting on lyric, bending the prose line as much as possible until it almost breaks.

The blank gaze of why; condescending faces at education conferences; hostile faces of academic physicians in hospitals; puzzled (and sometimes intimidated) faces of narrativists in health humanities spaces; sympathetic faces of colleagues who practice arts-based methods. For their part, our expressions do not matter, save when writing poems themselves, a look of intense concentration, our faces seized by an imagined unity, a synthesis of tenses, visualizing almighty images, straining for novel metaphors. And then revisions of our face as we ourselves revise, slightly frowning, no this will not do.

Our contributors seem much more intelligent than we are, interested in so many avenues and tributaries. They venerate certain poets themselves, which we celebrate; to bring physician-poets and disabled poets into greater resolution, we did not dream that the book would feature such pieces! To closely consider the work of poets is to venerate the art. And then the substantiations, the pieces that narrate the teaching of poetry in medical contexts, clearing the way for other educators to consider poetry as an option for their learning objectives, to use the biomedical parlance, and should such happen, then poetry is granted greater purchase in the profession, advancing the cause of deepening aesthetic sensibility. The poetic revolution called for in psychiatry – we stand at the barricades.

 DOI: 10.4324/9781003341796-39

Always the advice prevailing upon editors who seek to publish a book: what is the intended audience? The ideal reader? Somewhat ridiculously in this context – *psst*, don't tell Routledge – the market?

1. Our intended audience includes medical educators; all physicians who are poetry-curious, poetry initiates, and practiced poets; and health humanities scholars interested in new directions for their research, poetry in medicine being under-developed. This book provides a theoretical base upon which to explore the milieu further.
2. Our ideal reader's profile is simple and multiple in number. Hopefully, our ideal reader is you. Our ideal reader feels joy when reading poetry, feels moved. That's it. That's the only prerequisite to enjoy this book and – to us – a great indicator that, should you be a physician, you will practice medicine poetically. Should you be an educator, you will teach poetry poetically.
3. The market is admittedly small in the context of the health humanities readership, currently under the hegemony of narrative. Part of the problem faced by poetry in medical contexts has been its subsumption under narrative, its usurpation, not to mention the fact that despite sporadic articles offering theory that appear in the literature, there has been a lack of texts establishing a beachhead for poetics in medicine. We therefore claim, in a Spencerian fashion, that the market for this book is growing and perhaps will be called into being because of it.

The pleasure of correspondence with some of our heroines and heroes, mighty figures in the field; approaching them trepidatiously, and to receive their positive responses, followed by the honour of their work. The pleasure of reviewing new and innovative investigations. The pleasure of resisting narrative's impositions and demands, our editorial cause reified in front of our eyes by our contributors.

To be strange, different; to bring into print voices that are strange and different but also consider the strange and different; to honour one editor's (SN) community of the mad. To have found a lifelong friend in another poet (AB) who is also a scholar, who believes in the cause, who has suffered under narrative and also who has suffered for not being understood, because all of our lives are poetic too, narrative being the hermeneutic that only comes latterly, poetry our ontology in the moment when teaching or when practicing, respectively.

To have co-authored a book (SN and AB) that was the first of its kind, *Poetry in the Clinic*, a book that did the work of this book albeit in a more limited fashion, the product of two minds in conversation; to have built on the earlier book with this book, the product of a diverse range of scholars all part of the larger cause, bringing their lives and experiences with poetry to the fore; and, finally, to imagine what will come, the further developments of others in the field, and the dream: for people to appreciate poetry in medical contexts, and for poetry itself to deepen its reach and possibility.

Conclusion as prelude

Alan Bleakley

First, thanks must go to my co-editor, colleague, and friend Shane Neilson, for whom I have deep admiration. Shane is a polymath – physician, poet, critic, editor, academic, literary scholar, amateur historian. It has been such a pleasure to work on this collection with him. He brings an eagle eye and deep intelligence. I look forward to future collaborations.

It is easy to be pessimistic about life under the shadow of the 'big four' apocalyptic scenarios: climate change disaster, rogue artificial intelligence, nuclear threat, and another devastating pandemic. Surely the future of medicine is bleak under this cloud, mobilized in the capacity of fire-fighting rather than care? Such pessimism is however misplaced, where quality of life is improving globally despite such gloomy spectres. Facts show that global poverty is receding despite widespread misperception that poverty is on the increase. Longevity is improving worldwide.

While big-picture pessimism may be going against the grain of reality, ironically at a personal level optimism may reign; for example, as Simon Kuper (2023) drily observes, 'few newlyweds expect to get divorced'. Kuper further points to a 'main reason for planetary optimism' that is 'medical breakthroughs'. The public puts huge faith in medical research, and it is largely rewarded. Look how quickly a vaccine for COVID-19 was produced. The first-ever malaria vaccination will be available across African nations by late 2023. There are breakthroughs in drug therapies to slow progression of Alzheimer's. Through greater knowledge of messenger RNA dynamics, a range of cancer treatments are rapidly progressing. These are surely reasons to be cheerful and to applaud 21st-century biomedicine.

However, our concern in this book has been with the translation of such medical research into face-to-face clinical practice with individual patients. Here, there is always room for improvement, for learning is lifelong. Learning medicine is not just about storing facts (in any case, much medical knowledge is outdated in a very short space of time) but about depth, intensity, and quality of *being* as a physician. Medical education is about identity formation – where this book shows, through every chapter, how such identity formation can be viewed as an ethical, political, transcendental, and aesthetic practice. Indeed, a *poetic* practice. Good medicine, like a well-lived life, is an admixture of sprung rhythm, choice metaphors, lyricism, and alliteration (not for effect – the best diagnoses are *on point* and echoic). The making of a physician can be like the crafting of a poem.

So, as 'big picture' medical research is progressing, we should be worried about how the yield of such research is delivered on the ground. Is everyday medical practice, shaped by the way that doctors are educated, in step with the big successes of medical research? For example, while new drugs are developed, what are their patterns of use in clinical practice? In worst-case scenarios, how do we avoid another opioid crisis? How do physicians best negotiate political intrusions upon health care decisions such as the fallout from the repeal of *Roe vs Wade* in America? Is medicine ready for rogue Artificial Intelligence (AI)?

Additionally, while increasing life expectancy is seen as a win for medicine, it also creates increasing pressure on health care resources. Members of burgeoning elderly populations invite careful, integrated management by health and social care professionals. 'Careful' is the key word here. Teams must work in an integrated way around patients, with an eye to rhythm, meshing like a string quartet sticking to a score or a jazz quintet allowing long periods of improvisation grounded in tight ensemble playing.

Mozart supposedly said of his work that 'The music is not in the notes, but in the silence between'. It is this kind of 'sprung' or 'sideways' thinking that surely marks out quality in medical work, and inventive medical educators know how difficult it is to 'teach' such creative apprehension. A recent text on new ideas in evolutionary biology by David Haig (2020) suggests that Aristotle's material and efficient causes (the matter out of which something is made and the forces that set such matter in motion) are secondary to formal and final causes (why is something made from this matter and not another matter, and what is the purpose of all matter?). For now, we are in an era of culturally driven evolution. Haig suggests that evolution must be seen as the making of *meanings* (note, in the plural), but more, meanings can only be grasped through metaphor, where 'All that we know about the world is metaphor', or, gnomically, 'Phenomena are metaphors used to comprehend things'. Are 'things' themselves not 'phenomena'? Yes, they are. So, metaphors must be employed to comprehend metaphors. Now we are deep into the territory of poetry. Here, evolutionary biology is not reduced to poetry; rather, it *is* poetry, just as good medicine and medical education are forms of poetry, repeated over and over in our contributors' fine chapters.

From the chapters in this handbook that precede our conclusions, we can then read such educated patterns of care as displaying intrinsic rhythms, while inviting innovation and shaping of practices through metaphor. By this, we mean inhabiting a life of imagination beyond technical competence. Clinical practice is not cold mechanics, the body is not a machine in need of maintenance – we are unpredictable warm animals in need of imaginative care. Our emotional worlds are as important as our calculating cognition. Such patterning of clinical practice can then – once more – be seen as poetic, where poetry is also a primary medium for both expression and shaping of affect. Central to this, as my co-editor Shane Neilson insists, is *revision, revision, revision* based on the mantra 'no this will not do'. Also, for clinical practice, 'mostly I'm doing fine, but there's always room for improvement'. As for medical education, well, many of us believe a deep overhaul is needed – again, 'no this will not do'. We can, and will, always do better. It is a matter of formulating new and improved pedagogies; following Haig, medical education shaping medicine is in an arc of incremental evolutionary deepening, seeking 'meanings' beyond mere information. Again, the template must be the face-to-face consultation prior to diagnosis and treatment plan: tolerating silences as meaningful, the sudden eruption of descriptive language, insights forming, the collapsing of matter into forceful densities, a moment of mastery of rhythm, and then surprising disclosures.

There is a saying in Paris that 'you never own a Parisian flat, you just look after it for future generations'. While we have been the architects of this collection – the first of its kind – we gladly pass on the documentation resting in this house of medicine and poetry to future generations, for careful habitation and curation. This, of course, is the development of archive (and we have emphasized the value of this with our return to EP Scarlett's seminal 'Medicine and Poetry' from 1936/7) and processional history. No doubt there will be mainstream additions as well as radical innovations in the field long after we, the editors, have gone. This conclusion, then, must act as prelude to what is to come.

References

Haig D. 2020. *From Darwin to Derrida: Selfish Genes, Social Selves, and the Meanings of Life*. Cambridge, MA: MIT Press.

Kuper S. 2023. Why So Sad? The World Could Have a Very Good Decade Ahead. *Financial Times Weekend Magazine*, July 22/23.

ACKNOWLEDGEMENTS

Chapter 4: 'Medicine and Poetry' by EP Scarlett

Transcribed from the original articles in the *Canadian Medical Association Journal* December 1936 (Part I) and January 1937 (Part II).
Permission gained (thanks to Holly Bodger, publisher of *CMAJ*).

Chapter 5: 'Medicine as poetry' by John Launer

Transcribed from the original article in the *Postgraduate Medical Journal* and reproduced here with permission from the publisher *British Medical Journal*.
Launer J. *Postgraduate Medical Journal*. 2014; 90: 302.

Chapter 7: 'Poetry and medicine' by Audrey Shafer

Reprinted from *Anesthesiology Clinics*. 2022; 40: 359–72, with permission from Elsevier.

Chapter 9: 'Positive negative' by Daisy G Bassen

'In the Midrash, Lot's wife is called Edith' first appeared in *Bodega Magazine*.
'Domina' first appeared in *So to Speak*.
'My abortions' first appeared in *Harpur Palate*.
'Tansy' first appeared in *Ilanot Review*.
'Catherine-Wheel' first appeared in *The Delmarva Review*.
'Folie à deux' first appeared in *Wards Lit*.
'Kenoma' first appeared in *The Rail*.
'Training for Death Certificate Completion' first appeared in *Sheila-ng-Gig*.

Chapter 12: 'Nourished by experiences: meaning without metaphysics in the poetry of Dannie Abse' by W Richard Bowen

This chapter first appeared as an article in the *International Journal of Welsh Writing* in English (University of Wales Press): Bowen WR. Nourished by Experiences: Meaning without Metaphysics in the Poetry of Dannie Abse. *International Journal of Welsh Writing in English*. 2019; 6: 1. The article is reproduced here with permission of the author, who retains the publication rights.

Chapter 13: 'Debriding the moral injury' by Tolu Oloruntoba

'Medical Séances' Palimpsest Press, 2021. From *The Junta of Happenstance*.
'Divination' first appeared in *The Ampersand Review of Writing & Publishing*.
'In Fetu' Palimpsest Press, 2021. From *The Junta of Happenstance*.
'Bloodletting' Palimpsest Press, 2021. From *The Junta of Happenstance*.
'Kneecap' first appeared in *The Ampersand Review of Writing & Publishing*.
'a coast is not the same as a land' with permission from Alan Bleakley.
Rights to remaining poems retained by the author.

Chapter 21: 'Oncology and poetry: the case of Patrick Kavanagh' by Martin Dyar

'The Hospital' by Patrick Kavanagh is here reproduced in its entirety with permission from the Patrick Kavanagh Foundation. The quotations from poems by Patrick Kavanagh are reprinted from *Collected Poems*, edited by Antoinette Quinn (Lane 2004), with the kind permission of the Trustees of the Estate of the late Katherine B. Kavanagh, through the Jonathan Williams Literary Agency.

Chapter 28: 'Creative writing in medical education' by Michael Hanne

Permissions for poems quoted have been obtained from Art Nahill, Glenn Colquhoun, Johanna Emeney, and Greg Judkins, with thanks to the authors.

BIOGRAPHIES

Marta Arnaldi

Dr Marta Arnaldi is Lecturer in Italian at the University of Oxford and Postdoctoral Research Fellow at the University of Oslo. She is the author of five books, including a monograph and three award-winning poetry collections. A scholar of Italian and comparative literature, Marta has an interdisciplinary background including medical training. She is the founder and leader of *Translating Illness*, a medical humanities research project and international network of scholars, health and policy professionals, and artists.

Iain Bamforth

Dr Iain Bamforth's publications include five volumes of poetry, an anthology of medical literature *The Body in the Library*, collections of essays on modern European writers and philosophers, and many articles on dealings between medicine and the wider world of ideas. Some of these were published in *A Doctor's Dictionary* (2015) and *Scattered Limbs* (2020) – described in *Literary Review* as a 'disturbing, brilliant and wildly original dreambook'. He has worked in hospital medicine in several countries, as a GP in the UK and France, and for EC-funded health projects in Asia as well as in literary journalism. He lives in Strasbourg.

Daisy G Bassen

Dr Daisy G Bassen is a child psychiatrist located in Warwick, Rhode Island, where she is also the medical director of a community health centre. Having first studied English at Princeton University (graduating *magna cum laude* 1998), she studied medicine at the University of Rochester, specialising in child and adolescent psychiatry (Butler Hospital/Brown University). She has been in practice for over 20 years and is a widely published poet.

Alan Bleakley

Dr Alan Bleakley is Emeritus Professor of Medical Education and Medical Humanities at Plymouth Peninsula School of Medicine, University of Plymouth, UK. He was instrumental in setting up an innovative medical humanities curriculum and medical education research centre at Peninsula Medical School (established in 2002) and is a leading international figure in the fields of medical education and medical humanities. He has published 20 academic books, seven collections of poetry, and many academic articles and book chapters. Educated as a zoologist, psychologist, and psychotherapist, he has focused much of his work on employing radical pedagogies within health care.

W Richard Bowen

Professor W Richard Bowen is a Fellow of the Royal Academy of Engineering. He also holds degrees in physical sciences (Oxford) and theology (Wales). He has special interests in understanding across conceptual schemes. His publications on poetry include studies of Dannie Abse, Vernon Watkins, John Ormond, and Anne Cluysenaar. He has published extensively on the relationship between faith and science. A Chinese language edition of his book *Engineering Ethics: Challenges and Opportunities* (Springer 2014) has been published by Zhejiang University Press (2020). He is strongly committed to the use of engineering for the promotion of peace, health, and wellbeing.

Megan EL Brown

Dr Megan EL Brown is a Senior Research Associate in Medical Education at Newcastle University, where her research focuses on workforce sustainability and equity. She is an amateur poet and has upcoming publications in *Consilience* and *Wishbone Words Review*. Megan has a clinical background but is non-practicing, working full-time in medical education teaching and research. She is interested in poetic inquiry in the context of research across broad topics with health professions learners.

Jessica Chaytor

Jessica Chaytor, MEd, is a Student Success elementary teacher living in Mi'Kma'ki (Nova Scotia). She works in the public school system, and her research background includes language development in children. She is currently enrolled in a second master of education programme (inclusive education).

Sarah de Leeuw

Dr Sarah de Leeuw, a professor and Canada Research Chair (Humanities and Health Inequities) with the Northern Medical Program (a distributed site of UBC's Faculty of Medicine) is an award-winning researcher, creative writer (poetry and literary non-fiction), and multidisciplinary scholar studying why some people and places have better health than others. Her research, activism, and creative practices have for more than 30 years focused on anticolonial, feminist, and queer-informed understandings of overlooked people, communities, and geographies. She grew up in Haida Gwaii and Terrace (Kitsumkalum territory) and now divides her time between Lheidli T'enneh/Dakelh Territory (Prince George) and Syilx Territory (Okanagan Centre).

Martin Dyar

Dr Martin Dyar is an Irish poet and medical educator. He is presently Adjunct Professor in Medical Humanities and Ethics in the School of Medicine, Trinity College, Dublin. He has published two collections of poems, *Maiden Names* (Arlen House), and *The Meek* (Wake Forest University Press), and is the editor of the anthology *Vital Signs: Poems of Illness and Healing* (Poetry Ireland). He has held fellowships in Creative Writing, including at the University of Iowa, the University of Limerick, the Washington Ireland Program, and the Jackie Clarke Collection. He holds a PhD in English from Trinity College Dublin.

Johanna Emeney

Dr Johanna Emeney was educated at Pembroke College, Cambridge, where she read English Literature and Japanese. She gained her PhD in Creative Writing at Massey University, Auckland. She has published three collections of poetry and a nonfiction book, *The Rise of Autobiographical*

Medical Poetry and the Medical Humanities (*ibid*em 2018), in addition to a children's book, co-authored with Sarah Laing called *Sylvia and the Birds* (Massey University Press 2022). She has worked as a senior school teacher, university tutor, writer, and editor.

Sarah Fraser

Dr Sarah Fraser (MSc, MD, CCFP) is a general practitioner living in Mi'Kma'ki (Nova Scotia). She is Co-Director of the Medical Humanities Program at Dalhousie University and Deputy Editor for *Canadian Family Physician*.

Michael Hanne

Retired from directing the Comparative Literature Programme he founded in 1995 at the University of Auckland, New Zealand, Michael Hanne still teaches a medical humanities course to 3rd-year medical students at the same university. He also continues to research and convene conferences around the crucial role of narrative and metaphor in medicine and other disciplines. His articles on the part these rhetorical devices play in doctor–patient communication, diagnosis, medical research, and media coverage of health and sickness and along the boundary between medicine and criminology can be found at narrativemetaphornexus.weebly.com.

Michael Hulse

Professor Michael Hulse, described by Gwyneth Lewis as 'a formidable poet', has won firsts in the National Poetry Competition and the Bridport Prize (twice) and honours including a Cholmondeley Award. Reading invitations have taken him to Canada, the US, and Mexico; Australia and New Zealand; India; and several European countries. He has translated from the German (Goethe, Rilke, Nietzsche, Jelinek, Sebald) and has worked with the Nobel Foundation, Goethe Institute, British Council. and Günter Grass Foundation. His co-edited anthology *The Twentieth Century in Poetry* was described by *The Guardian* as 'magnificent', and his collection *Half-Life* was a Book of the Year in the *Australian Book Review*.

Martina Ann Kelly

Dr Martina Ann Kelly is an Irish family physician and Professor of Family Medicine and Community Health Sciences, Cumming School of Medicine, University of Calgary, Alberta, Canada. She is interested in how doctors and patients understand and relate to each other (intersubjectivity), which she explores drawing on ideas from hermeneutic phenomenology.

Monica Kidd

Dr Monica Kidd has written several books of poetry, fiction, and non-fiction, most recently *Chance Encounters with Wild Animals* (Gaspereau Press 2019). She practices family medicine with low-risk obstetrics in Alberta and works as a freelance journalist as well. She is an associate editor of humanities at the *Canadian Medical Association Journal*.

Laurence J Kirmayer

Dr Laurence J Kirmayer is James McGill Professor and Director, Division of Social and Transcultural Psychiatry, McGill University. He directs the Culture & Mental Health Research Unit at the Institute of Community and Family Psychiatry, Jewish General Hospital, in Montreal, where he conducts research on culturally responsive mental health services, psychiatric anthropology, and the philosophy of psychiatry. His publications include the co-edited volumes *Re-Visioning Psychiatry: Cultural Phenomenology, Critical Neuroscience, and Global Mental Health* (Cambridge 2015) and *Culture, Mind and Brain: Emerging Concepts, Methods, and Applications* (Cambridge 2020). He is a Fellow of the Canadian Academy of Health Sciences and the Royal Society of Canada.

Elisabeth Kumar

Elisabeth Kumar is a lecturer in the University of Auckland School of Medicine's medical human- ities programme, co-teaching (with Michael Hanne) a course called Unexamined Metaphors, Uncharted Stories. She practices as an occupational therapist in forensic psychiatry. She is par- ticularly interested in literature around disability, madness, and dialogue.

John Launer

Dr John Launer is an educator and writer with a background as a GP and family therapist. His books include *Narrative-Based Practice in Health and Social Care: Conversations Inviting Change* (Routledge 2018) and *How Not To Be A Doctor: And Other Essays* (Duckworth 2018). He is an honorary consultant at the Tavistock and Portman NHS Trust and an honorary associate clini- cal professor at University College London. John writes a regular column for the *British Medical Journal*.

Alastair Morrison

Dr Alastair Morrison is a medical student at McMaster University's DeGroote School of Medi- cine. He holds a PhD in English and comparative literature from Columbia University, and he has taught at universities in Canada, the United States, and Denmark. His academic work deals with relationships between literature and mental and neurological illness, as well as with literary stud- ies in medical education. His articles have appeared in *Medical Humanities*, *Criticism*, and other journals, and his poems have recently appeared or are forthcoming in *Canadian Literature*, *The Literary Review of Canada*, *Pidgeonholes*, and elsewhere. He lives in Hamilton, Ontario, with his spouse and two children.

Thirusha Naidu

Professor Thirusha Naidu is a clinical psychologist and researcher in mental health, medical edu- cation, and global health. Her writing and research in academic prose and poetry focus on the health humanities. Using geopolitics and diversity lenses, she explores decoloniality, antiracism, equity, and the lived experiences of marginalized people, especially women. Her academic aims include disrupting dominant epistemology and methods. Her poetry and academic writing have appeared in *Academic Medicine, BMJ Humanities, The Lancet*, and *The Lancet Global Health*. She is an Associate Professor in Behavioural Medicine at the University of KwaZulu-Natal and a Senior Honorary Visiting Fellow at Cambridge University Department of Public Health and Primary Care.

Shane Neilson

Dr Shane Neilson (mad; autistic) is a poet and physician from New Brunswick, Canada. He prac- tises family medicine in Guelph and is an adjunct assistant professor of family medicine attached to the Waterloo Regional Campus of McMaster University. His dissertation on the representations of pain received the Gold Medal from the Governor-General, and he was awarded SSHRC's Talent Award given to a single Canadian PhD candidate per year. He published *Canadian Literature and Medicine: Carelanding* with Routledge in 2023 and co-authored *Poetry in the Clinic: Towards a Lyrical Medicine* (Routledge) with Alan Bleakley in 2021. In 2025, he will publish *The Reign*, the second volume in his New Brunswick trilogy, with Goose Lane Editions.

Tolu Oloruntoba

Dr Tolu Oloruntoba was born in Ibadan, Nigeria, where he also practiced medicine. He is the author of *The Junta of Happenstance* (Palimpsest Press/Anstruther Books), winner of the Canadian Grif- fin Poetry Prize and Governor General's Literary Award, and *Each One a Furnace* (McClelland &

Stewart/Penguin Random House Canada), a Dorothy Livesay Poetry Prize finalist. His poetry has also appeared in *Harvard Divinity Review*, *Columbia Journal*, *Canadian Literature*, and elsewhere. He was the 2022 League of Canadian Poets Anne Szumigalski Lecturer and is a Civitella Ranieri fellow. He lives on Coast Salish lands in Surrey, western Canada.

Bahar Orang

Dr Bahar Orang is a writer and psychiatrist living in Toronto. Her first book, *Where Things Touch: A Meditation On Beauty* (Book*hug Press, 2020), was shortlisted for the Gerald Lampert Memorial Award and was named a best book of the year by CBC and NPR. She is currently completing a PhD in cultural studies and a clinical fellowship in reproductive life stages psychiatry.

Sophie Ratcliffe

Dr Sophie Ratcliffe is Professor of Literature and Creative Criticism at the Faculty of English, University of Oxford. Her research focuses on histories of feeling and reading. Her publications include *On Sympathy* (OUP 2008) and the autocritical work *The Lost Properties of Love* (William Collins, 2019) – forthcoming in the USA as *Loss, a Love Story* (Northwestern UP, 2024). Her current book project on children and libraries makes a special study of the value of children's hospital libraries and considers the idea of 'curative reading'. She has recently partnered with Oxford's Department of Psychiatry to develop resources to communicate with children about serious illness within their families: www.psych.ox.ac.uk/research/covid_comms_support. More details about her research and publications can be found at www.sophieratcliffe.com.

Lynne Richards

Ms Lynne Richards is a young South African woman of colour pursuing a career in mental health. She is currently completing her master of social science in clinical psychology, cultivating a career as a lecturer and researcher. Her areas of interest in the field of psychology include the neuropsychological effect of trauma and violence, as well as critical feminism and intersectionality. She is committed to providing mentorship to students in the field of health sciences.

Daniel A Romero Suarez

Dr Daniel Antonio Romero Suarez (PhD – Vanderbilt University) is a Professor of Literature and Literary Theory at the Pontifical Catholic University of Peru (PUCP). With a focus on medical humanities and contemporary poetry, his articles feature in journals such as *Modern Language Notes*, *Romance Notes*, and *Boletín de la Academia Peruana de la Lengua*. His current research explores environmental fictions, the portrayal of COVID-19, and the intersection of disease and memory. He is also interested in developing new ways to teach literature courses through digital humanities.

Alfonso Santarpia

Dr Alfonso Santarpia is an associate professor of clinical psychology (Université de Sherbrooke, QC, Canada). His research is principally concerned with approaches in the humanistic–existential traditions, adopting quali-quantitative mixed methods. He has observed effects of the arts on the metaphors of the body. In particular, he is interested in the role of poetry in psycho-oncology. He invented two poetic protocols termed SADUPA. His publications include the French manual (2020 2nd ed) *Introduction to Humanistic Psychotherapies*.

EP Scarlett

Dr Earle Parkhill Scarlett (1896–1982) was a celebrated Canadian physician who served as Chancellor of the University of Alberta from 1952–58. He gained his medicine degree from the University of Toronto, practiced in the United States, and returned to Calgary, where he established a reputation as a physician, educator, and champion of what we now call the medical or health humanities.

Andrew Schuman

Dr Andrew Schuman is a GP partner at 19 Beaumont St, Oxford, and a Clinical Tutor at the University of Oxford. He combines his medical work with literary interests and for the past 20 years has been using literature (and poetry in particular) as a vital part of his educational work with medical students and doctors. Andrew was shortlisted for the 2010 International Hippocrates Prize for Poetry & Medicine. He is the co-founder of the Poetry of Medicine initiative, and he co-edited the anthology *Stressed Unstressed: Classic Poems to Ease the Mind* (2016). His article on the history of bibliotherapy, written with the academic Jonathan Bate, was published in *The Lancet* in 2016.

Audrey Shafer

Audrey Shafer MD is Professor Emeritum of Anesthesiology, Perioperative and Pain Medicine, Stanford University School of Medicine/Veterans Affairs Palo Alto Health Care System; founder, Stanford Medicine & the Muse Program, Stanford Center for Biomedical Ethics; founder, Biomedical Ethics and Medical Humanities Scholarly Concentration; and co-founder of Pegasus Physician Writers. She completed her undergraduate studies at Harvard University, medical school at Stanford, anaesthesiology training at University of Pennsylvania, and her research fellowship at Stanford. She is the author of *The Mailbox*, a children's novel on posttraumatic stress disorder in veterans. Her poetry has been published in journals and anthologies.

Erin Soros

A mad settler living in Vancouver, Erin Soros writes poetry, fiction, nonfiction, and theory. She was a postdoctoral fellow at Cornell University and a visiting writer at Cambridge. She researches psychosis and the psychiatric and police response to it. Recent articles have appeared in *Topia* and *Sociologica*. Her poetry received *The Malahat Review* Long Poem Prize and inclusion in *Best Canadian Poetry*. Her fiction received the CBC Literary Award and the Commonwealth Award for the Short Story. Her essays received the Writers' Union of Canada Short Prose Award and Gold at the National Magazine Awards for 'One of a Kind Storytelling'.

Christie Stilwell

Christie Stilwell is a PhD candidate at Dalhousie University and a recipient of a Frederick Banting and Charles Best Canada Graduate Doctoral Scholarship from the Canadian Institutes of Health Research. Her doctoral research explores mental wellness and ageing well among Inuit in south and central Labrador. She is also involved in studies on health and support services for women experiencing intimate partner violence/interpersonal violence and ageism directed at social admissions in tertiary health care centres. Christie is the co-founder and co-Editor-in-Chief of the student-run *Healthy Populations Journal*, which aims to reduce barriers to peer-reviewed publishing for emerging scholars.

Peter Stilwell

Dr Peter Stilwell is a postdoctoral researcher at McGill University in the Faculty of Medicine and Health Sciences – School of Physical & Occupational Therapy. Most of his research is on pain and person-centred care. He is especially interested in pain theory and medical humanities. He currently holds a fellowship from the Canadian Institutes of Health Research. Previously, he was the Ronald Melzack Fellow in Chronic Pain Research at the Alan Edwards Centre for Research on Pain at McGill. He was recently awarded a Marie Skłodowska-Curie Actions Fellowship to conduct pain research at the University of Southern Denmark starting in 2024.

Jiameng Xu

Dr Jiameng Xu is a psychiatry resident at the University of British Columbia. She graduated from the MD-PhD programme at McGill University in 2021. She completed her PhD dissertation, *Practices of Being Near: An Ethnographic Study of Family Members and Persons with Lived Experience of Mental Illness*, in 2019. She has been involved in initiatives to create a space for the arts and humanities within health professional training and settings of health care delivery, including *Journeys Through Health*, an exhibition of artworks by persons with lived and living experience of illness. Her poetry and essays have appeared in *ROOM* and *The COVID Journals*.

INDEX

Note: Page numbers in *italics* indicate a figure and page numbers in **bold** indicate a table on the corresponding page. Page numbers followed by "n" with numbers refer to notes.

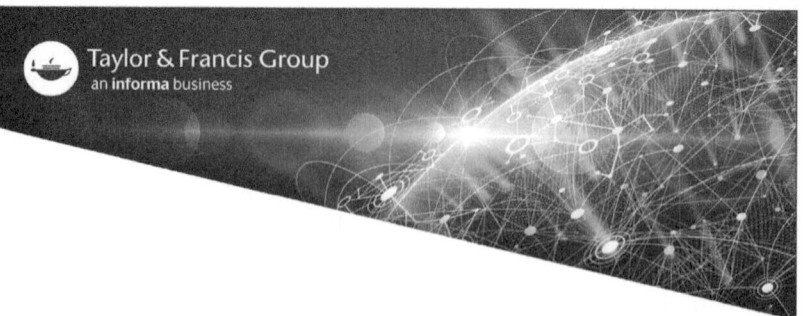
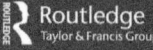
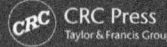